Sexual Behaviour and HIV/AIDS in Europe

GW00372510

Social Aspects of AIDS
Series Editor: Peter Aggleton
Institute of Education, University of London

Editorial Advisory Board

Sexual Behaviour and HIV/AIDS in Europe

Comparisons of National Surveys

Edited by

Michel Hubert, Nathalie Bajos and Theo Sandfort

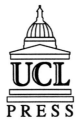

PRESS

First published in 1998 by UCL Press

UCL Press
1 Gunpowder Square
London EC4A 3DE
UK

and

1900 Frost Road, Suite 101
Bristol
Pennsylvania 19007-1598
USA

The name of University College London (UCL) is a registered trade mark used by UCL Press with the consent of the owner.

British Library Cataloguing-in-Publication Data
A CIP catalogue record for this book is available from the British Library.

Library of Congress Cataloging-in-Publication Data are available

ISBN: 1-85728-818-1 (cased)
ISBN: 1-85728-819-X (paperback)

Typeset in 10/12pt Baskerville by Best-set Typesetter Ltd., Hong Kong
Printed and bound by T.J. International Ltd, Padstow, UK

Contents

Contents

Tables

Tables

Figures

Preface

The aim of this volume is to present cross-national analyses of key data on sexual behaviour and attitudes towards HIV/AIDS from 16 population surveys carried out in 11 European countries between 1989 and 1993. It is the second book to come out of a European Concerted Action on sexual behaviour and the risks of HIV infection supported by the EU Biomedical and Health Research Programme (BIOMED). The first volume, *Sexual Interactions and HIV Risk* (L. Van Campenhoudt, M. Cohen, G. Guizzardi and D. Hausser, Eds), published in 1997 in this same series examined new conceptual perspectives for understanding risk behaviour.

In order to understand how the authors were able to bring together such a large diversity of survey contents and methods and performed their cross-national analyses, the reader should start with the first chapter of this book, which also presents the main characteristics of the surveys under comparison. The different contributions are then divided into four parts. The first part provides basic information on sexual behaviour in Europe in the era of AIDS. Whereas AIDS provides the context rather than the focus of analysis in this first section, Part 2 is primarily epidemiological and is devoted to the measurement of exposure to sexual transmission of HIV using survey data. Part 3 focuses on preventive practices and the normative context that surrounds them. Finally, Part 4 discusses the specific issues of knowledge and representations of HIV/AIDS and their relation to discrimination against people with HIV/AIDS. The book closes with a chapter that summarizes some of the findings and brings together some of the lessons for HIV/AIDS prevention and future research that may be drawn from the various comparative analyses.

Designing, processing and publishing such comparative analyses was a long-running project that started in 1991. Three main stages were needed to develop the analyses described in this book. First, the objectives, tasks and working procedures for the project were determined by the Centre d'études sociologiques (CES) of the Brussels-based Facultés universitaires Saint-Louis, which coordinated this project, aided by a steering committee. Then, the investigators who carried out the different surveys were asked to act as data providers and/or authors to design and process cross-national analyses. They were helped in these tasks by the CES, which provided them with all the necessary information about the surveys and survey questions and served as a hub for data exchange. Writing and editing the chapters was the final phase, during which the book was shaped to a standardized and consistent format. This does not mean, however, that differences in styles and scopes of analyses do not remain among the various chapters, or that additional cross-national analyses are not still possible.

Although we were conscious of the enormous challenge we had set ourselves from the very outset, the undertaking has gone well beyond what we expected and represented many more working hours than an average collectively written book. But we believe that this work was a necessary step in creating a community of researchers exploring sexual behaviour and attitudes to HIV/AIDS in Europe, and think it makes an important contribution to building up the empirical knowledge that is needed not only for HIV/AIDS prevention and epidemiology but also for other sexual health problems (STDs, abortion, and so on). We thus warmly thank all those who were engaged in this adventure. The following list of names is a way of acknowledging their work, but also gives the reader an idea of the many tasks that were necessary to realize this project.

First of all, we should like to thank the individual authors who worked with us and will hopefully enjoy the outcome. They include sociologists, psychologists, demographers, epidemiologists and medical doctors all involved with national surveys. We are particularly grateful to Jacques Marquet, who contributed to the writing of several chapters of the book. We should also like to thank Osmo Kontula, who wrote a chapter on attitudes towards sexual norms that unfortunately could not be included for lack of comparable data.

Not all those who contributed to this project actually participated in writing the various chapters. Several survey investigators, namely, Gerhard Christiansen, Meni Malliori, Dario Paez, João Santos Lucas and Ricardo Usieto, agreed to provide their data without being included as authors. Several data analysts did the same. Our gratitude goes to them, particularly to Jean-Claude Deheneffe, who took charge of the analyses that were to be made in Brussels on several data files and provided comparative tables of the 'common variables' created in all the data files to serve as independent variables throughout the book. Philippe Huynen performed analyses of several data files too, as did Ernest de Vroome. Osma Ahvenlapi, Ioseba Iraurgi, George Koulierakis, Ann Petruckevitch, Stefano Campostrini and Reiner Trometer analyzed their own national data for us.

Nathalie Bajos, Michel Hubert, Casimiro Marques Balsa, David McQueen, Theo Sandfort, Peter Stringer and Kaye Wellings participated in the steering committee that advised on the structure of this book. Michel Hubert was the leader of the whole project. Casimiro Marques Balsa was in charge of designing and setting up the 'bank of indicators' that was created to analyze the contents of the questionnaires and to select the survey questions to be compared.

Michel Vanderkelen was in charge of programming the 'bank of indicators' and several collaborators – Luc Hachez, Sylvie Jamet and Jackie Balsa – had the tedious task of encoding all the questionnaires.

Beckie Field and Kaye Wellings collected a set of relevant demographic, social and cultural indicators to help the authors interpret differences and similarities in data across Europe. Ester Zantedeschi provided all the authors with a selection of publications on the topics they were addressing.

The secretariat of the Concerted Action consisted of Josette Jamet and Françoise Paulus, who prepared the final layouts of both texts and tables. Véronique Eloy and Pascale Malice assisted in organizing meetings and workshops on several occasions.

Gaby Leyden has been more than an English editor throughout this project. She was a colleague who corrected our mistakes, translated some of the chapters and re-read the whole book.

Finally, we want to stress the fact that this project would not have been possible without the support of the European Commission, particularly Dr André Baert, whose support for the project was enduring, and the late Gaston Everard. We should also like to thank the Facultés universitaires Saint-Louis, which housed and encouraged our collective efforts.

Last, we thank our colleagues and families for their support and for having borne with us throughout what occasionally seemed to be a never-ending project.

Michel Hubert, Nathalie Bajos and Theo Sandfort

Series Editor's Preface

When the epidemics of HIV and AIDS were first detected little was known about patterns of sexual behaviour in different European countries beyond that attributable to conjecture and stereotype. Relatively few countries had conducted population surveys of young people's and adult's sexual behaviour, and the data that was available was most usually non-comparable. This was unfortunate in so far as forward planning for the prevention of HIV was concerned. It also posed problems for the development of a European strategy against AIDS sensitive to the needs of particular countries and areas. Thankfully, the European Concerted Action on sexual behaviour and the risk of HIV infection, whose work is reported in this book, took place, since for the first time it allowed a comparative analysis of data collected in 11 countries. Here we find the fruits of over seven years labour. Scientific information about the prevalence of different kinds of sexual behaviour is analyzed in ways relevant to a better understanding of the epidemic and its dynamics. Among the issues examined are sexual debut, the reported prevalence of different sexual practices, patterns of homosexuality and bisexuality, reported rates of sexually transmitted diseases, reported condom use and other forms of prevention. Behavioural data is complemented by an analysis of social representations of HIV and AIDS, attitudes towards the syndrome, and factors influencing discrimination and stigmatization. In a significant number of respects therefore, this is a truly remarkable book. The challenge now lies in developing programmes and interventions that build upon what we have learned, and in focusing our work so as to meet the real, rather than the imagined, needs of different countries, communities and groups.

Peter Aggleton

Introduction

Chapter 1

Studying and Comparing Sexual Behaviour and HIV/AIDS in Europe

*Michel Hubert**

Introduction

Concern about AIDS appeared in most European countries soon after this new disease was discovered in 1981. In Europe, as in North America, gay communities were the first to be affected and to engage in the fight against AIDS. Because of the seriousness of the epidemic and fear of discrimination, they quickly mobilized to disseminate preventive messages, take care of people with HIV/AIDS, call for treatments, and so on. The spread of the pandemic was paralleled by a wealth of research on sexual behaviour, risk practices and prevention among gay men (Pollak *et al.*, 1994) and, later, injecting drug users (Rezza *et al.*, 1994). The need for general population campaigns was not felt in most European countries until 1985 (Wellings and Field, 1996). Based on the idea that everyone should be concerned about HIV/AIDS prevention, these campaigns targeted the entire population due to fear that HIV might have spread widely beyond the primary 'risk' groups and a desire to avoid stigmatizing these same risk groups.

In this context, many European countries realized that, outside specific studies on gay men and injecting drug users, little was known about the prevalence of various types of HIV/AIDS risk-related behaviour, or indeed sexual behaviour in general, in their national populations. They thus decided to fill the information gap by engaging in large-scale population surveys for the first time.[1] Exceptional investments were made in such surveys in Europe,

*I should like to thank Casimiro Marques Balsa who coordinated with me the European Concerted Action of which this book is one of the outcomes and took an active part in designing and running the project. Many thanks to all the survey investigators who kindly provided access to their research material and information about their surveys. The members of the Research Network for Comparative Research in Europe (Rencore) also provided numerous references and advice to help place the studies reported here in the larger tradition of comparative research.

3

as well as on other continents (Cleland and Ferry, 1995; Catania *et al.*, 1996), from 1987 on. Because data were needed urgently, researchers and funding bodies could not spend much time harmonizing their approaches with other countries. This was also difficult because of the variety of research objectives that had to be fulfilled (each country having its own priorities), the diversity of research strategies that could be followed to survey such sensitive topics, and the multitude of perspectives that were available.[2]

In this chapter, we shall describe the surveys that will be compared in the book, with special attention given to the diversity of questionnaire orientations and contents and the sampling and data collection techniques involved. We shall make explicit what the consequences of this diversity were for the comparability of data. Then we shall describe how we proceeded with our cross-national analyses.

The main purpose of the cross-national analyses was to describe and interpret differences and similarities across Europe in basic aspects of sexual behaviour, such as sexual initiation, sexual orientation, sexual practices or number of partners, as well as in other features linked directly to HIV transmission and prevention (risk factors and indicators *vis-à-vis* HIV, preventive practices, knowledge and discrimination against people with HIV/AIDS, and so on). Adopting a cross-national perspective on sexual behaviour and HIV/AIDS was all the more necessary to make national data more meaningful and base future policies on this information. It was the first time that such systematic comparisons had been undertaken in Europe. The cross-cultural analyses that then existed were either highly specific in terms of problems (for example contraception, see Leridon *et al.*, 1987; Ketting, 1990) or populations studied (for example homo/bisexuals, see Pollak *et al.*, 1994) or focused more on the differences between our societies and other societies (Davenport, 1976; Davis and Whitten, 1987; Lavee, 1991), with particular emphasis on primitive societies, or between different periods of history within our societies (Ariès and Béjin, 1985; Gregersen, 1994) rather than on differences among current European societies. These anthropological and historical approaches were, however, particularly important in drawing attention to the fact that the meaning, range and contents of what we class as sexual, are far from shared by all the societies and that, therefore, we should spend time deconstructing definitions of sexual behaviour. We should wonder, too, whether any constants lie embedded within this variety (Reiss, 1986).

Sixteen Surveys from 11 European Countries

As shown in Table 1.1, 16 surveys from 11 European countries were included in our comparisons. The British, Danish and Icelandic surveys were the only Western European national surveys that were not included systematically in

Table 1.1 *European surveys under comparison*

Survey identification*	Field period	Study name	Principal investigators	Funding bodies	Language	Special characteristics
Athens–KABP 1989	3–4/89	Knowledge, Attitudes, Beliefs and Practices in relation to HIV Infection and AIDS	D. Agrafiotis	World Health Organization (WHO)	Greek	
Athens–PR 1990	3–10/90	Partner Relations and Risk of HIV Infection	M. Malliori A. Rabavilas C. Stefanis N. Vaidakis	World Health Organization (WHO)	Greek	
Belgium 1993	4–6/93	National Survey of Sexual Behaviour and Attitudes to the Risk of AIDS	M. Hubert J. Marquet	Fonds de la recherche scientifique médicale (Programme de recherche Sida), Fonds national de la recherche scientifique, Brussels – Capital Region, European Union (DG V)	French, Dutch	
Finland 1992	11/91–2/92	The National Study of Human Relations, Sexual Attitudes and Lifestyles in Finland (FINSEX)	E. Haavio-Mannila O. Kontula	Research Council of Social Sciences of the Academy of Finland, National Agency for Welfare and Health	Finnish, Swedish	About one-third of the questions asked were the same as in a comparable survey carried out in 1971.

Table 1.1 *(cont.)*

Survey identification*	Field period	Study name	Principal investigators	Funding bodies	Language	Special characteristics
France–ACSF 1992	9/91–2/92	Analysis of Sexual Behaviour in France (ACSF)	A. Spira N. Bajos	Agence nationale de recherche sur le sida, Direction générale de la santé, Agence française de lutte contre le sida, Comité français d'éducation à la santé	French	A joint ACSF–KABP follow-up survey has been carried out in 1994
France–KABP 1992	10/91–3/92	National Survey of Knowledge, Beliefs, Attitudes and Practices towards HIV (KABP)	J.-P. Moatti N. Beltzer	Agence nationale de recherche sur le sida, Agence française de lutte contre le sida	French	Similar surveys carried out in 1990 and 1992 using a different sampling method. A joint ACSF–KABP follow-up survey carried out in 1994
Germany (East) 1990	7–9/90	AIDS '90 Study	M. Haeder	Zentral Institut für Hygiene, Mikrobiologie und Epidemiologie	German	Former Democratic Republic of Germany
Germany (West) 1990	1990	Sexual Behaviour of Men and Women in the Federal Republic of Germany	H. Jung	Bundesministerium für Gesundheit	German	Federal Republic of Germany (before reunification)
Germany (East & West) 1993	10–12/93	AIDS in the Public Awareness of the Federal Republic	G. Christiansen J. Töppich	Bundesministerium für Gesundheit	German	Reunified Germany. Annual survey since 1987 in the former Federal Republic of Germany

Country/year	Date	Survey	Authors	Organization	Language	Notes
Great Britain 1991	5/90–12/91	National Survey of Sexual Attitudes and Lifestyles (NATSAL)	J. Field, A. Johnson, J. Wadsworth, K. Wellings	Wellcome Trust	English	
Netherlands 1989	7–8/89	Health and Relationships	T. Sandfort, G. van Zessen	Ministry of Health and Netherlands Foundation for Preventive Medicine	Dutch	
Norway 1992	11/92	The Norwegian Sexual Behaviour Study	P. Magnus, J.M. Sundet	Ministry of Health	Norwegian	Survey carried out by post. Similar survey in 1987.
Portugal 1991	12/90–2/91	Partner Relations and Risk of HIV Infection	J. Santos Lucas	Comissão Nacional de Luta contra a SIDA, World Health Organization (WHO)	Portuguese	Survey limited to localities of at least 10000 inhabitants
Scotland 1992	7/91–4/92	Study of Lifestyle and Health (LAH–AIDS)	D. McQueen, B. Robertson, D. Uitenbroek	Scottish Home and Health Department	English	Continuous data collection (5 days a week) since July 1987
Spain 1990	2/90	Risk Practices and AIDS among the Spanish Population	R. Usieto Atondo, J. Sastre Espada	Universidad Internacional Menendez Pelayo – Centro de Analisis social, Distrex Iberica	Spanish	
Switzerland 1992	10/92	Survey of AIDS Prevention Behaviour	F. Dubois-Arber, A. Jeannin, F. Paccaud	Office fédéral de la santé publique	German, French, Italian	Annual survey since 1987, every two years after 1992

* This identification will be used throughout the book. It comprises 1) the country or area of investigation, 2) an additional qualification if two surveys were carried out in the same country or area at the same period, 3) the year data collection ended. The abbreviations used for the same surveys in some tables or figures in the book are: ATH89, ATH90, B93, FIN92, FR92 (ACSF or KABP is added if the two French surveys are used in the same chapter), EG90, WG90, EG93, WG93, GB91, NL89, N92, P91, CH92, SP90.

the comparisons,[3] but specific analyses from these surveys were completed for Chapter 2 (and Chapter 5 for the British data). Former communist countries (except former East Germany) were not included because their participation was not allowed at the time by the EU programme under which this project was funded.[4] Northern, central and southern Europe are, however, equally represented. The first surveys included in our comparisons were carried out in 1989 and the last one in 1993. Additional surveys have been carried out more recently, for example, the French, German and Swiss follow-up surveys and the Swedish national survey in 1996, but it was not possible to include them at the time our cross-national analyses were made.[5] All the surveys compared in this book are cross-sectional studies. Some – Switzerland, Germany, Norway, France and Scotland – were repeated once or several times, partly or fully. For these surveys only the latest investigation at our disposal was taken into account in our comparisons, although the first ones were conducted in 1987. Thus, two of the 16 surveys compared in this book were carried out in 1989, four in 1990, two in 1991, six in 1992 and two in 1993.

All the surveys except two of the three German ones were carried out by universities or research institutes, which often commissioned a private market research agency to collect the data. They were all publicly funded, except the British one, which, like the American survey (Laumann, Gagnon and Michael, 1994a), received a political veto after first having received the agreement of national bodies responsible for public health and research (Johnson and Wellings, 1994). Three surveys (Portugal and the two Athens surveys) were partly or fully sponsored by the World Health Organization. The others were financed mostly by national ministries of health, specific AIDS research or prevention programmes, or national research councils. In one-third of the cases, several bodies financed the surveys jointly.

The survey identifications used in Table 1.1 will be used accordingly throughout the book (the dates are the years when data collection ended). The abbreviations used for the same surveys in some tables or figures in the book are presented in the note in Table 1.1.

Questionnaire Orientations and Contents

Social scientists have been discouraged from studying sexuality by pre-conceptions, normative discourses and beliefs that no reliable information on this intimate topic can or should be obtained from the population, to name just a few of the obstacles that have made research in this field difficult (Laumann *et al.*, 1994b; Bozon, 1995). A large number of researchers, however (Gagnon and Simon, 1973; Carballo *et al.*, 1989; Johnson and Wellings, 1994; Bozon and Leridon, 1996) that think like any other basic human activity (such as eating), sexuality is a social product. That is to say that while it is rooted in biological capacities and processes, its expression is multiple and varies historically and socio-culturally within and across societies. Therefore, there is no scientifically acceptable reason not to study sexuality and sexual behaviour. Moreover, by providing a better knowledge of sexuality, the social sciences can contribute to the understanding and solving of the problems that are sometimes associated with this activity (such as violence and diseases).

The approaches taken to the study of sexuality in the surveys compared in this book are diverse, as suggested by the variety of research contexts mentioned before. This is shown even better by the questionnaires' orientations and contents, which we shall now turn to.

All these surveys were prompted by the AIDS epidemic. This was explicitly stated in most survey reports and publications (Sundet *et al.*, 1988, 1990; Athens School of Public Health, 1990; Basisresearch, 1990; Stefanis, 1991; van Zessen and Sandfort, 1991; Moatti, Dab and Pollak, 1992; Bajos *et al.*, 1994; Giami, 1996; Hubert *et al.*, 1993; Santos Lucas, 1993; Dubois-Arber *et al.*, 1996; Statens Institutt for Folkehelse, 1993; Bundeszentrale für Gesundheitliche Aufklärung, 1994; Johnson and Wellings, 1994). The researchers' aims were to measure to various extents the prevalence of some behaviour and attitudes and to understand risky practices better so as to inform preventive policies and the modelling of the epidemic. The only exception was the Finnish survey, carried out in 1992, which clung resolutely to a tradition of research into sexuality that goes back to the late nineteenth century and is closely connected to sexological research conducted in the other Scandinavian countries and the USA. This survey, one of the aims of which was to assess behavioural changes occurring since a 1971 survey, paid almost no attention to AIDS prevention (Kontula and Haavio-Mannila, 1995).[6]

In a sense, HIV/AIDS prevention and epidemiology have legitimized research on sexuality, which was somewhat devalued and under-developed in the past. But it is also true that many survey investigators who had no background in sex research (but rather in social sciences in general, public health or epidemiology) did not place their work in this tradition. Many surveys that are part of our comparisons are not sex surveys as such but primarily health studies. Examples are the Scottish survey (Robertson, McQueen and Nisbet, 1993), KABP[7] surveys (Athens 1989, France–KABP 1992), AIDS prevention evaluation surveys (Germany 1993, Switzerland 1992) or surveys on aspects of sexual behaviour defined as being strictly relevant to HIV/AIDS (Athens 1990, Belgium 1993, West Germany 1990, Norway 1992, Portugal 1991). The Dutch (1989), British (1991), Finnish (1992) and French ACSF (1992) surveys are probably the only European surveys that were more straightforwardly in the tradition of sex research, even though AIDS prevention was the focus of these investigations (except for Finland) and other influences were acting too (for example, the epidemiological influence in the French survey, as noted by

Giami (1996), or the sexual health influence for the British and Finnish surveys – see below).

Although any research is contingent on the way problems are posed in a society at a given time, some authors (di Mauro, 1995; Bozon, 1995) consider that nowadays, because research on sexuality is driven almost exclusively by HIV risk, a large part of the sexual activity of the population, even some aspects that may be relevant in the context of HIV/AIDS prevention, have not been studied – or too little – and thus remain widely unknown. Bozon (1995) cites the example of masturbation, which was taken out of many questionnaires because HIV cannot be transmitted by this practice and embarrassment from respondents was feared.

In taking note of the various influences that had some impact on the way the European surveys were designed, we must emphasize the important role played by the World Health Organization (WHO), which in the early stages of this field of research (1987–9) provided some European researchers[8] with the opportunity to meet, exchange ideas and contribute to the design of a survey protocol that was used in several developing countries (Cleland and Ferry, 1995) and adapted in four European surveys (namely, Athens–KABP 1989, Athens–PR 1990, Portugal 1991, West Germany 1990). Some European survey investigators followed with great interest the preparation of the US survey on health and sexual behaviour (Laumann *et al.*, 1994b), particularly its network approach, and also Catania, Coates and Stall's (1992) study on AIDS-related risk factors. Classical sex surveys, like Kinsey's (Kinsey *et al.*, 1948, 1953) or, in France, Simon's (Simon *et al.*, 1972), were also taken into account, but sometimes to oppose the current approach.

A count of the questions on a few key topics asked in each survey gives us an idea of the importance of some influences or informs us at least about the predominance of some topics (Hubert and Marques Balsa, 1995). Table 1.2 does not tell us the number of respondents who received the different questions (there were multiple filters) but informs us about the weight (in terms of percentages) given to different topics in each survey questionnaire.[9]

The sizes of the questionnaires in our review range from 83 questions in the Norwegian survey to more than 668 in the Dutch questionnaire. Two-thirds of the questionnaires contain more than 200 questions. This information is important to remember when analyzing Table 1.2, for the shorter a questionnaire, the fewer the number of topics that can be tackled, but also the fewer the number of questions for each topic. The consequences of this are that, first, the shortest questionnaires should be easier to characterize and, second, the percentages presented in our table should be used mainly to study the relative predominance of certain topics within the different questionnaires rather than to evaluate how extensively a topic has been studied in the different surveys, since a smaller percentage in a large questionnaire may cover a larger number of questions than a higher percentage in a smaller questionnaire.

Table 1.2 Proportions of questions on different topics in the various surveys under comparison*

	ATH KABP 1989	ATH PR 1990	B 1993	FIN 1992	FR ACSF 1992	FR KABP 1992	EG 1990	WG 1990	GB 1991	NL 1989	N 1992	P 1991	SCOT 1992	CH 1992
Knowledge, perception, attitudes towards HIV risk and prevention	32.5	6.3	7.9	1.4	8.6	46.2	29.0	7.5	3.9	12.1	0.0	39.0	19.4	13.2
Condom use and representations	10.7	14.1	8.2	0.0	10.2	8.4	16.9	4.6	1.6	5.8	4.8	8.2	3.0	21.9
Number of sexual partners	3.8	9.7	1.1	4.2	3.8	2.9	2.4	5.2	10.7	7.8	16.5	7.1	3.0	7.0
Characteristics of the partners, the meeting places and the relations between partners	0.5	13.0	34.5	8.7	10.6	0.3	2.4	7.5	18.3	24.1	17.3	4.5	2.2	5.3
Sexual practices	0.0	8.4	1.5	8.7	19.6	0.0	0.0	21.5	5.0	21.1	2.4	10.8	0.0	0.0
Past and current family life	25.7	2.9	2.6	13.6	2.3	2.9	0.8	5.6	12.8	0.3	2.4	0.4	0.8	0.9
Contraception and abortion	1.0	3.7	4.6	5.6	1.1	0.5	0.0	0.3	8.9	2.1	4.8	3.7	0.0	0.9
N	206	241	609	426	416	381	124	303	382	668	83	269	131	114

Note:
The column totals are not equal to 100% since all the topics are not presented
*Germany 1993 and Spain 1990 have not been included in this comparison.

We shall first evaluate how central the AIDS-related questions were in the different questionnaires. Then we shall focus on sexual partners and practices. We shall finish with the importance given in the different surveys to family planning and sexual health issues.

The proportions of questions about knowledge of modes of transmission and means of protection, risk perception, and attitudes towards prevention and information sources confirm the predominance of this topic in not only the KABP surveys (Athens and France) but the East German and Portuguese surveys as well. The absence of questions on this topic in the Norwegian questionnaire, just as on all other topics related to attitudes and representations, reveals the authors' assumption that 'it is difficult to get reliable and valid information about feelings and attitudes by means of a self-administered questionnaire' (Sundet *et al.*, 1990, p. 81). The small percentages in the Finnish and, to a lesser extent, British questionnaires tell us that, as the next counts will show as well, these surveys were less directly focused on HIV/AIDS.

The number of questions on condom use and opinions about condoms is also a good indicator of the importance given to HIV risk and prevention in a survey. One out of five questions in the Swiss survey was about this matter, but six other surveys asked between 8 and 16 per cent of their questions on this topic as well. Here again the Finnish and British questionnaires stand out from the others by containing no, or very few, questions on condoms. It is also interesting to note that the Swiss questionnaire has the highest proportion of questions on voluntary HIV testing (data not shown). This reveals a growing interest in recent years in this practice, both as a way of dealing with HIV risk and as an important issue in the context of the development of new treatments, which require early testing.

Questions on number and types of sexual partners (that is, recording and counting sexual experiences according to different types of partners and periods) were asked in all the surveys. This was an inevitable piece of information, whatever the approach taken by the authors. The Norwegian questionnaire, which was designed mainly by epidemiologists, is the one that has the highest proportion of questions on partners (16.5 per cent of all questions), but the two questionnaires (Athens–PR and Portugal) that were derived from the WHO questionnaires on partners' relations, and the British, Dutch and Swiss surveys also have a fairly high rate of questions on this issue.

Studying how partners negotiate over sexual risk by asking questions about the characteristics of the partners and the relations between them is a new direction of research that the Belgian survey has pursued much more than the others. Close to a quarter of the questions in the Belgian survey dealt with the characterization of the relationships in which the respondents were involved. Several other surveys (Athens–PR, France–ACSF, Great Britain, the Netherlands, Norway) asked a significant proportion of questions on this issue as well.

Questions about sexual practices, to measure the prevalence of vaginal, anal and oral sex, sex without penetration, masturbation, and so on, but also to try to grasp the variety of sexual activity in the population (including practices such as sado-masochism or voyeurism, for example), are highly prevalent (one out of five questions) in just a few surveys (the French ACSF, West German and Dutch surveys) and totally absent from KABP surveys and AIDS prevention evaluation surveys.

The differences in the proportions of questions in the different questionnaires about respondents' past and current family lives can be explained by the researchers' backgrounds and past concerns for family planning and sexual health issues. Thus, the Finnish and British questionnaires, which both presented themselves as surveys on 'sexual attitudes and lifestyles', contained many more questions pertaining to the respondents' family lives and conjugal experiences than the other surveys (the Athens–KABP questionnaire also contained a lot of questions on that topic, but they were used mainly to describe the profile and composition of the household for methodological purposes). The Finnish and British surveys also included higher percentages of questions on attitudes towards sexuality and sexual norms than most of the other surveys (the Belgian, Dutch and French ACSF included this concern as well) (data not shown).

The British investigators' concern to place HIV risk in the broader context of sexual health and to examine other sexual risks is confirmed by a larger proportion of questions in these surveys on contraception and abortion, for example, which were studied in some other surveys too (such as the Finnish and Belgian ones).[10] These issues were nearly non-existent in several other surveys.

Catania *et al.* (1996) also compared the contents of the questionnaires used in different countries to survey sexual behaviour and attitudes towards HIV risk. They did it in a different way than we did by determining whether relevant indicators for modelling HIV spread or mapping risk behaviour were present in or absent from each questionnaire. Their conclusion was that most surveys in their global review – including the surveys we are examining in this book – provided insufficient information for modelling HIV spread but adequate information for identifying levels of various risk factors (behavioural mapping).

A Wide Diversity of Data Collection and Sampling Techniques

There were important differences in the interview techniques used by different European investigators (Table 1.3). Face-to-face interviews predominate (in eight surveys) but the telephone was used widely (in six surveys), while self-completion was used in many surveys, either as the sole survey technique (in three surveys) or more often to complement face-to-face interviews (in five surveys).

Table 1.3 *Methodological characteristics of the surveys under comparison*

Survey ident.	Age range	Interview mode	Sampling method	Sample size (total)	Sample size (18–49)
Athens–KABP 1989	15–64	FTF + SAQ	Two-stage clustered sampling: selection of 150 clusters; random-route selection of households; selection of one individual in each household according to age and gender criteria	1200	952
Athens–PR 1990	15–49	FTF	Two-stage clustered sampling: selection of three area units in 40 clusters; random-route selection of households; selection of one or more individuals in each household according to age and gender criteria	1980	1777
Belgium 1993	15–59	CATI	Multi-stage stratified random sampling of individuals in the population registry (*)	3733	2789
Finland 1992	18–74	FTF + SAQ	Random sampling in the population registry	2248	1529
France–ACSF 1992	18–69	CATI	Stratified random sampling of households in the telephone directory; selection of individuals according to their birthday (*)(**)	20055 (4820 'long' questionnaires only)	3379 ('long' questionnaires only)
France–KABP 1992	18–69	CATI	Stratified random sampling of households in the telephone directory; selection of individuals according to their birthday (*)(**)	1927	1320
Germany (East) 1990	16–74	SAQ	Random sampling of 40 'Kreise' of former EG; random-route selection of the households; selection of individuals according to their birthday (**)	1319	822
Germany (West) 1990	18–69	FTF + SAQ	Quota sampling of German nationals (criteria: gender, age, profession, marital status, state, town size)	3014	2405

	Age range	Method	Sampling		
Germany (East & West) 1993	16–74	CATI in WG FTF in EG	Random sampling (**). In WG: sample of phone numbers in systematically selected communities; randomized-last-digit procedure; selection of individuals according to their birthday. In EG: sample of 40 'Kreise' of former EG; random-route selection of the households; selection of individuals according to their birthday	4662	2776
Great Britain 1991	16–59	FTF + SAQ	Multi-stage stratified random sampling of addresses in the Post Office's PAF; selection of individuals according to a variant of the Kish Grid (*)	18876	15027
Netherlands 1989	18–50	FTF	Multi-stage stratified random sampling of addresses in the housing registry; selection of individuals according to their birthday	1001	990
Norway 1992	18–60	SAQ postal	Random sampling in the population registry	4760	4029
Portugal 1991	18–49	FTF + SAQ	Multi-stage stratified sampling at region and habitat levels; quota sampling (based on age, gender and education) at locality level[1] (*)	2471	2471
Scotland 1992	18–60	CATI	Random digit dialling; random selection of the respondent in the household (**)	5880	4674
Spain 1990	14+	SAQ	Random sample of national registry	1103	859
Switzerland 1992	17–45	CATI	Random sampling of households in the telephone directory; selection of individuals according to gender and age quotas (*)	2800	2685[2]

Abbreviations:
CATI = Computer-assisted telephone interview
FTF = Face-to-face
SAQ = Self-administered questionnaire
(*): sample weighted to correct for differential probabilities
(**): sample weighted to adjust to external data
Notes:
[1] Survey limited to localities of at least 10000 inhabitants
[2] The age range is 18–45 in Switzerland

The advantages and drawbacks of the various data collection techniques were much debated among the researchers. The investigators of only one of the surveys in our review (ACSF investigators, 1992a) compared the effects of different modes of interviewing (telephone and face-to-face). According to this study, the participation rates for the two techniques were equivalent. The authors noted great consistency in answers to questions on sexual behaviour, but more answers to attitudinal questions that were in accordance with dominant social norms in telephone than face-to-face interviews. They also wrote that the main advantage of the telephone, apart from its lower cost, is the possibility of creating the 'right distance' between interviewer and interviewee and a more continuous and homogenous follow-up of interviewers. There is extensive literature (for a review, see Bradburn and Sudman, 1979; Groves *et al.*, 1988) on how the properties of different modes of data collection influence measurement error. The capacity of the different modes to increase the credibility of the study and the anonymity of the answers is a special focus of the assessment of the different modes. But as Catania *et al.* (1990) suggested, we should not only consider the impact of the different modes of data collection as such, but also the effect of varying properties within a particular mode. On the other hand, it is clear that the type of research objective pursued is often decisive in the choice of the data collection technique (Tielman, 1990). It is not surprising, for instance, that the telephone has been used widely in repeated surveys (such as the German, Swiss and Scottish), the aims of which are to provide policy makers and AIDS prevention workers continuously and relatively cheaply with needed information on knowledge, attitudes and reported behaviour.

The surveys compared in this book were aimed at populations spread across their respective national territories (or at least those who master sufficiently the national languages). The exceptions were Scotland, the two Greek surveys, which were limited to greater Athens, and the Portuguese survey, in which only localities of at least 10 000 inhabitants were included.[11] The lower age limit was 18 years old in half the surveys[12] whereas it ranged from 14 to 17 in the other surveys. The upper limit ranged from 45 to 74 (no limit for Spain).

All but three of the surveys used probability samples of the population (Table 1.3). Quotas were used at some stage of the procedure in the West German survey (1990), as well as in the Portuguese and Swiss surveys. The sampling strategies differed from one country to the next according to the availability and access of sampling bases, the data collection technique and the local research tradition. For these reasons participation rates are difficult to compare, as discussed by Field, Wadsworth and Bradshaw (1994) and Laumann *et al.* (1994b). The participation rates of those with whom a contact was achieved with an interviewer appear to be particularly high (between 60 and 75 per cent in most surveys). This is in contradiction to the previously expressed fears that people would not agree to talk about their intimate lives by telephone.

It is important to stress that sending an advance letter to the respondents increased the participation rate, as shown by the French investigators (ACSF Investigators, 1992b). But the contents of this letter, as these authors said, can become controversial when scientific and ethical arguments compete, in particular about how far we should go in divulging the topic of the survey (public health, sex and/or AIDS?) and obtaining respondents' informed consent. When we compare various experiences, however, the topic of the survey, as announced in the advance letter, seems to have less impact on the participation rate than the degree of trust that surrounds surveys and polls in a country or the incentives given by the investigators to motivate the respondents (Hubert, forthcoming).[13]

In contrast, the subject chosen to announce the survey may have great impact on the quality and nature of the responses. Placing a survey on sexuality under the sign of AIDS, for example, inevitably calls forth certain images of sexuality and can undermine the reliability of certain responses, such as those concerning condom use (Giami, 1996) or sexual experience and number of partners. On the latter, a pilot survey conducted in Belgium showed that some married respondents did not consider their spouses to be sexual partners. This reflected their belief that only extramarital sex was of interest to the investigators in connection with AIDS (Peto, Marquet and Hubert, 1995).

The mode of data collection is also a factor that may produce some bias and skew the actual distribution of the populations under study. These biases are specific to the telephone and self-administered surveys. The former are restricted to telephone subscribers. The impact of this restriction on the samples' characteristics will depend on the overall telephone coverage in the countries where this technique was used, and the inequalities in coverage among the different social categories. On the other hand, self-administered questionnaires likewise introduce biases that are not equally distributed in the social structure. They require socio-cultural skills to be able to read and understand the questions properly, as well as to write the answers. In addition, in the absence of an interviewer, the respondents are more free to skip questions. This explains the higher 'no answer' rates observed for the questions about the number of partners, for example (see Chapter 5 of this book).

On the whole, quite different numbers of people were surveyed from one European country to the next (Table 1.3). The French and British surveys had similar sample sizes (close to 20000 respondents)[14] while the other surveys ranged from about 1000 to 5000 respondents. Altogether more than 80000 Europeans[15] were interviewed about their sex lives, which gives an idea of the importance of the investment made in these investigations in a short period of time.

In nine of the 16 surveys under review the samples have been weighted, that is to say that some individuals have been multiplied by a coefficient so that the socio-demographic characteristics of the samples are closer to those of the populations under study. Two different types of weighting have to be distinguished (see the asterisks in Table 1.3). The first, to correct for differential probabilities, is an integral part of the sample design. It was used in the French and British surveys to take the size of the household into account, since only one individual was selected per household (Leridon, 1994; Field, Wadsworth and Bradshaw, 1994), and in the Belgian, Portuguese and Swiss surveys to give to the regions that compose the country and were oversampled their proportionate sizes (Hubert *et al.*, 1993; Santos Lucas, 1993; Institut universitaire de médecine sociale et préventive, 1993). The second type of weighting consists in applying to some individuals a coefficient calculated from information that is external to the samples themselves, such as census data. Five of the nine weighted samples (the two French, East German (1990), German (1993) and Scottish) have been adjusted in such a way by comparing the distribution of variables such as age, gender and civil status with external sources.[16] This procedure relies on the assumption that the behaviour of the 'missing' individuals in a category is closer to the mean of the respondents of the same category than to the mean of the whole (unadjusted) sample (Leridon, 1994). Thus, among the group of weighted samples, the British, Belgian, Portuguese and Swiss investigators did not share this assumption[17] and weighted their samples to correct for differential probabilities only. No weighting at all was applied to the Athenian, Finnish, Dutch, Norwegian and Spanish samples, which were all probability samples. The investigators of all these surveys thought that the biases in participation could not be fully explained by the limited external socio-demographic data available and considered that one had to take the samples as they were, knowing which categories were under- or over-represented.

The samples' age and gender profiles as drawn from the information available in each survey report[18] are summarized in Table 1.4 for all the probability samples[19] that were not weighted for age and gender, as the weighting process itself eliminated any deviation in this respect. This does not mean, however, that the latter or the samples presented in Table 1.4 do not deviate from external data with regard to other variables.

The probability samples that were not weighted by age and gender show a male deficit when they are compared with external data. As Field, Wadsworth and Bradshaw (1994, p. 57) say, 'This appears to be due to greater difficulty in contacting selected male respondents and to proxy refusals rather than to higher rates of direct refusal.' Relatively small differences were observed when the samples were broken down by age, but the most marked under-representation is in older age groups and over-representation in younger age groups (which vary from one survey to the next).

Table 1.4 *Comparison of the probability samples with external data on age and gender (only samples not weighted for age and gender)*

Athens–KABP[1] 1989	Correspondence of overall gender breakdown with census data; large under-representation (−5%), especially among men, of people over 40, and large over-representation (+5%) of 15–30
Athens–PR[2] 1990	Total deficit of about 2% of males; under-representation of older respondents, balanced by over-representation of younger
Belgium[3] 1993	Total deficit of about 3% of males; slight under-representation of men over 50 and women over 55, but also of men aged 30–39, partly balanced by a slight over-representation of 15–19 and 45–49
Finland[4] 1992	Slight total deficit of males; under-representation of people aged 35–44, balanced by over-representation of people aged under 25
Great Britain[5] 1991	Total deficit of about 5% of males, deficit present in all age groups; slight under-representation of men over 50 and women over 55, balanced by a slight over-representation of younger age groups (men aged 16–24 and 35–39, women aged 16–19 and 25–39)
Netherlands[6] 1989	Total deficit of about 9% of males, deficit mainly present over 40; slight under-representation of people aged 45–49, balanced by a slight over-representation of 30–34
Norway[7] 1992	Total deficit of males deficit present in all age groups; under-representation of older respondents, balanced by over-representation of younger (continuous lower participation rates from younger to older respondents)
Spain 1990	(survey report not communicated)

Sources:
[1] Athens School of Public Health, 1990
[2] No information available in Stefanis, 1991. Conclusions drawn from census data provided by the Athens School of Public Health (1990)
[3] Hubert and Marquet, 1993
[4] Kontula and Haavio-Mannila, 1995
[5] Field *et al.*, 1994
[6] Van Zessen and Sandfort, 1991
[7] Statens Institutt for Folkehelse, 1993

How Did We Deal with This Diversity?

In many cross-national projects, a 'juxtaposition approach' (Hantrais, 1996) is often taken to carry out comparative studies. In such an approach, national experts are required to provide descriptive accounts from national data sources according to agreed criteria, and these accounts are presented side by side (one chapter for each country). In this book we took the opposite tack, for we wanted to conduct systematic comparisons of the available surveys. To reach this goal the steering committee[20] that led this project and, later, the three co-editors of the book had to set up a complex working procedure to deal with the just-mentioned diversity in questionnaires' orientations and contents, on the one hand, and sampling and data collection techniques, on the other. In this section, we shall present the consequences of this diversity on the comparability of data and the working procedure that was set up accordingly.

Comparing Questions

The fact that all the authors in this book had to compare data from questionnaires designed according to different orientations and used in different contexts is not a problem as such. As Alwin *et al.* noted (1994), it is mainly a problem of 'functional equivalence', that is, do the questions asked in the different countries stand in identical relationships to the intended theoretical dimensions? In other words, how do we capture the same concept or a similar phenomenon in the face of very different social realities? This problem is thus often not simply a problem of 'literal replication', as the same question asked in different socio-cultural and linguistic contexts may not have the same meaning.[21] It is impossible, for example, to measure the level of education of the populations of various European countries with the same question, for the education systems are very different. Or an identical attitudinal question about HIV/AIDS prevention policy may be interpreted very differently from one country to the next if the financial means allocated to such prevention are high or low, the policy much debated or not, and so on. In such cases, one would stress the importance of achieving 'conceptual replication', that is, constructing items that differ in their manifest content but are equivalent with regard to their theoretical dimensions. Thus, depending on the context, either literal or conceptual replication may be valid approaches to establishing functional equivalence.

The issue of functional equivalence is not specific to multinational surveys, but affects national studies as well. Some of the surveys compared in this volume (such as the Belgian, Finnish and Swiss ones) were administered in several languages and all surveys had to deal with a more or less wide spectrum of socio-culturally differentiated subpopulations. Typically, any single-country survey is based on the assumption that standardized questions can be asked and understood the same way by all, and thus answers can be summed. Differing interpretations of survey questions are usually conceptualized in terms of measurement errors. Multinational survey measurement just adds more complexity to this problem.

The members of the steering committee had no miraculous solution to propose to the authors for assessing the functional equivalence of the questions to be used to make their cross-national comparisons. They dealt with this problem by developing a series of working procedures to enhance 'intersubjectivity'[22] among the authors, that is, the possibility of sharing key information about the surveys, comparing ideas and, in a later step, checking the validity of the interpretations.

The steering committee first set a few author eligibility requirements. Apart from being a specialist in the field, the first condition was to have taken an active part in the design, data collection and analysis of one of the surveys involved in the comparisons. Although all the survey investigators could not be authors, all the authors were survey investigators and were thus aware, from the inside, of the specific problems of collecting data on sexual behaviour and HIV/AIDS and able to share relevant information about their own surveys (meanings of some question wordings, peculiarities of field work, and so on). Another condition for becoming an author was to have conducted cross-national analyses of data with one or more co-authors from different countries.[23] This condition, together with participating in the meetings we organized and the possibility of exchanging qualitative information among survey investigators, guaranteed that even if it were impossible for each survey investigator to participate in the work of all the working parties, the national specificities could be taken into account.

Another important aspect is the way the items to be compared were selected and their comparability analyzed. Direct access to survey questions was organized by the coordinating team at the Centre d'études sociologiques (CES) of Facultés universitaires Saint-Louis (Brussels).[24] Sets of relevant survey questions were selected in a 'bank of indicators' for all the proposed topics and provided to the authors of each chapter. This 'bank of indicators' (see Hubert and Marques Balsa, 1995) – the term 'bank of questions' would be more appropriate – was a computerized database in which the approximately 5000 questions asked in the different surveys were stored, summarized and classified to allow different types of searches. The authors of each chapter were then asked to select in the set of questions provided to them the survey questions they wanted to compare, and to assess the comparability of the different survey questions they finally used. That is why each chapter contains a large 'methods' section devoted to the analysis of the differences in question wordings and time periods, and of the national and survey context of the selected questions. These methodological considerations led in some chapters to interesting observations about, for example, differences in frequencies depending on types of question formulations or on 'no answer' rates according to interview modes.

A last opportunity for mutual control and exchange of information, on question wordings in particular, was when the authors had to address their data requests (cross-tabulations, statistics, and so on) to the investigators of the surveys they wanted to include in their comparisons. Centralizing all of the original data files at the CES in Brussels was out of the question. These data files were sometimes so complex that only the researchers who produced them truly knew them. What is more, it is not certain that all of the survey investigators would have accepted or been allowed to release their data files to others. That is why we opted for a data exchange procedure in which each survey investigator received and processed the data requests put to him/her by the authors.[25] The advantage of such a procedure was that the data were processed primarily by the investigators who had generated them and thus who knew them best. The disadvantages were that this required myriad written, phone and electronic exchanges and considerable shuttling between the working parties and the survey investigators before the right analyses were obtained. In addition, this generated a considerable amount of work for the survey investigators.

These working procedures were interesting to describe since such close-to-the-field collaborative enterprises are becoming rarer in a context where the volume of studies has been swelling and the availability of research data for secondary analysis, away from field work, is increasing (Alwin *et al.*, 1994).

Comparing Samples

Given the variations in age ranges covered by each survey, we decided to limit the comparisons to the 18- to 49-year-old age group, which was the only age span common to all the surveys but one, Switzerland, where the upper limit was 45.[26] Table 1.3 above gives the exact size of all the samples when restricted to the age group 18–49. Four surveys – Athens–KABP, East Germany (1990), the Netherlands and Spain – contained fewer than 1000 respondents when restricted in this manner.

We also had to deal with the considerable diversity in sampling and data collection techniques. Because these were drawn up before the project could start, we had no way of influencing the survey designs. Thus, we have to assume that the researchers in charge of these surveys made the best sampling and mode of data collection choices in light of the available sampling bases and funding, as well as doing their best to attain the highest possible participation rate. As Kish (1994) noted, it is better to allow a certain flexibility of choice in sampling design for multinational comparisons because the sampling resources differ greatly between countries. This is particularly defensible if probability sampling is used. We must say that this was not completely the case in three of the surveys under comparison, that is West Germany (1990), Portugal (1991) and Switzerland (1992), where quotas were used at some stage of the procedure.

What denominators are looked at in the different chapters? Whereas in some chapters (Chapters 5 and 12 for example) the authors compared the 'no answer' rates to some questions in the different surveys as a preliminary result to inform the reader about issues like question sensitiveness or impact of

Table 1.5 *Confidence intervals for various sample sizes*

Sample size	p = 2%	p = 5%	p = 10%	p = 25%
100	0–4.7	0.7–9.3	4.1–15.9	16.5–33.5
400	0.6–3.4	2.9–7.1	7.1–12.9	20.8–29.2
1000	1.1–2.9	3.6–6.4	8.1–11.9	22.3–27.7
6000	1.6–2.4	4.4–5.6	9.3–10.7	24.1–25.9

interview mode on response rate, most analyses concerned only the population who replied. In addition, in many chapters the analyses were restricted to those who reported having ever had sex.

Adjusting the survey data in line with external data is a scientifically debated type of weighting. Here again we must say that we had no other possibility than to compare weighted and unweighted samples together because we had no influence on the investigators' choices. Of course, it would have been better if each sample had been weighted according to the same criteria to avoid bias specific to certain countries. Although the deficit in older respondents that was observed in all the surveys is less damageable since the samples were restricted to 49, it remains that the youngest age groups and females are still slightly over-represented in unweighted probability samples (listed in Table 1.4). This is why the data have been controlled for age and gender in all the chapters.[27] Other key socio-demographic variables (such as level of education or size of the place of residence) have also been used throughout the book as control variables.

The above limitations in sampling equivalence made it even more important to take into account the confidence intervals within which the measurements lie. In the tables presented in the book, particularly those with numerous cells, where these intervals are not provided, they can easily be estimated by the usual formula.[28] In weighted samples, the denominators (Ns) are provided unweighted but the percentages are weighted. Table 1.5 gives some useful 95 per cent confidence interval values.

Making Cross-national Analyses

Nations can be compared by considering them either as *units* of analysis or *contexts* of analysis (Kohn, 1989). When the nation is the unit of analysis, dependent variables will be measured as similarly as possible across different countries and researchers will try to interpret the observed differences and similarities. When comparative research focuses on testing hypotheses, for example on whether predictive relationships found in one country hold up in other countries, the nation is often treated as a 'context' variable and may not

Table 1.6 *Socio-demographic characteristics of the samples[1]*

	ATH89 KABP	B93	FIN92	FR92 ACSF	EG90	WG90	EG93	WG93	GB91	NL89	N92	P91	SCOT92	CH92[2]
MEN														
Age														
18–19	8.3	7.2	5.8	6.2	5.3	6.1	3.8	5.1	6.8	7.9	7.2	11.0	4.6	9.9
20–24	19.6	17.6	14.5	17.3	14.5	19.4	15.0	14.0	17.3	18.2	17.6	19.6	13.0	16.6
25–29	18.3	13.7	15.9	15.8	12.6	22.4	18.5	19.3	17.1	16.3	17.6	10.2	18.6	17.4
30–39	37.3	30.5	33.4	31.9	37.7	29.2	35.8	34.4	30.4	35.9	31.4	33.5	34.7	37.5
40–49	16.5	31.0	30.4	28.8	29.9	22.8	26.9	27.2	28.5	21.8	26.2	25.8	29.1	18.6
Cohabitation														
Cohabiting	83.5	63.9	66.5	66.2	75.5	51.2	72.2	59.3	64.0	56.5	61.3	52.7	45.6	53.9
Not cohabiting	10.2	22.4	33.5	33.8	24.5	21.0	26.8	40.4	36.0	16.3	38.6	46.9	61.0	46.1
No answer	6.3	13.7	0.0	0.1		27.8	0.9	0.4	0.0	27.3	0.2	0.4	39.0	0.0
Place of residence														
Rural		3.2	38.1	32.2	19.8	31.7	27.9	14.2	n.p.	2.4	31.3	n.p.	n.a.	40.2
Small towns		66.7	36.3	23.0	51.9	16.9	32.5	55.3	n.p.	73.2	45.9	n.p.	n.a.	44.5
Towns		18.4	25.0	27.4	21.2	21.7	28.7	22.9	n.p.	24.4	22.3	n.p.	n.a.	14.9
Large cities		11.8		17.4	7.2	28.8	10.9	7.6	n.p.			n.p.	n.a.	
No answer			0.5			1.0			n.p.		0.4	n.p.		0.5
Education														
Low	25.4	23.0	23.0	31.2	11.9	27.8	12.4	34.4	n.p.	5.0	41.1	37.8	57.9	4.5
Medium	37.3	39.3	54.0	45.4	54.1	56.3	51.1	26.9	n.p.	59.8	21.3	38.9	11.4	82.3
High	37.3	37.4	22.9	23.3	34.1	15.7	35.4	38.1	n.p.	34.2	37.0	23.1	30.7	13.0
No answer		0.3	0.1	0.1		0.2	1.1	0.6	n.p.	1.0	0.5	0.2		0.2
N	480	1334	787	1696	405	1126	579	840	6669	418	1787	1221	2130	1362

WOMEN

Age														
18–19	7.0	5.5	5.7	6.1	4.6	4.9	5.3	4.6	6.3	7.5	6.4	11.0	3.3	9.9
20–24	16.3	14.6	16.4	17.7	15.8	19.1	14.6	14.2	15.1	15.9	17.8	17.2	13.3	18.0
25–29	18.2	16.1	15.1	15.2	19.0	17.4	18.0	19.0	18.4	18.2	17.9	11.9	18.8	17.4
30–39	38.8	34.4	33.6	32.6	34.5	34.8	34.9	34.3	31.6	32.5	32.7	32.7	34.7	36.9
40–49	19.7	29.5	29.2	28.5	26.1	23.8	27.2	27.9	28.6	25.9	25.2	27.2	29.9	17.8
Cohabitation														
Cohabiting	84.5	72.9	68.6	67.8	89.5	64.5	77.1	67.7	70.6	69.2	71.7	58.4	61.1	62.3
Not cohabiting	9.3	15.6	31.4	32.2	10.5	17.4	22.8	31.8	29.4	11.5	28.0	41.3	38.9	37.6
No answer	6.1	11.5	0.0	0.0		18.1	0.2	0.5	0.1	19.2	0.4	0.4		0.1
Place of residence														
Rural		2.9	34.5	28.1	20.1	30.0	32.0	16.5	n.p.	5.2	29.1	n.p.	n.a.	42.3
Small towns		66.2	36.8	23.4	49.2	16.7	34.5	52.8	n.p.	68.7	46.0	n.p.	n.a.	45.1
Towns		17.6	28.7	30.9	22.8	23.0	23.6	23.1	n.p.	26.0	23.1	n.p.	n.a.	12.3
Large cities	100	13.3		17.5	8.0	29.7	9.9	7.6	n.p.			n.p.	n.a.	
No answer			0.0			0.6			n.p.		1.7			0.3
Education														
Low	36.0	20.7	21.2	33.2	7.6	43.2	13.9	37.6	n.p.	4.4	38.6	42	63.2	9.9
Medium	37.3	39.2	49.7	41.4	67.1	48.6	50.1	36.8	n.p.	70.8	22.8	34.1	12.1	82.8
High	41.3	39.7	29.1	25.4	25.3	7.9	34.6	25.2	n.p.	23.4	38.4	24	24.6	7.0
No answer		0.4	0.0	0.0		0.4	1.3	0.3	n.p.	1.4	0.2	0		0.2
N	472	1455	742	1682	368	1279	567	790	8358	572	2242	1246	2544	1323

Base: All respondents (18–49 years) who ever had sex

Abbreviations:

n.a. = not available

n.p. = not provided by the survey investigators

Notes:

[1] Athens PR 1990 France–KABP 1992 and Spain 1990 have not been included in this table

[2] Switzerland: the age range is 18–45

be of interest *per se.* In that case, taking into account as many nations as possible is the means to enlarge the empirical base in which these predictive relationships can be tested.

A few chapters (Chapter 11 on social networks and normative contexts and Chapter 14 on knowledge and discrimination) can be viewed as following the second approach (testing the generality of some hypotheses). But most authors followed the first approach primarily. First, they made country-to-country comparisons of the frequencies of their dependent variables, paying attention to the importance, as mentioned earlier, of taking the confidence intervals into account in order to keep statistically significant differences only. Index construction (that is, creating new synthesis variables with several indicators) was only possible in Chapters 12 and 14, because in the other chapters where it would have been relevant to do so, too, there were not enough comparable questions to be included in an index. This was also made difficult by the fact that all the data files were not centralized in Brussels. The second stage usually consisted of cross-tabulating the dependent variables with socio-demographic or other independent variables, the purpose being to discover trends common to all countries or groups of countries in Europe through co-variations between the independent and dependent variables. We thought that the existence of such trends, more than correlations within one single country, would draw our attention to issues that might be of particular importance for the problems under study, but we did not believe this would demonstrate any causal relationship between the associated variables, which could be explored by multivariate analyses only.

The frequencies of some of the main variables used in this book as independent variables are presented in Table 1.6 above. The cohabitation variable is the current cohabiting status, that is, whether one is living or not with a *sexual* partner. Thus, people who cohabit with somebody else (parents, sister or brother, friends, and so on) are classified as *not* cohabiting. The residence variable covers the size of the locality where the respondent lived. Four categories were chosen: under 5000 inhabitants (rural), between 5000 and 100 000 (small towns), between 100 000 and 999 999 (towns), and over one million (large cities). Level of education was broken down in three categories to try to fit the large diversity in education systems and survey questions. 'Low education' ranges from no education to secondary school not completed. 'Medium education' is defined as secondary school completed. Students currently in secondary school are also put in this category. 'High education' means post-secondary school education, whether this education has been completed or not. Of course, such a definition is somewhat arbitrary. We must say that in this study we were interested not in education systems as such, but in building a functionally equivalent education variable that could be used as an independent variable and cross-tabulated with some dependent variables to determine whether or not common trends could be detected across countries.

To help them interpret differences and similarities between countries, all the authors received a set of relevant demographic, social and cultural indicators selected by J. Field and K. Wellings (1993) for our Concerted Action. In Chapter 3, for instance, the countries were classified on the basis of such external information (for example from less to more tolerant on sexual matters) and this classification was compared with the frequencies of some dependent variables (for example, the declaration of some homosexual experience) to determine if this external information could in a way 'explain' the dependent variables (in this example, whether the social climate influences the expression of homosexuality). Such an approach, which Hantrais (1996) calls the 'societal approach', could lead to more systematic characterization of the nations under study. In some cases, it may also be desirable (and possible) to measure the variables that differentiate nations directly and enter these variables into the analysis (Rokkan, 1964; Przeworski and Teune, 1970, quoted by Alwin *et al.*, 1994). But such an approach faces at least two important difficulties. The first – and this is a criticism already levelled at Durkheim's study on suicide (as recalled by Boudon, 1969) – is that the more complex a society, the more difficult it is to identify the factors of similarity and dissimilarity and give the observed statistical relationships unequivocal meaning. As Loriaux (1995) points out, the principle of *ceteris paribus* is not applicable when comparing nations that are characterized by many different variables. The second difficulty is that most European countries are not homogeneous entities. The overlap in geographical border areas, for example, can be quite substantial. Divisions along linguistic and cultural lines are another powerful factor. Therefore other units of analysis than nations, such as regions for instance, should be considered when making further comparative analyses.

Conclusion

The surveys that have been taken into account in each chapter are listed in Table 1.7. The selection of surveys was made by the authors according to the availability and comparability of data for the topics under study. Data from at least three to 12 countries were compared in each chapter. The Athens–KABP, France–KABP and Scottish surveys are considered in one or two chapters only, whereas data from the Belgian, Dutch and French surveys are present in most chapters. Due to co-ordination problems, the British survey data are present in Chapters 2 and 5 only, although they could have been processed for more chapters.

Having three co-editors from different countries (Belgium, France and the Netherlands) and backgrounds (sociology, socio-demography and

Table 1.7 Surveys represented in each chapter

	ATH KABP 1989	ATH PR 1990	B 1993	FIN 1992	FR ACSF 1992	FR KABP 1992	EG 1990	WG 1990	G 1993	GB 1991	NL 1989	N 1992	P 1991	SCOT 1992	SP 1990	CH 1992
Sexual initiation*		x	x	x	x			x		x	x	x	x			x
Homo- and bisexual behaviour		x	x	x	x			x			x	x	x		x	x
Sexual practices		x	x	x	x			x			x	x			x	x
Sexual partners		x	x	x	x			x		x	x	x	x		x	x
Risk behaviour		x	x	x	x	x	x	x	x		x	x	x		x	x
STDs			x	x	x		x	x			x	x				
Adaption to HIV		x	x	x	x	x	x	x	x		x		x		x	x
Condom use	x	x	x		x		x		x		x		x			x
HIV testing			x	x	x	x	x				x	x				x
Social networks			x		x						x					
Knowledge		x	x	x		x	x		x		x		x	x	x	
Discrimination	x		x			x	x									
Knowledge and discrimination	x		x	x		x	x		x		x					

Blank cells mean that data was not available
*In this chapter, data from Denmark and Iceland have been included as well

psychology) was important in drawing authors' attention to some of the pitfalls of comparative analysis and helping them go as far as possible in the interpretation of data. But we were conscious that the problems and limitations of conducting cross-national analyses of data on such a large range of countries were not overcome by such an approach.

Because it makes the experiences of the various survey investigators more accessible and presents results that were not discernable by looking separately at the different national surveys, this book aims to provide an empirical source of information for further European research and policy development.

Notes

1   A few large-scale sex surveys had been carried out in some European countries – Finland (Sievers, Koskelainen and Leppo, 1974), France (Simon *et al.*, 1972) and Sweden (Zetterberg, 1969) – long before the outbreak of AIDS.

2   A WHO survey protocol (Carballo *et al.*, 1989; WHO, 1990), designed for the developing countries in which WHO itself funded the surveys, served as a starting point and common basis for discussion in Europe.

3   The Icelandic survey was identified too late to be included. We failed to have continuing collaboration with the Danish and British investigators.

4   Data from some non-EU countries (the 'COST' countries), like Norway and Switzerland, with which the European Union had some co-operation agreement, could be included in this project.

5   Except the 1994 Swiss data in Chapter 9 on condom use.

6   The title of Kontula and Haavio-Mannila's book – *Sexual Pleasures* – reflects this sexological orientation.

7   AIDS-related knowledge, attitudes, beliefs and practices.

8   Mainly the survey investigators from Belgium, France, Great Britain, Greece, Portugal, the Netherlands and Switzerland.

9   This analysis was not possible for two surveys (Germany 1993 and Spain 1990) because they were included in our comparisons at a later stage.

10   In the case of the Belgian survey, this was studied in relation to the first sexual experiences only.

11   Specific restrictions were imposed on the national territory in some other surveys, too. Thus, the French surveys were limited to continental France (an additional survey was conducted in the French Antilles and Guyana), while the British survey excluded the Orkneys, Shetlands, Western Isles and part of the Highland region north of the Caledonian Canal.

12   This lower limit was set at 18 years of age most often for legal reasons, as parental consent is necessary in some countries to ask younger people about certain

things. In some countries, it was decided to carry out specific surveys on young people.

13 Number of contact attempts, reminder letters, ability of the interviewers to convince the selected people to take part in the survey or, as in the Dutch (van Zessen and Sandfort, 1991) and US (Laumann *et al.*, 1994b) surveys, the money given to respondents who would have been hard to involve otherwise.

14 In the French survey, only 4820 respondents received a 'long' questionnaire, after a 'short' questionnaire was used to select them (because of their at-risk behaviour or as part of a control group).

15 This figure would have been much higher if we had taken into account all the surveys that have been replicated several times.

16 The French surveys weighted the samples for the following variables: age, gender, marital status, occupation, region of residence; the East German survey (1990) weighted for age, gender and marital status; the German survey (1993) weighted for age and gender; and the Scottish survey weighted for occupation and phone ownership.

17 The situations of the Portuguese and Swiss samples were rather different, since quotas were used to select the individuals (see later).

18 Information on other key socio-demographic variables is available in the Dutch (van Zessen and Sandfort, 1991) and British (Field, Wadsworth and Bradshaw, 1994) publications.

19 The quota samples were all built on age and gender criteria.

20 Nathalie Bajos, Michel Hubert (project leader), Casimiro Marques Balsa, David McQueen, Theo Sandfort, Peter Stringer and Kaye Wellings were part of this Steering Committee.

21 Problems of translation are at stake here too, for these are not only technical problems but also have to do with socio-cultural differences in meanings. For example, in some cultures, preference may be given to one or another of the expressions 'having sex', 'sexual intercourse', 'sexual relation' or 'making love', each of which does not have exactly the same meaning, whereas in other cultures these terms may be used interchangeably.

22 See Quéré (1996) for an explanation of this concept developed by Habermas.

23 This condition was met in all the chapters except Chapters 3, 6 and 7, which had one author only.

24 C. Marques Balsa played a key role in this task.

25 Only three survey investigators preferred to give CES their data files and have CES handle the requests addressed to them. The surveys in question were Athens PR (1990), West Germany (1990) and Portugal (1991).

26 For Spain we were obliged to study the population aged 19–50 because of precoded categories. Some of the analyses presented in Chapter 2 took the whole sample into account so as to study age at first intercourse across as many generations as possible.

27 Except in Chapter 10 on HIV testing.

28 With a 95 per cent coefficient: $p \pm 1.96 \, [p(1 - p)/N]^{1/2}$ or, for the French ACSF survey, due to sample design specificities: $p \pm 1.96 \, [2p(1 - p)/N]^{1/2}$.

References

ACSF INVESTIGATORS (1992a) 'A comparison between two modes of investigation, telephone survey and face-to-face survey', *AIDS*, **6**, pp. 315–23.

ACSF INVESTIGATORS (1992b) 'Analysis of sexual behaviour in France (ACSF): what kind of advance letter increases the acceptance rate in a telephone survey on sexual behaviour?', in *Bulletin de méthodologie sociologique*, **35**, pp. 46–54.

ALWIN, D.F. *et al.* (1994) 'Measurement in multi-national surveys', in BORG, I. and MOHLER, P.PH. (Eds) *Trends and Perspectives in Empirical Social Research*, Berlin and New York: Walter de Gruyter.

ARIÈS, PH. and BÉJIN, A. (1985) *Western Sexuality*, Oxford: Blackwell.

ATHENS SCHOOL OF PUBLIC HEALTH (1990) *Knowledge, Attitudes, Beliefs and Practices in Relation to HIV Infection and AIDS: The case of the city of Athens (Greece)*, Athens: Department of Sociology.

BAJOS, N., BOZON, M., GIAMI, A. and FERRAND, A. (1994) 'Orientating the research procedure', in SPIRA, A., BAJOS, N. and the ACSF GROUP, *Sexual Behaviour and AIDS*, Aldershot: Avebury (French edition: 1993).

BASISRESEARCH GMBH (1990) *Repräsentative Untersuchung zum Sexual-verhalten von Männern und Frauen in der Bundesrepublik Deutschland*, Frankfurt (unpublished report).

BOUDON, R. (1969) *Les méthodes en sociologie*, Paris: PUF, coll. 'Que sais-je?'

BOZON, M. (1995) 'Observer l'inobservable: la description et l'analyse de l'activité sexuelle', in BAJOS, N., BOZON, M. and GIAMI, A., *Sexualité et Sida. Recherches en sciences sociales*, Paris: ANRS.

BOZON, M. and LERIDON, H. (1996) 'The social constructions of sexuality', in BOZON, M. and LERIDON, H. (Eds) *Sexuality and the Social Sciences. The French Survey on Sexual Behaviour*, Aldershot: Dartmouth (French edition: 1993).

BRADBURN, N. and SUDMAN, S. (1979) *Improving interview method and questionnaire design*, San Francisco: Jossey-Bass.

BUNDESZENTRALE FÜR GESUNDHEITLICHE AUFKLÄRUNG (1994) *Aids im öffentlichen Bewusstsein der Bundesrepublik.*, Wiederholungsbefragung 1993, Köln: Referat 2–25.

CARBALLO, M., CLELAND, J., CARAËL, M. and ALBRECHT, G. (1989) 'A cross-national survey of patterns of sexual behaviour', *Journal of Sex Research*, **26**, pp. 287–99.

CATANIA, J., COATES, T. and STALL, R. (1992) 'Prevalence of AIDS-related risk factors and condom use in the United States', *Science*, **258 (5085)**, pp. 1101–6.

CATANIA, J., GIBSON, D., CHITWOOD, D. and COATES, T. (1990) 'Methodological problems in AIDS behavioral research: influences on measurement error and participation bias in studies of sexual behavior', *Psychological Bulletin*, **108**, 3, pp. 339–62.

CATANIA, J.A., MOSKOWITZ, J.T., RUIZ, M. and CLELAND, J. (1996) 'A review of national AIDS-related behavioural surveys', *AIDS*, **10** (suppl. A), S183–S190.

CLELAND, J. and FERRY, B. (Eds) (1995) *Sexual Behaviour and AIDS in the Developing World*, London: Taylor and Francis.

DAVENPORT, W.H. (1976) 'Sex in cross-cultural perspective', in BEACH, F.A., *Human Sexuality in Four Perspectives*, Baltimore and London: The Johns Hopkins University Press.

DAVIS, D.L. and WHITTEN, R.G. (1987) 'The cross-cultural study of human sexuality', *Annual Review of Anthropology*, **16**, pp. 69–98.

DI MAURO, D. (1995) *Sexuality Research in the United States. An Assessment of the Social and Behavioral Sciences*, New York: The Social Science Research Council.

DUBOIS-ARBER, F., JEANNIN, A., MEYSTRE-AGUSTONI, G., MOREAU-GRUET, F., HAOUR-KNIPE, M., SPENCER, B. and PACCAUD, F. (1996) *Evaluation of AIDS-prevention strategy in Switzerland mandated by the Federal Office of Public Health. Fifth synthesis report 1993–1995*, Lausanne: Institut universitaire de médecine sociale et préventive.

FIELD, R. and WELLINGS, K. (1993) *Context of Sexual Behaviour in Europe. Selected Indices Relating to Demographic, Social and Cultural Variables*, Prepared for the EC Concerted Action on 'Sexual Behaviour and Risks of HIV Infection', London: Academic Department of Public Health, St Mary's Hospital Medical School.

FIELD, J., WADSWORTH, J. and BRADSHAW, S. (1994) 'Survey methods and sample characteristics', in JOHNSON, A. *et al.*, *Sexual Attitudes and Lifestyles*, Oxford: Blackwell Scientific Publications.

GAGNON, J.H. and SIMON, W. (1973) *Sexual Conduct. The Social Sources of Human Sexuality*, Chicago: Aldine.

GIAMI, A. (1996) 'The ACSF Survey Questionnaire: the influence of an epidemiological representation of sexuality', in BOZON, M. and LERIDON, H. (Eds), *Sexuality and the Social Sciences. The French Survey on Sexual Behaviour*, Aldershot: Avebury (French version: 1993).

GREGERSEN, E. (Ed.) (1994) *The World of Human Sexuality. Behaviors, Customs and Beliefs*, New York: Irving Publishers.

GROVES, R., BIEMER, P., LYBERG, L., MASSEY, J., NICHOLLS, W. and WAKSBERG, J. (Eds) (1988) *Telephone survey methodology*, New York: Wiley.

HANTRAIS, L. (1996) 'Comparative research methods', *Social Research Update*, Issue 13 (electronic journal).

HUBERT, M. (1995) 'Studying sexual behaviour and HIV risk: towards a pan-European approach', in FRIEDRICH, D. and HECKMANN, W. (Eds) *AIDS in Europe – The Behavioural Aspect. Vol. 1: General Aspects*, Berlin: Editions Sigma.

HUBERT, M. (forthcoming) 'Les enquêtes sur les comportements sexuels. Quelques controverses à propos et autour de leur mise en oeuvre', in RIANDEY, B. (Ed), *Démographie, statistique et vie privée*, Paris: INED.

HUBERT, M. and MARQUES BALSA, C. (1995) 'EU Concerted Action on Sexual Behaviour and Risks of HIV Infection. Final Report', Brussels: Centre d'études sociologiques, Facultés universitaires Saint-Louis.

HUBERT, M. and MARQUET, J. (co-ordinators), DELCHAMBRE, J.P., PETO, D., SCHAUT, C. and VAN CAMPENHOUDT, L. (1993) *Comportements sexuels et réactions au risque du sida en Belgique*, Brussels: Centre d'études sociologiques, Facultés universitaires Saint-Louis.

INSTITUT UNIVERSITAIRE DE MÉDECINE SOCIALE ET PRÉVENTIVE (1993) *Kampagne zur*

Aids-Prävention. Repräsentative Befragung zur Kondom-Benützung (Bericht t6, 1992), Lausanne: Cahiers de recherches et de documentation, **82.6**.

JOHNSON, A. and WELLINGS, K. (1994) 'Studying sexual lifestyles', in JOHNSON, A. *et al.*, *Sexual Attitudes and Lifestyles*, Oxford: Blackwell Scientific Publications.

KETTING, E. (1990) *Contraception in Western Europe. A Current Appraisal*, Carnforth: Partenon.

KINSEY, A.C., POMEROY, W.P. and MARTIN, C.E. (1948) *Sexual Behaviour in the Human Male*, Philadelphia: W.B. Saunders.

KINSEY, A.C., POMEROY, W.P., MARTIN, C.E. and GEBHARD, P.H. (1953) *Sexual Behaviour in the Human Female*, Philadelphia: W.B. Saunders.

KISH, L. (1994) 'Multipopulation survey designs: five types with seven shared aspects', *International Statistical Review*, **62**, 2, pp. 167–86.

KOHN, M.L. (1989) 'Cross-national research as an analytic strategy', in KOHN, M.L. (Ed.) *Cross-national Research in Sociology*, Newbury Park: Sage.

KONTULA, O. and HAAVIO-MANNILA, E. (1995) *Sexual Pleasures. Enhancement of Sex Life in Finland, 1971–1992*, Aldershot: Dartmouth Publishing Company.

LAUMANN, E., GAGNON, J. and MICHAEL, R. (1994a) 'A political history of the National Sex Survey of Adults', *Family Planning Perspectives*, **26**, 1 (January/February), pp. 34–8.

LAUMANN, E., GAGNON, J., MICHAEL, R. and MICHAELS, S. (1994b) *The Social Organization of Sexuality. Sexual Practices in the United States*, Chicago: University of Chicago Press.

LAVEE, Y. (1991) 'Western and non-western human sexuality: implications for clinical practice', *Journal of Sex and Marital Therapy*, **17**, pp. 203–13.

LERIDON, H. (1994) 'Sample obtained: characteristics and adjustment', in SPIRA, A., BAJOS, N. and the ACSF GROUP, *Sexual Behaviour and AIDS*, Aldershot: Avebury, 69–76 (French edition: 1993).

LERIDON, H., CHARBIT, Y., COLLOMB, P. *et al.* (1987) *La seconde révolution contraceptive: la régulation des naissances en France de 1950 à 1985*, Paris: INED-PUF.

LORIAUX, M. (1995) 'L'analyse comparative: avantages et limites', in DUCHÊNE, J. and WUNSCH, G. (Eds) *Collecte et comparabilité des données démographiques et sociales en Europe*, Chaire Quetelet 1991, Louvain-la-Neuve: Academia, Paris: L'Harmattan.

MOATTI, J.-P., DAB, W. and POLLAK, M. (1992) 'Les Français et le SIDA', *La Recherche*, **23**, 247, pp. 1202–11.

PETO, D., MARQUET, J. and HUBERT, M. (1995) 'Elements of evaluation of the Belgian questionnaire on sexual behaviour and attitudes to HIV risk', in FRIEDRICH, D. and HECKMANN, W. (Eds) *Aids in Europe – The Behavioural Aspect, Vol. 4: Determinants of Behaviour Change*, Berlin: Editions Sigma.

POLLAK, M. *et al.* (1994) 'Evaluating AIDS prevention for men having sex with men: the West European experience', *Social and Preventive Medicine*, **39**, Suppl. 1, S47–60.

PRZEWORSKI, A. and TEUNE, H. (1970) *The Logic of Comparative Social Inquiry*, New York: Wiley.

QUÉRÉ, L. (1996) 'Vers une anthropologie alternative pour les sciences sociales?', in *Habermas, la raison, la critique*, Paris: Cerf.

REISS, I.L. (1986) 'A sociological journey into sexuality', *Journal of Marriage and Family*, **48**, pp. 233–42.

REZZA, G. *et al.* (1994) 'Assessing HIV prevention among injecting drug users in European Community countries: a review', *Social and Preventive Medicine*, **39**, Suppl. 1, S61–78.

ROBERTSON, B.J., McQUEEN, D.V. and NISBET, L. (1991) *AIDS-related Behaviours, Knowledge and Attitudes; Provisional Data from the RUHBC Cati Survey*, Edinburgh: Research Unit in Health and Behavioural Change (RUHBC).

ROKKAN, S. (1964) 'Comparative cross-national research: the context of current efforts', in MERRIT, R.L. and ROKKAN, S. (Eds) *Comparing Nations: The Use of Quantitative Data in Cross-national Research*, New Haven, CT: Yale University Press.

SANTOS LUCAS, J. (1993) *A sexualidade desprevenida dos Portugueses*, Lisbon: McGraw-Hill.

SIEVERS, K., KOSKELAINEN, O. and LEPPO, K. (1974) *Suomalaisten sukupuolielämä (Sex life of the Finns)*, Porvoo: WSOY.

SIMON, P., GONDONNEAU, J., MIRONER, L. and DORLEN-ROLLIER, A.-M. (1972) *Rapport sur le comportement sexuel des Français*, Paris: Julliard, Charron.

STATENS INSTITUTT FOR FOLKEHELSE (1993) *Rapport fra seksualvaneundersokelsene i 1987 og 1992*, Seksjon for epidemiologi, Oslo.

STEFANIS, C. (1991) *Relations, Patterns and Risk of HIV Infection*, Athens: Athens University Medical School, Department of Psychiatry.

SUNDET, J.-M., KVALEM, I.-L., MAGNUS, P. and BAKKETEIG, L.S. (1988) 'Prevalence of risk-prone sexual behaviour in the general population of Norway', in FLEMING, A.F., CARBALIV, M. and FITZSIMONS, D.F. (Eds) *The Global Impact of AIDS*, London: Alan R. Liss.

SUNDET, J.M., MAGNUS, P., KVALEM, I. and BAKKETEIG, L. (1990) 'Self-administered anonymous questionnaires in sexual behaviour research: the Norwegian experience', in HUBERT, M. (Ed.) *Sexual Behaviour and Risks of HIV Infection*, Brussels: Publications des Facultés universitaires Saint-Louis, collection Travaux et recherches.

TIELMAN, R.A.P. (1990) 'Telephone surveys and comparisons with other methods in psycho-social AIDS research', in HUBERT, M. (Ed.) *Sexual Behaviour and Risks of HIV Infection. Proceedings of an international workshop supported by the European Communities*, Brussels: Publications des Facultés universitaires Saint-Louis.

VAN ZESSEN, G. and SANDFORT, TH.G.M. (1991) *Seksualiteit in Nederland; seksueel gedrag, risico en preventie van aids*, Amsterdam/Lisse: Swets and Zeitlinger.

WELLINGS, K. and FIELD, B. (1996) *Stopping AIDS. AIDS/HIV Public Education and the Mass Media in Europe*, London and New York: Longman.

WORLD HEALTH ORGANIZATION (1990) *Research Protocol: partners' relations and risk of HIV infection (phase 2)*, Geneva: Global Programme on AIDS, Social and Behavioural Research Unit.

ZETTERBERG, H. (1969) *Om sexuallivet i Sverige (On sex life in Sweden)*, Stockholm: SOU.

Part 1

Sexual Behaviour in the Era of HIV/AIDS

Sexual Initiation and Gender in Europe: A Cross-cultural Analysis of Trends in the Twentieth Century

Michel Bozon and Osmo Kontula

Introduction

The regulation and supervision of the access of young people (especially young women) to sex have always been considered critical issues. All societies, at every period of their history, have striven to have control over sexual initiation,[1] given the key role of sex in biological and social reproduction[2] (Kontula, 1991; Loyola, 1992). Sexual debut remains a moment of great significance, for social norms and representations, cultural scripts, institutional arrangements and legal constraints come together with physical practices to give this memorable event its full meaning (Gagnon and Simon, 1973).

The timing and conditions of sexual initiation in developed societies have followed secular trends that are related to the overall social and cultural transformations that have taken place in recent decades (Roussel, 1987; Van de Kaa, 1987; Trost, 1990). In Europe for instance, a general trend towards a relaxation of social mores has been observed, since the 1960s, against a background of a weakening in the influence of religion. Patterns of marital and family behaviour have likewise undergone radical changes involving such major shifts as lower fertility rates, the postponement of and reduction in the number of marriages, a rise in births out of wedlock, an increase in informal cohabitation, especially at the start of unions, and higher divorce rates. These reflect mainly young women's changing attitudes, also expressed in the dramatic spread of reliable birth control methods, the rise in women's level of education and women's rapidly growing participation in the labour force. All this caused a notable increase in female autonomy by reducing parental control, male economic domination and the fear (and reality) of unwanted pregnancy. Changes in cultural attitudes and wider opportunities of choice for women may have modified the transition to adult sexuality more for females than for males. It is often assumed that the onset of the HIV pandemic in the 1980s ran counter to this trend towards looser constraints; the timing and conditions of sexual initiation may have been especially affected, with a possible postponement of first intercourse, since AIDS prevention policies have targeted mainly the youngest. However, the effects of the pandemic on norms and behaviours should be measured, not just assumed. A cross-national analysis is useful to assess the extent and factors of the fall in the debut age over the generations and the potential effects of AIDS on sexual initiation in different countries.

First sexual experience and intercourse have always been considered a crucial stage in the individual's life history and self-construction. Over the centuries, this step was perceived and interpreted differently according to country, period and gender. Traditionally, female sexual initiation was closely linked with marriage. Special emphasis was laid on virginity and continence, and women were supposed to be initiated into sex by their husbands, especially in southern European countries (Peristiany, 1966). This close association between marriage and sexual initiation for women has lost ground everywhere, all the more so as marriage has also been declining. Nevertheless, female and male notions of what first intercourse means have never totally converged. There is a tendency among young males to consider sexual initiation an uncommitted teenage experience, whereas for women this experience tends more to require a steady relationship or a strong emotional commitment (Kontula, Rimpelä and Ojanlatva, 1992; Traeen, Lewin and Sundet, 1992; Bozon, 1996). The special health implications of sexual initiation, formerly linked with the risk of unplanned pregnancy, which was a risk for women when birth control methods were less common and reliable, have been renewed by the concern about HIV transmission, which may be shared more equally by both partners. Cross-national data may be used to assess the divergence or convergence of men's and women's attitudes, which must be taken into account in designing more adequate preventive strategies.

It has been shown in several countries that age at first intercourse is a powerful indicator of the characteristics of adult sex life (Johnson and Wadsworth, 1994; Bozon, 1996). In each generation, there are individuals who start their sex lives early and others for whom initiation occurs later. Early and late starters differ in terms of their attitudes, sexual behaviours and adaptability to risk from the very beginning and throughout their lives (Bajos *et al.*, 1998). This may be a major issue for sex education, which should start early enough to be effective and be adapted to normative and behavioural diversity. Cross-national data can thus be used to check whether behavioural differences with respect to timing of initiation are found in men and women and in all countries.

After a presentation of the methodology used in this analysis, the paper describes the trends of coital début age of men and women by generation, with special reference to the first cohorts who began their sex lives under the threat of the AIDS pandemic. The influence of level of education on age at first intercourse is assessed. The relationship with first partner and the connection of sexual initiation with first union are analyzed. Differences in the timing of initiation are related to differences in adult behaviours. The conclusion addresses the issue of European sex culture by mapping gender convergence or differences in sexual initiation and suggests possible consequences for educational and preventive strategies.

Methods

The analysis covers surveys carried out in 12 countries between 1989 and 1993. In this chapter we were able to include the data of Great Britain and two additional countries where mail surveys on sexual behaviour and HIV risk were organized, namely, Denmark and Iceland (Meldbye and Biggar, 1992; Jónsdóttir, 1996).[3] All the surveys included questions of very similar wording on age at first intercourse. In seven countries, the question asked was 'How old were you when you had your first (sexual) intercourse?' In two countries (Great Britain, Netherlands) the question was split into one on first intercourse with the opposite sex and another on first intercourse with the same sex. In three more countries, sexual intercourse was specified as first intercourse with (oral, vaginal or anal) penetration (Belgium) or full sexual intercourse for the first time (Portugal and Greece (Athens),[4] which borrowed the phrase from the WHO–Partner Relations questionnaire). Very few surveys defined intercourse precisely. This lack of definition is by no means an obstacle to comparison. We assume that, in its plain form, this wording was understood in the same way in all countries as implying penetration. First experiences of bodily contact without penetration (petting, kissing, and so on) are not generally termed first time or first intercourse. As it is perceived as marking a passage, first coitus is deeply and unambiguously rooted in the memory. The 'first time' is not easily forgotten.

In addition to first intercourse, several questionnaires included questions on age at the time of previous events, such as first kiss or first sexual experience (Finland, Netherlands, Great Britain) or asked for some detail about the first partner, such as age (Finland, France, Norway, Great Britain) and relationship (Athens, Finland, Germany, Great Britain), or other circumstances surrounding the event, such as feelings (Belgium, Finland, France, Great Britain), initiative (Belgium, Finland, Great Britain), contraception or protection (Finland, Great Britain). The Finnish and British questionnaires were the most detailed with regard to sexual initiation.

To describe this century's trends of coital debut, we divided the population investigated into seven groups or 'generations', each of which combined several cohorts (see Table 2.1). There was a four-year gap between the earliest (Netherlands 1989) and latest (Belgium 1993) surveys. To be able to bring out a potential 'HIV generation effect', we needed a strictly similar definition of generations from one country to another. The generations were consequently defined by year of birth rather than by age at interview. As the age ranges were not the same in all surveys, we have two countries with data on seven generations, seven with six generations and three with five generations.

Another point of view on age at first intercourse was taken in the section addressing the influence of timing of sexual initiation on adult behaviour. Instead of being the described variable, age at first intercourse becomes a descriptive variable. Population aged 20 to 49 is divided into four groups of identical sexual precocity, early (first intercourse at 16 or before), intermediate (17 or 18), late (19 or 20) and very late (21 and over). This classification is not totally satisfactory. It has been shown (Bozon, 1996) that the notion of sexual precocity is relative, pertinent only when referring to a given generation in a given country, and not necessarily gender-neutral. By mixing together people belonging to generations with specific sexual profiles, we consequently introduced a bias.[5] We know, for instance, that the 'very late' will belong mostly to the older generations. In-depth analysis should obviously restrict itself to the data of one generation in a given country. Cross-cultural analysis may be more modest because it has the advantage of drawing attention to converging or diverging trends between countries.

In this chapter, no distinction is made between homosexual and heterosexual first intercourse. A specific question on first homosexual intercourse (if ever) was asked in only two surveys. In other countries, only one first intercourse was considered, and it might have been with a partner of the same sex. Actually, the majority of homo/bisexuals report having had heterosexual intercourse first, with the 'coming-out' process starting later (Pollak, 1985; Wellings, Wadsworth and Johnson, 1994; Messiah and Mouret-Fourme, 1996). Eventually, we decided to leave aside the difficult question of the construction of sexual identity among homosexuals, which needed a specific approach (see in this volume Chapter 3 on homosexual behaviour), and to refer simply to first sexual intercourse.

Trends of Age at First Intercourse

The reduction in age at sexual initiation that occurred over the second half of the twentieth century was more marked for women than for men. The initial gender gap tended to narrow and ages at first intercourse to converge. The data from the successive generations are summed up in three complementary indicators: the median, the interquartile range of ages at first intercourse, and the percentages of respondents who had intercourse before age 16, 18 or 20 (Tables 2.1 and 2.2).

Decrease in Age of Female Debut

A lowering of female début age has been a distinctive trend all over Europe, even though initial differences between women of different countries have not vanished, for there are still countries with 'early' women and these countries are the same in 1990 as the ones in 1950. Between women who started their sex lives in the 1950s (that is, Generation 2, born in the 1930s), and those who started in the 1990s (that is, Generation 7, born in 1972–3), age at first intercourse has fallen by at least two years in all countries (Table 2.1). Everywhere, there was a dramatic fall in the percentage of late starters (Table 2.2). In Belgium and Great Britain, for instance, 62 per cent of the women in the second generation (1932–41 cohorts) had their first intercourse at 20 or later, and only 31 and 15 per cent, respectively, in the sixth generation (1967–71 cohorts). The more 'advanced' countries are Denmark, Iceland and Norway, where female debut age in the 1950s was already 19. The Nordic countries have kept their lead, reaching a median age of female initiation of 17 in the 1990s. Icelandic women have remained the most precocious among European women, with a record debut age of 16.3 in the 1972–3 cohorts. Quite a different pattern is observed in southern Europe, for which only two surveys are available, one for Portugal and the other for Athens. Entry into adult sexual life, which was not experienced by half of women before 23 in the 1950s, took place at 19 in the 1990s. Despite a dramatic four-year decline in three decades, the women of these countries remain the latest starters in Europe, as far as we know. Even if we have no data from Italy or Spain, we may assume that these countries followed a similar trend, as they did for demographic behaviour (nuptiality, fertility) and other socio-economic factors (lower female participation in the workforce) (Barrère-Maurisson and Marchand, 1990; Sardon, 1993). At least the starting points should be close. Finally, a third intermediate profile can be discerned including all the remaining countries (such as France, West Germany and Great Britain) and characterized by a rather high median age of women at first sexual encounter in the 1950s (20 or more) and a marked fall to 18 or below in the 1990s.

Other contrasts appear if we examine in which decades the decline was steepest, or, in other words, when and in what socio-historical context changes really started. The Nordic countries (except Finland) may have experienced a sharp fall in women's age at sexual initiation earlier, probably from the 1950s, given the rather low age at first intercourse in these countries in the 1950s. This hypothesis ought to be checked against other data. Unfortunately, our

Table 2.1 *Age at first intercourse by gender and generation (median and interquartile range of ages, in years)*

Generations (by year of birth)		Athens[1] 1990 Men	Athens[1] 1990 Women	Belgium 1993 Men	Belgium 1993 Women	Denmark[2] 1989 Men	Denmark[2] 1989 Women	Finland 1992 Men	Finland 1992 Women	France ACSF 1992 Men	France ACSF 1992 Women	Germany West 1990 Men	Germany West 1990 Women
G1 (1922–31)	Median							18.8 (148)	20.7 (187)	18.0 (140)	21.1 (100)	20.2 (125)	20.9 (161)
	Q3–Q1							4.3	6.0	3.8	5.7	6.5	7.0
G2 (1932–41)	Median	17.3 (54)	22.8 (57)	20.4 (245)	20.9 (252)	18.4 (232)	19.0 (295)	18.7 (134)	20.0 (149)	18.4 (200)	20.6 (161)	19.0 (203)	19.7 (237)
	Q3–Q1	2.7	5.1	4.5	3.9	3.5	3.2	3.0	4.7	3.8	5.4	3.3	3.3
G3 (1942–51)	Median	17.3 (213)	20.6 (258)	19.0 (385)	20.0 (408)	18.2 (269)	18.3 (351)	18.2 (227)	19.0 (209)	18.1 (432)	19.3 (341)	18.4 (263)	18.6 (325)
	Q3–Q1	2.8	5.7	4.1	3.7	2.6	2.3	3.6	3.1	3.6	3.2	3.3	2.9
G4 (1952–61)	Median	17.5 (259)	19.5 (322)	18.5 (411)	18.8 (509)	17.8 (328)	17.7 (390)	18.0 (256)	17.7 (246)	17.6 (679)	18.3 (560)	18.0 (362)	17.5 (454)
	Q3–Q1	2.3	3.4	3.8	3.3	2.8	2.3	3.1	2.7	2.5	2.7	3.1	2.3
G5 (1962–6)	Median	17.6 (136)	19.2 (163)	18.0 (199)	18.6 (240)	17.1 (179)	16.8 (199)	17.3 (123)	17.8 (109)	17.4 (502)	18.2 (386)	17.7 (263)	17.6 (241)
	Q3–Q1	2.5	3.9	4.3	4.1	3.7	2.6	2.7	3.3	2.5	2.4	3.2	2.5
G6 (1967–71)	Median	17.5 (152)	19.0 (155)	18.1 (216)	18.7 (229)	17.5 (178)	17.0 (206)	18.0 (113)	18.0 (121)	17.7 (539)	18.3 (471)	17.7 (182)	17.7 (198)
	Q3–Q1	3.2	3.1	3.3	3.3	3.1	2.5	2.3	2.4	2.4	3.1	3.2	3.0
G7 (1972–3)	Median			17.4 (105)	18.0 (90)	17.4 (164)	16.7 (202)	18.0* (46)	16.6* (40)	17.0 (150)	18.1 (159)		
	Q3–Q1			2.3	3.3	–	2.4	–	–	–	–		

Notes:
Q3–Q1 is the difference in years between the 3rd quartile and the 1st quartile of the distribution of ages at first intercourse. It is a measure of dispersion
* N in the cell is between 15 and 50
[1] Athens: G2 = 1940–1
[2] Denmark: the generation boundaries are different: G2 (1930–9), G3 (1940–9), G4 (1950–9), G5 (1960–4), G6 (1965–9), G7 (1970–1)

Table 2.1 *(cont.)*

Generations (by year of birth)		Great Britain 1991		Iceland[3] 1992		Netherlands[4] 1989		Norway 1992		Portugal[5] 1991		Switzerland[6] 1992	
		Men	Women	Men	Women	Men	Women	Men	Women	Men	Women	Men	Women
G1 (1922–31)	Median												
	Q3–Q1												
G2 (1932–41)	Median	19.1 (1318)	20.9 (1980)	17.8* (33)	18.7* (39)	21.2* (28)	21.6* (39)	19.3 (256)	19.5 (271)	16.4* (29)	24.3* (39)		
	Q3–Q1	*5.2*	*3.8*	*3.7*	*3.9*	*6.0*	*4.4*	*6.1*	*4.3*	*3.2*	*4.7*		
G3 (1942–51)	Median	18.3 (1924)	19.5 (2306)	17.5 (85)	18.0 (100)	19.1 (94)	19.7 (162)	18.8 (442)	18.8 (536)	16.8 (383)	21.9 (334)	19.2 (239)	19.5 (229)
	Q3–Q1	*4.3*	*3.6*	*4.3*	*2.4*	*4.2*	*3.6*	*3.9*	*3.6*	*3.4*	*4.6*	*4.1*	*2.9*
G4 (1952–61)	Median	17.5 (2268)	18.2 (3031)	16.9 (143)	17.2 (143)	18.2 (154)	18.4 (195)	18.3 (548)	17.7 (714)	16.5 (379)	20.3 (394)	18.5 (495)	18.7 (478)
	Q3–Q1	*3.3*	*2.9*	*2.6*	*2.1*	*4.6*	*3.1*	*4.0*	*3.0*	*2.9*	*4.1*	*3.2*	*3.1*
G5 (1962–6)	Median	17.2 (1202)	17.9 (1629)	16.8 (67)	17.1 (87)	17.8 (73)	17.8 (93)	18.4 (308)	17.5 (392)	16.8 (142)	19.8 (147)	18.7 (237)	18.5 (224)
	Q3–Q1	*2.9*	*2.8*	*2.0*	*2.0*	*4.3*	*2.7*	*4.3*	*3.0*	*3.1*	*4.4*	*3.8*	*3.4*
G6 (1967–71)	Median	17.1 (864)	17.4 (1125)	16.8 (56)	16.9 (76)	18.3 (52)	18.3 (74)	18.3 (311)	17.6 (396)	17.1 (256)	19.9 (234)	18.1 (227)	18.4 (233)
	Q3–Q1	*2.9*	*2.4*	*3.0*	*2.1*	–	*3.4*	*4.0*	*2.9*	*3.1*	–	*3.5*	*2.7*
G7 (1972–3)	Median	17.0 (288)	17.3 (350)	16.4* (49)	16.3 (63)			18.1 (125)	17.5 (143)	16.2 (66)	>19 (68)	18.2 (128)	18.4 (123)
	Q3–Q1	–	–	–				–	–	*3.1*	–	–	–

Notes:
Q3–Q1 is the difference in years between the 3rd quartile and the 1st quartile of the distribution of ages at first intercourse. It is a measure of dispersion
* N in the cell is between 15 and 50
[3] Iceland: G7 = 1972–5
[4] Netherlands: G2 = 1939–41
[5] Portugal: G2 limited to 1941
[6] Switzerland: G3 = 1946–51

Table 2.2 Proportions of men and women having had their first intercourse before the age of 16, 18, and 20, by generation / %

First intercourse before the age	Athens[1] 1990		Belgium 1993		Denmark[2] 1989		Finland 1992		France ACSF 1992		Germany West 1990		Great Britain 1991		Iceland[3] 1992		Netherlands[4] 1989		Norway 1992		Portugal[5] 1991		Switzerland[6] 1992	
	M	W	M	W	M	W	M	W	M	W	M	W	M	W	M	W	M	W	M	W	M	W	M	W
G1 (1922–31) 16							11	1	27	2	6	2												
18							35	10	50	16	25	12												
20							57	44	77	42	48	39												
G2 (1932–41) 16	19	2	5	2	10	7	10	7	18	0	8	1	11	2	21*	8*	7*	0*	9	3	40*	0*	9	1
18	59	11	20	15	37	40	31	26	42	12	31	18	33	12	52*	39*	21*	3*	39	26	78*	6*	30	19
20	83	19	47	38	72	71	68	53	71	36	65	56	56	38	76*	64*	39*	33*	59	63	93*	19*	58	61
G3 (1942–51) 16	28	4	7	2	18	7	18	4	21		11	7	19	6	33	16	8	4	12	6	37	2	12	6
18	64	13	28	19	51	44	47	33	48	24	38	33	46	27	55	50	29	20	39	38	67	10	39	38
20	88	42	57	48	82	82	74	69	75	61	70	71	69	57	77	88	59	56	68	68	88	23	73	68
G4 (1952–61) 16	21	8	11	4	23	23	16	20	19	10	13	14	25	9	29	18	18	10	17	19	42	4	14	9
18	62	25	39	32	59	62	49	56	60	42	49	59	58	46	72	69	47	41	45	57	76	17	37	39
20	90	57	69	66	85	84	77	84	87	78	77	86	80	77	87	92	71	75	74	83	89	45	68	71
G5 (1962–6) 16	18	6	14	10	31	36	24	19	21	10	17	16	25	11	33	35	22	14	19	21	32	7	12	9
18	58	27	51	38	64	74	63	53	63	43	54	61	63	51	85	85	53	54	43	59	69	26	49	40
20	89	59	78	69	84	91	82	78	87	77	79	86	83	81	94	95	69	85	70	83	91	52	73	76
G6 (1967–71) 16	27	5	15	9	27	32	20	18	22	13	15	18	25	16	38	22	17	12	19	22	30	7	15	4
18	59	24	49	36	59	71	50	50	57	46	54	56	66	63	73	72	46	45	45	59	68	26	46	41
20	–	–	75	69	82	90	78	84	84	76	74	69	83	85	88	88	–	–	73	84	82	51	–	–
G7 (1972–3) 16			18	18	26	34	15*	35*	23	7			32	20	45*	40			18	22	43*	12		
18			66	49	57	72	50*	68*	68	49			65	62	–	–			48	60	–	–		
20			–	–	–	–	–	–	–	–			–	–	–	–			–	–	–	–		

Notes:
* N in the cell is between 15 and 50
For the sizes of each generation, see Table 2.1
[1] Athens: G2 = 1940–1
[2] Denmark: the generation boundaries are different: G2 (1930–9), G3 (1940–9), G4 (1950–9), G5 (1960–4), G6 (1965–9), G7 (1970–1)
[3] Iceland: G7 = 1972–5
[4] Netherlands: G2 = 1939–41
[5] Portugal: G2 limited to 1941
[6] Switzerland: G3 = 1946–51

data for these countries are truncated, as we do not have information on the generations who became sexually active in the 1940s. We do know that in Sweden – a neighbouring country for which survey data on sexual behaviour are not yet available[6] – informal cohabitation had started to rise as early as the 1950s, and the weakening of marriage is generally related to changes in sexual initiation (Hoem and Rennermalm, 1985). What about countries for which we have sufficient historical depth? Little change is observed between the 1940s and 1950s in Finland and in France, whereas a marked decline (from 20.9 to 19.7 years) linked to a sharp decrease in age at marriage can already be noted in West Germany (Sardon, 1993).

The 1960s (the third generation) are the decade when great changes start for a majority of countries, which follow the path of the forerunners of the 1950s. This is the case in Finland, France, the Netherlands, and Great Britain, but also Greece (Athens) and Portugal. Yet a decline in age at first intercourse does not necessarily mean a radical change in the sexual behaviour of youth. If it goes together with an earlier age at marriage and a high and stable nuptiality rate it may be interpreted as merely an aspect of earlier marriage. This is what happened in Europe in the 1950s. Mean age at marriage fell steadily from the 1950s until the mid-1960s in the Nordic countries, the mid-1970s in France, Germany and Great Britain, and the beginning of the 1980s in southern Europe (Sardon, 1993). The trend subsequently reversed in all countries, as marriage was postponed and the marriage rate declined. A decrease in age at first intercourse can be interpreted as a marker of a relaxation in sexual mores only when sexual initiation and marriage are clearly disconnected, that is, when age at marriage starts rising, in different periods in the different regions of the continent.

The decline in age at first intercourse continued in the 1970s for the countries that had started to change in the former decade, whereas it was just beginning for Belgium and Switzerland (at Generation 4). The 1980s, for their part, were a period of general stabilization of timing of sexual initiation. Between Generations 4 (1952–61 cohorts) and 5 (1962–6 cohorts), the age of women at first intercourse did not drop any more, except in Denmark and (to a lesser extent) the Netherlands. This slowing down of the pace of change took place before the onset of AIDS. Generation 6 (1967–71 cohorts) women, who were sexually initiated in the second half of the 1980s, did not have their first intercourse sooner or later than the preceding generation, despite the threat of the epidemic. Here, again, there are two exceptions, namely the Netherlands, where age at first intercourse went up in the second half of the decade (Generation 6), and Great Britain, where it went down. Still, these variations are rather small. The overriding impression is that AIDS did not affect the timing of sexual initiation for women, as its onset coincided with a period of stagnation. In the nine countries for which we have data on a seventh generation (1972–3 cohorts), it appears that a new decrease took place in a minority of countries only (Belgium, Finland, Iceland). AIDS may then have contributed to a relative stabilization of age at first intercourse, but cannot be the only cause of this lasting pause, which preceded the pandemic.

Male behaviour has changed less in the second half of the century than female behaviour. In the southern European countries, male initiation occurred at the same very early age in the 1950s and early 1990s (16.4 and 16.2 years of age respectively, for young Portuguese males, for instance). In Belgium, Germany, and the Netherlands, on the contrary, the age at first intercourse of young men, who used to become sexually active rather late (at age 20 or older) in the 1940s and 1950s, dropped to 18 or less. In other countries, such as France or the Nordic countries, the downward trend over these 40 or 50 years was less marked (about one year). In spite of the spread of AIDS, the difference between the first and second halves of the 1980s is again very small, with a small rise in age at first intercourse in the 1967–71 generation in Finland and the Netherlands and very small rises in France and Portugal. In the 1990s, the decline in age at first intercourse resumed only in Belgium, France, Iceland, and Portugal. The main impression is that there has been very little change over the last two decades, Switzerland and Great Britain being two good examples. On the whole, the effect of AIDS on the timing of first intercourse is hardly more noticeable for men than for women.

The non-use of contraception at first intercourse has been declining steadily from the 1970s onwards. In 1991, 'non-use of contraception at first intercourse in Great Britain was reported by fewer than a quarter of women (24%) and fewer than a third of men (31%) aged 16–24' (Wellings and Bradshaw, 1994, p. 87). In Finland in 1992, entirely unprotected first intercourse was even lower, with only 13 per cent of women and 17 per cent of men aged 18–24 reporting no contraception at all (Kontula and Haavio-Mannila, 1995). In France, 30 per cent of women reported non-use of contraception during first-time sex in 1988, but the proportion had fallen to 16 per cent in 1993 (Toulemon and Leridon, 1995). This rise in the level of contraceptive use occurred together with a major shift in methods, for there is evidence of a strong revival of condom use at first intercourse in all countries from the second half of the 1980s that may be linked to AIDS prevention policies. This is true for Great Britain, where the prevalence of condom use rose to more than 60 per cent in the early 1990s after several decades of stable, routine use at first intercourse (approximately 40 per cent of women reported using the condom in the 1960s and 1970s). In Finland, 65 per cent of women aged 18–24 in 1992 reported using the condom during their first intercourse. 'The use of a condom has clearly been increasing among young people since the mid-1960s . . . Use . . . declined slightly during the 1970s, but picked up again in the 1980s, probably due to the condom campaigns' (Kontula and Haavio-Mannila, 1995, p. 58). In France, condom use, which declined steadily in the 1970s and 1980s as oral contraceptives gained ground, has started to rise dramatically (it jumped from 8 per cent in first intercourse in 1987 to 45 per cent and above in 1993 and is still on the increase) (Toulemon and Leridon, 1995). In all countries, the rise in condom use took place at the expense of the pill.

Dynamics of Gender Gap Patterns

The gap between the ages of men and women at sexual initiation and changes therein over the past century are powerful indicators of how gender and sexual behaviour interrelate in the different countries. Two clear-cut profiles stand out sharply, namely, the double standard of the south and the egalitarianism of the north and of some other countries. The southern European countries are characterized by a strong gender-based double standard. For example, the gender-based age difference at initiation in Portugal and in Athens, which used to be six or more years in the 1950s, has narrowed but by no means disappeared (at the end of the 1980s there remained a three-year difference in Portugal and a two-year difference in Athens). This pattern is close to those observed in some developing countries (Thailand, Manila, Rio de Janeiro), where the difference is interpreted as an indication that young men have sex with older experienced women or sex workers (Caraël, 1995). This was probably the case in southern Europe too, where female premarital intercourse was strictly controlled. The gradual closing of the gap over time means that a growing proportion of young women do have premarital sex (one out of four had intercourse before 18 in Portugal and Athens in the 1980s). This consequently modifies slowly the conditions (not the age) of sexual initiation for young males, as sex workers become less needed.

Another pattern is shared by a group of countries – the Nordic countries, forerunners in the liberalization of sexual morals (except Finland, where behaviours converged only later), and also less permissive countries like Belgium, the Netherlands, Switzerland, and West Germany – where, as early as the 1950s, men and women had their first sexual encounters at roughly the same age. This 'egalitarianism' persisted until the 1990s, and the fall in age at first intercourse followed a parallel course between men and women. Within this context, debut age tended to be slightly earlier for women than for men in the youngest cohorts in Denmark and Norway. This was interpreted as an effect of a 'relatively advanced female emancipation' in the Scandinavian countries (Sundet *et al.*, 1992, p. 251). Yet even in these countries, there is an age gap between partners at first intercourse and between married men and women in favour of men that remains to be explained (see later).

Finally, the British, Finnish, and French trends do not fit either pattern. In the 1940s, the gap between the ages of men and women at sexual initiation was rather large in France (three years) and Finland (two years). For Great

Britain, we have data only for the 1950s, at which time the difference was two years. The ages converged in the 1970s in Finland and in the 1980s in Great Britain. The gap has shrunk greatly in France to less than one year due to a sharp drop in women's age at first intercourse, but the difference has not yet totally disappeared.

Other contrasts between countries and between men and women stand out if we examine the variability of age at first intercourse. This can be estimated by means of several indicators, for example, the proportions of very early starters (aged 15 or under), the proportions of late starters (aged 20 or above), and the interquartile range of ages at first intercourse (that is the difference in years between the third and first quartiles of the distribution) (see Tables 2.1 and 2.2). If we look at the younger generations (Generation 6), more than one quarter of the male respondents in five countries belonging to both northern and southern Europe (Denmark, Iceland, Great Britain, but also Athens and Portugal) are very precocious. Higher proportions of male late starters (more than 25 per cent starting after 19) are found in Belgium, Germany, the Netherlands, Norway, and Switzerland. The proportions of women late starters are markedly inferior to those of men in several northern European countries (Denmark, Finland, the Netherlands, Norway). Women seem to have their first experience of intercourse within a shorter time span, as shown by the lower interquartile range for women, even when the median age equals that of men (Denmark, the Netherlands, Norway). In these 'egalitarian' countries, there is a greater homogeneity of ages at sexual initiation for women and a greater variability among men. This has been interpreted as a marker of 'the importance of norms and roles for [female] sexual behaviour' (Sundet *et al.*, 1992, p. 250). It may also indicate a greater diversity in male sexual lifestyles from the start.

Level of Education and Age at First Intercourse

Several factors, such as social class, religion and educational level, are known to influence age at first intercourse. In each country, religious affiliation and degree of religious participation were identified as important factors connected with internalized personal values. Late sexual initiation is generally associated with a high degree of practice and participation in religious activities, whatever the generation, whereas people without any religious affiliation tend to be early starters. Another common finding in European surveys (Finland, France, Great Britain and others) is that first intercourse occurs earlier among working-class men and women (Kontula and Haavio-Mannila, 1995; Wellings and Bradshaw, 1994; Sundet *et al.*, 1992; Bozon, 1996). Nevertheless, because of the difficulty of having truly comparable definitions of socio-economic groups, we preferred not to publish any cross-national data on

Table 2.3 Proportions of respondents (under 39) who had their first sexual intercourse before the age of 18, by gender and level of education / %

Level of education	Athens[1] 1990	Belgium 1993	Finland 1992	France 1992	Germany West 1990	Great Britain 1991	Netherlands 1989	Norway[2] 1992	Portugal 1991
MEN									
Low	69.6 (92)	53.8 (145)	66.7 (87)	66.3 (249)	53.5 (217)	71.3 (737)	58.2 (67)	70.9 (412)	75.1 (269)
Medium	67.2 (174)	59.5 (274)	57.6 (290)	61.5 (421)	51.0 (453)	66.6 (1310)	46.0 (111)	67.2 (299)	76.5 (289)
High	44.0 (125)	39.1 (333)	43.6 (133)	51.5 (237)	40.0 (130)	53.3 (2267)	42.6 (47)	54.2 (450)	68.1 (163)
WOMEN									
Low	43.0 (151)	62.8 (153)	68.8 (77)	55.2 (270)	62.9 (385)	56.6 (1259)	61.8 (76)	88.6 (482)	22.6 (270)
Medium	19.1 (209)	41.5 (290)	60.8 (240)	43.2 (412)	57.9 (444)	55.0 (2432)	38.9 (157)	78.1 (406)	26.1 (245)
High	14.9 (121)	27.8 (411)	48.9 (176)	39.4 (259)	43.8 (80)	41.0 (2047)	39.2 (51)	61.1 (611)	20.3 (153)

Base: all respondents (20–39 years), except in Athens (23–37) and the Netherlands (22–36)
Notes:
[1] Athens: here low = low + medium–low
[2] Norway: first intercourse before the age of 19

sexual intercourse and social class. In this cross-cultural analysis, we shall thus focus on education alone.

Educational level clearly influences age at sexual initiation (Table 2.3). Because of the dramatic rise in levels of education over this century, we have presented cross-national data on people under 40 only. All over Europe, men and women graduates have their sexual initiation later than early school-leavers. The gap between the proportions of early school-leavers and graduates who had intercourse before 18 is more marked (20 per cent difference or more) in Finland, Greece (Athens), Great Britain and among Dutch and German women. The difference is smaller in France, Norway and among Dutch and German men. Portugal is the only country where graduates do not behave differently from non-graduates, whether male or female. In several countries, poorly educated women are much more 'advanced' than their male counterparts (Belgium, Germany, Norway) or slightly so (Finland, the Netherlands). In these cases, early sexual initiation may be related to a preference for union and raising a family rather than a career. On the whole, the strong, general trend towards spending more years in the academic system may be one of the major factors behind the stabilization of age at first intercourse all over Europe in the 1980s.

Embarking on long courses of study does not prevent students from getting sexual experience, for most young people experience their first intercourse before completing their studies. Nevertheless, the prolonged dependence that a longer stay in the academic universe implies may delay the appropriation of attributes of independence, such as sexual initiation. In spite of the probable availability of partners of the other sex in the school environment, the future graduates have an attitude and a lifestyle in which sexual initiation is not a priority, at least during secondary education (Kontula and Haavio-Manila, 1995). Things may change as soon as they enter college. In Athens, for instance, only 44 per cent of male graduates reported having had first intercourse at 17 or before (against 70 per cent of the non-graduates), but 33 per cent had had their sexual initiation when they were 18, the age which marks the end of secondary education. Early school-leavers, on the contrary, are in a position to take independent decisions and initiatives much earlier, free from parental control and from the constraints of school. Immediately entering the world of adult sexuality is, for some of them, a way of making the most of their youth and for others a way of acceding early to a stable relationship outside their respective families.

Age Difference with First Partner

In four countries, respondents were asked the age of the person with whom they had first intercourse (Table 2.4). It must be remembered that first

Table 2.4 *Age difference between interviewee and partner at first intercourse, by gender and age of the interviewee*

Age difference between interviewee and partner at first intercourse (%)	Finland 1992 Age of the interviewees		France 1992 Age of the interviewees		Great Britain 1991 Age of the interviewees		Norway 1992 Age of the interviewees	
	18–29	30–49	18–29	30–49	18–29	30–49	18–29	30–49
MEN								
First partner was younger	48.3	41.7	21.7	19.2	23.3	32.8	41.6	41.5
First partner had same age	36.3	29.9	37.0	41.4	40.2	41.1	28.4	30.2
First partner was older	15.4	28.4	38.4	36.0	34.4	23.8	28.1	24.3
(*older: 3 years' difference or more*)	*(8.5)*	*(8.9)*	*(16.0)*	*(19.7)*	*(13.2)*	*(10.1)*	*(10.4)*	*(9.6)*
No answer	–	–	2.9	3.4	2.1	2.3	2.0	4.0
Total	100	100	100	100	100	100	100	100
N	259	472	1089	1081	2171	3640	652	997
WOMEN								
First partner was younger	3.6	3.6	5.3	6.8	4.4	5.3	4.3	4.1
First partner had same age	11.6	13.6	16.8	15.8	21.6	21.8	16.7	14.5
First partner was older	84.8	82.8	76.8	75.7	73.2	71.8	77.6	77.5
(*older: 3 years' difference or more*)	*(47.2)*	*(37.1)*	*(44.1)*	*(43.6)*	*(37.5)*	*(37.6)*	*(45.3)*	*(40.2)*
No answer	–	–	1.1	1.7	0.8	1.1	1.4	3.8
Total	100	100	100	100	100	100	100	100
N	250	448	997	901	2974	4851	863	1283

intercourse is not necessarily an initiation for both, as the first partner may be experienced. It is sometimes assumed that first intercourse between equally inexperienced partners has become more common in the younger generations. This was checked by observing two groups of generations: the younger cohorts (between 18 and 29 at the beginning of 1992) and middle-aged cohorts (between 30 and 49). In spite of the general trend of men and women towards earlier initiation, the pattern of age gap with first partner at first intercourse has remained the same from one group of cohorts to the other. There are no such things as convergence and egalitarianism if we examine what takes place between two partners.

The age difference between a woman and her first partner is remarkably stable over time in all countries, and is about the same in the different countries. Three-quarters of the female respondents in France, Norway and Great Britain, and even more (85 per cent) in Finland, had their first intercourse with an older partner. Only a small minority (5 per cent) started with a younger partner. Moreover, studies in several countries show that the latter may take place only when sexual initiation occurs late (Kontula and Haavio-Mannila, 1995; Bozon, 1996). In France, age difference between partners at the first intercourse of women is comparable to the age gap that exists between spouses in married or cohabiting couples, with the same pattern of male/female domination through age[7] (Bozon, 1991).

If we consider the ages of men's first partners, different patterns seem to emerge. In the Finnish pattern, one out of two men had his first intercourse with a younger woman, and one out of three with a same-age partner. Older partners are rather uncommon, even more and more so. In France, conversely, more than one out of three men (38 per cent) had his first intercourse with an older woman, 37 per cent with a partner of the same age, and only one out of five with a younger partner. French men are apparently not so keen on having their sexual initiation with inexperienced women and seem to prefer older initiators. Another explanation may be that women in this country avoid inexperienced men for the 'first time'. Although young women are now much more available for premarital sex than in the past, this male attitude may well be the cultural legacy of a time when men had little choice and had to turn to older women. We assume that this pattern is found in southern Europe, even though the data are not currently available in these countries. Norway has very much in common with Finland, but with more men having first experiences with older women than in the latter country. Finally, men in Great Britain behave like French men in the younger generations: the proportion of men turning to older women for sexual initiation is on the increase in this country (34 per cent versus 24 per cent in the older generation). What must be stressed, even if some differences are observed between men of different countries, is the following permanent, typical feature of female first intercourse all over Europe: for a woman, sexual initiation still occurs typically with an older man, whatever the gender relations in the country.

Commitment and Relationship with First Partner

In the younger generations, men and women do not start their sex lives with the same type of partner. Differences in age gap and unequal commitments to the relationship suggest that sexual initiation and first partner still do not mean the same thing to young men and women, even if there are indications of a trend towards diminishing differences between male and female experiences, especially in northern Europe.

A few decades ago, male initiation through prostitution was not uncommon. In France, in cohorts born before 1937 (more than 55 years old in 1992), one man out of 10 had his first intercourse with a prostitute (Bozon, 1996). In the cohorts born in 1972 or 1973, this form of sexual initiation has almost disappeared. In Great Britain the frequency of prostitution at first intercourse was much lower than in France in older generations (3.4 per cent in cohorts born between 1931 and 1946) and has also disappeared in the new generations. Men in the southern countries have been very precocious for decades. This was possibly connected to a high prevalence of prostitution, although we cannot be totally certain about this, as the question was not asked in the surveys on Portugal and Athens. This hypothesis is supported indirectly in Portugal by the fact that the number of premarital partners of men has always been very high, with 16 per cent of men reporting more than 10 partners before marriage (Santos-Lucas, 1993). We hypothesize that sex workers are still playing a significant, although not central, role in male sexual initiation in these countries.

First intercourse is generally part of a steady relationship. What is more, this characteristic is always more accentuated among women (Table 2.5). Changes over the generations have taken place in opposite directions. In Athens, Germany, and Great Britain fewer men in the younger than in the older generations started their sexual activity with casual partners, whilst the proportion has not changed in Finland. In contrast, the proportion of women who had their first intercourse with a steady or regular partner (or a spouse) has tended to decrease slightly from a previously very high level, in line with decreasing age at first intercourse. In Germany for instance, men and women are experiencing the same kind of relationship in first intercourse. In Athens, on the contrary, sexual initiation still does not carry the same significance at all for males and females.

Significantly more women than men report being in love with their first partner. The proportion of women in love is two-thirds in Finland and France (deeply in love), whereas only half of the men in Finland and a third in France report the same feeling at first intercourse (Kontula and Haavio-Mannila, 1995; Bozon, 1996). In the British survey, the question was not asked in the same way. In this survey, 'I was in love' was one possible answer among the main factors for having a first intercourse, together with 'I was a bit drunk at the time', 'Most people in my age group seemed to be doing it', and six other

Table 2.5 *Proportions of respondents who had their first sexual intercourse with regular partner or spouse, by gender and age / %*

Age of interviewee	Athens[1] 1989		Finland 1992		Germany West 1990	
	Men	Women	Men	Women	Men	Women
20–24	34 (111)	79 (110)	51 (101)	74 (115)	51 (136)	55 (177)
25–29	35 (116)	80 (157)	50 (121)	64 (106)	48 (189)	55 (191)
30–39	20 (239)	85 (322)	45 (251)	68 (241)	38 (283)	52 (396)
40–49	23 (227)	88 (243)	52 (225)	85 (209)	39 (215)	61 (270)
50–59	–	–	53 (132)	89 (153)	39* (44)	65 (52)
60–69	–	–	48 (114)	88 (152)	–	–

Notes:
*N in the cell is between 15 and 50
[1] Athens: only married partner

answers (Wellings and Bradshaw, 1994, p. 99). Even so, a large gap is found between men and women (17.3 per cent of men and 44.9 per cent of women reporting love). The gender gap regarding love has tended to narrow over time in Finland and Great Britain, whereas it remains unchanged in France.

All in all, men who experienced their first intercourse early reported love for their first partner, who was less often a steady partner, less frequently. Late first intercourse is associated with the opposite characteristics, as observed in Finland, France, and Great Britain (same authors), but this does not always hold true for women. For instance, French women in all generations report being deeply in love, regardless of their age at first intercourse (Bozon, 1996).

Several surveys asked who had taken the initiative at first intercourse. Over the generations, there has been a shift from a predominantly male initiative to a mutual initiative, according to data from Finland and Great Britain. Being able to report mutual initiative is a sign of increasing desire among young women. Yet, as it might be expected, men and women's answers on this point do not correspond totally. This inconsistency can be interpreted, however, in terms of gender roles and of different attitudes to sexuality. In Finland, for instance, younger men are more likely than women to see first intercourse as the result of a shared initiative and even accept the idea of female initiative (15 per cent in the 18–24 cohorts); in contrast, younger women reject almost totally the idea that the initiative might have been theirs (3 per cent in the younger cohorts), without equal male participation; still, one in two (50 per cent) considered the man to have been the initiator. For women, desire, when it is not mutual, is still equated with masculinity (Kontula and Haavio-Mannila, 1995). In Great Britain, a very high proportion of the respondents tend to report that both they and their partners were equally willing at first intercourse, although a small gender difference subsisted (85 per cent of the men, 74 per cent of the women). In some cases, first intercourse was not a completely voluntary experience for women. Yet, over the generations, the proportion of those pressed or forced to have sex the first time has declined, according to British and Finnish data.

From First Partner to First Union

In older generations, it was common for a woman to be initiated sexually by her husband (Segalen, 1981) at the time of marriage (either on the wedding night or some time before). This situation has become very rare: in the 1990s, even cohabiting with the first partner has become an exception. On this issue, the behaviour of women has tended to look more like that of men. Thus, more than 60 per cent of Finnish women over 50 had their first intercourse with their spouse or future spouse. The corresponding figure for men was less than 30 per cent. In the younger cohorts, the first sexual partner is usually no longer the person one marries or starts to live with. In other words, first sexual partners are no longer future spouses. In France, age at first marriage coincided with that of first intercourse in one out of two women over 55 (born before 1937), while the proportion of men who had first intercourse and wed in the same year was much smaller (22 per cent). The proportions fell to 11 and 7 per cent, respectively, for women and men born after 1967.

A comparison between southern and northern countries shows that changes do not follow the same pace everywhere (Table 2.6). If we take women 25 to 49 years old, three out of four married or started cohabiting the year they had first intercourse in Portugal, but only one French or Athenian woman in three, one British woman in four, and only 7 per cent of Finnish women. For all these women, the weight and commitment of marital life loom on the horizon of first sexual relations from the outset. This is less common for men. Yet in both France and Portugal every fifth man gets engaged very soon after his first intercourse, while this happens very seldom in Athens, Finland, and Great Britain.

As a result, many men have the opportunity of being sexually active for quite a few years before any engagement. According to survey data, four-fifths of men in Athens, two-thirds in Finland, and half in Portugal and Great Britain were free to indulge in at least five years of premarital (in the broad sense) sex. During this time, these bachelors may have had a high turnover of partners. France is a surprising exception, with only 23 per cent of men enjoying the same 'freedom'. Only a small minority of women had the time and opportunity to have numerous experiences before their first union. The highest proportion is found in Finland (one-third), followed by only one out of six in

Table 2.6 *Proportions of respondents starting their first union (cohabitation or marriage) at the same age or at least five or more years later than the first sexual intercourse, by gender*

Timing of first union	Athens[1]	Finland	France ACSF	Great Britain	Portugal
	1989	1992	1992	1991	1991
MEN					
Same age as first intercourse (%)	4	4	20	9	20
At least five years later (%)	85	65	23	46	52
	(426)	(515)	(952)	(3862)	(779)
WOMEN					
Same age as first intercourse (%)	35	7	31	24	72
At least five years later (%)	18	37	9	17	6
	(644)	(503)	(1032)	(5493)	(837)

Base: all respondents (18–49 years) who ever had sex
Note:
[1] Athens: only marriage

Athens and Great Britain. The lowest figures are found in France and Portugal (less than one out of 10). Although first couple and first intercourse are no longer simultaneous, these events remain more closely connected for women than for men.

Age at First Intercourse and Subsequent Sex Life

European surveys on sexual behaviour bring to light links between age at first intercourse and the content of an individual's subsequent sexual experience. In the French case in particular, it was shown that age at first intercourse was a strong predictor of male adult sexuality (Bozon, 1996); in other words, early or late initiation is an indicator of a type of sexual lifestyle. This empirical observation should not be limited to one country. Cross-cultural data are helpful to check if the connection is also found in other countries of Europe (Tables 2.7 to 2.10).

Several aspects of sexual behaviour at the time of the survey were examined. They included the proportion of people with multiple partners in the last 12 months (Table 2.7) or the frequency of intercourse in the last month (Table 2.8). Early and late sexual initiation are connected to distinct subsequent behaviours in all countries, but the differences are not always as marked as with French males.

The respondents who started late (we shall leave out the 'very late' group, which corresponds mostly to an older generation (see above)) had fewer

Table 2.7 *Proportions of respondents with more than one partner in the last year, by gender and sexual precocity / %*

Sexual precocity[1]	Belgium 1993	Finland 1992	France 1992	Germany West 1990	Great Britain 1991	Netherlands 1989
MEN						
Early	27 (358)	43 (249)	18 (869)	15 (352)	22 (2774)	27 (116)
Intermediate	17 (460)	26 (262)	14 (881)	11 (394)	15 (1835)	20 (107)
Late	13 (191)	19 (117)	9 (296)	10 (189)	12 (760)	17 (64)
Very late	3 (178)	9 (74)	8 (156)	6 (99)	4 (840)	4 (88)
Total	16	29	14	12	16	18
WOMEN						
Early	13 (253)	25 (208)	10 (429)	7 (380)	13 (2434)	15 (116)
Intermediate	8 (497)	15 (261)	8 (775)	5 (495)	7 (2866)	8 (186)
Late	3 (312)	10 (132)	5 (380)	3 (197)	4 (1514)	3 (150)
Very late	2 (253)	3 (73)	4 (208)	3 (79)	2 (1269)	3 (90)
Total	6	18	7	5	8	7

Base: all respondents (18–49 years) who ever had sex
Note:
[1] Sexual precocity: men and women were divided into four groups depending on whether their first intercourse occurred early, at an intermediate age, late or very late. Early is 16 and before; intermediate = 17 or 18; late = 19 or 20; very late = 21 and over

Table 2.8 *Proportions of those having intercourse two or more times a week, by gender and sexual precocity / %*

Sexual precocity[1]	Finland 1992	France 1992	Germany West 1990	Great Britain 1991	Netherlands 1989	Switzerland 1992
MEN						
Early	55	59	62	32	55	50 (340)
Intermediate	41	54	60	27	46	45 (488)
Late	38	39	45	24	44	48 (256)
Very late	39	36	43	18	40	38 (157)
Total	45	53	56	28	43	46
WOMEN						
Early	41	48	59	31	55	52 (217)
Intermediate	40	53	50	29	52	45 (513)
Late	43	50	46	24	49	44 (307)
Very late	29	42	35	22	40	47 (176)
Total	40	50	51	28	47	46

Base: all respondents (18–49 years) who ever had sex
Note:
[1] Sexual precocity: see note to Table 2.7

Table 2.9 *Practice of anal sex (in life or in the last 12 months) by gender and sexual precocity / %*

Sexual precocity[1]	Belgium[2] 1993	Finland[3] 1992	France[3] 1992	Germany West[3] 1990	Great Britain[3] 1991	Netherlands[4] 1989
MEN						
Early	20	18	41	25	20	7
Intermediate	13	17	34	20	14	1
Late	16	12	25	14	14	–
Very late	16	11	17	11	9	1
Total	15	16	34	20	16	3
WOMEN						
Early	21	24	32	23	19	7
Intermediate	22	16	29	15	13	2
Late	16	12	21	15	11	4
Very late	13	7	22	12	9	6
Total	17	16	27	17	13	5

Base: all respondents (18–49 years) who ever had sex
Notes:
[1] Sexual precocity: see note to Table 2.7
[2] Belgium: at least once in one of the current relations
[3] Finland, France, West Germany, Great Britain: at least once in life
[4] Netherlands: at least once in the last 12 months

partners in the preceding year than the early starters, and this holds true for men and women. The study carried out in France revealed that even in the more limited population of those living in union at the time of the survey, the proportion of respondents with multiple partners (in the last year) continued to be higher in the subgroup of early starters than among 'late-comers' (Bozon, 1996). The frequency of sexual activity in the last month is also linked to the timing of first intercourse: the earlier the start of one's sex life, the higher the frequency of intercourse. Yet this tendency is less marked in Switzerland and in Great Britain, and disappears among French and Finnish women. Among French males, the connection holds across generations.

One way of assessing the diversity of sexual repertoires is by measuring the frequency of rather uncommon practices, such as anal sex (Table 2.9). It is very clear in all countries, whether the practice was frequent or not, that the more 'advanced' respondents were more likely to have had anal sex in their lifetimes than the latecomers. This is true for men and women alike. In the French example, this remains true within each generation. This greater diversity of repertoire may be related to a higher turnover of partners, especially at a young age, which may offer more opportunities to experiment with more practices and to develop a marked interest in sexuality in its own right (Bozon, 1996).

Table 2.10   *Non-acceptance of extramarital relations, by gender and sexual precocity / %*

Sexual precocity[1]	Belgium[2] 1993	Finland[3] 1992	France[4] 1992	Great Britain[5] 1991	Netherlands[6] 1989
MEN					
Early	46	60	56	72	42
Intermediate	40	61	54	74	63
Late	46	66	66	79	67
Very late	58	67	75	83	74
Total	47	62	58	75	59
WOMEN					
Early	46	62	67	77	65
Intermediate	49	64	69	81	70
Late	54	65	74	85	63
Very late	61	50	76	86	58
Total	53	62	71	82	66

Base: all respondents (18–49 years) who ever had sex
Notes:
[1] Sexual precocity: see note to Table 2.7
[2] Belgium: 'When you are married, having sexual relations with another partner than your spouse is not acceptable', Answer: 'agree'
[3] Finland: 'One must be able to accept a husband's temporary infidelity', Answer: 'disagree'
[4] France: 'A man may have a few affairs with someone else during his marriage', Answer: 'not acceptable'
[5] Great Britain: 'What about a married person having sexual relations with someone other than his or her partner?', Answer: It is 'always wrong' or 'mostly wrong'
[6] Netherlands: 'In a steady relationship, you should allow each other to be free to have sexual contact with a third person', Answer: 'completely disagree'

Differences in the timing of sexual initiation are not so markedly related to differences in normative attitudes (Table 2.10). Once again, we shall leave out the 'very late' group. Among French and Dutch men, late sexual initiation is linked to a low acceptance of extramarital affairs of spouses, whereas tolerance is more common when first intercourse is early. The link between tolerance and early initiation is less strong among British and Finnish males and does not exist among Belgian men. Among women, attitudes towards extramarital relations are independent from age at first intercourse in Finland and the Netherlands, whereas there is a weak link between precocity and tolerance in Belgium, France and Great Britain.

A cross-national comparison shows that sexually 'advanced' individuals all over Europe have obviously more complex and less 'tidy' lives. They may be keener on sexual activity. From the data we have analyzed, we cannot infer that they have a specific attitude to HIV risk. The normative attitudes of early and late starters seem to differ less than their degree of sexual activity. On the whole, the clear-cut profiles that were found among the French males are not so apparent in other countries. For women it seems that an early start is less often a marker of a specific attitude or behaviour in the field of sexuality than it is for men, as it may only announce an early union with an older man.

Concluding Remarks

A revolution in morals marked by the decrease in women's age at first intercourse, the spreading of reliable means of birth control and the fall in fertility took place in Europe in the 1960s and 1970s. This resulted from a deep change in women's aspirations and reflected the increase in their personal autonomy, which could be observed simultaneously in new family behaviours, the increase in female educational level and, above all, the growing participation of women in the labour market. This movement affected all of Europe, to a greater or lesser extent. In the north the changes started in the 1960s, whereas in the south the new trend dates back only to the 1980s. Liberated by the loosening of the supervision and constraints that used to weigh on them, women were given the opportunity of embarking on sexual experiences with a partner earlier, free from the obsessing perspective of unwanted pregnancy.

The 1980s and early 1990s have been a period of continuing yet slower change. Young people's transition to adult life has lengthened (Cavalli and Galland, 1993). Family behaviours have continued to change, with rising rates of divorce and births out of wedlock. Although the educational level has kept rising, the latest economic crisis and resistance from the social body (at private or general level) have kept women from catching up with men in terms of participation in the workforce and careers. The onset of AIDS in the 1980s has forced public authorities and individuals to take into account the new risk of infection as a result of the very first experience of sexual intercourse.

Sexual initiation in the 1980s and the early 1990s has been characterized by three major trends: a steady decline of non-use of contraception at first intercourse, a marked rise in condom use in all countries, and a relative stagnation of age at first intercourse after the steep decrease that took place in the preceding decades. This plateau, which started before the advent of AIDS, may have been reinforced by the onset of the epidemic, in response to AIDS public education, but there is no evidence of a postponement of sexual initiation due to the new epidemiological context.

Despite these common trends, it cannot be maintained that a European sex culture with regard to first sexual intercourse has arisen. From one country to the other, the starting points as well as the time and extent of changes have been variable, and, as a result, different patterns of relations between men and women at sexual initiation have been observed. In the southern group, which includes in our sample Greece (Athens) and Portugal, there remains a clear gender-based double standard, that is, a difference in ages at first intercourse, which, after having reached six years not long ago, has fallen dramatically without disappearing. Mediterranean men have always been precocious, starting their sex lives well before marriage, while women in these countries, who still experience the latest sexual initiation in Europe, have only recently gained limited access to premarital sex and to the formal labour market. These countries probably are still in the process of change. In contrast, a long-standing pronounced egalitarian trend has been observed in the social, occupational and sexual spheres in the Nordic group, which in this study includes Denmark, Finland, Iceland, and Norway. For instance, these societies have long tolerated premarital relationships (Trost, 1978; Hofsten, 1978). The female employment rate has also long been high, as the Welfare State provided many opportunities for the care of young children. In most of these countries, men and women had their first intercourse at the same age (about 19) as early as the 1950s, and the subsequent fall in debut age followed a parallel course for both sexes, with female initiation occurring even earlier than that for men in some cases. Sexual liberalism is reflected, for instance, in the media, where sexual issues were gradually brought out into the open (Kontula and Kosonen, 1996). Yet the trend towards equalization meets insurmountable obstacles. Thus it remains a rule, in practice, that women should have their sexual initiation with older and more experienced men.

A third, albeit less homogeneous, set includes most of the remaining countries, that is Belgium, the Netherlands, Switzerland, and West Germany. These countries were characterized by rather late sexual initiation for both sexes (20 or over) in the not very remote past. We assume that some strong controls weighed on men and women alike until the 1950s (even later in some cases). The changes in morals and behaviours were sudden: moral pressure gave way to widespread tolerance, bringing age at first intercourse to 18.

France and Great Britain are more difficult to classify. These countries have in common clear gender inequality at the start and a very sharp change in women's behaviours. The French pattern is reminiscent of the course of events in southern countries, yet with attenuated features, whereas Great Britain, where male and female behaviours converged more rapidly, draws closer to the Nordic pattern.

In spite of the general reduction in gender differences, men and women still differ in all countries by the value they attach to first intercourse and first partner. Although sexual initiation has become largely disconnected from first union and the fear of unwanted pregnancy has decreased very much, women still take this stage very seriously, considering intercourse to be part of a relationship in which love for the partner is a normal component. The reflective female attitude is in stark contrast to that of men, who still tend to consider first intercourse to be an experience. Sexual initiation used to be a more serious concern to women because of its potentially major consequences. With the spread of HIV, protection against risk might become a common sexual health issue for men and women, promoting communication between partners.

Nevertheless, even with the broad spread of reliable contraception, it must be noted that teenage pregnancy has not disappeared (Eurostat, 1993) and even remains a major public health issue in several countries (Greece, Portugal and Great Britain). In Great Britain, the early starters (first intercourse before 16) have a very low rate of contraceptive use at first intercourse, which 'emphasizes the particular vulnerability of this group to unplanned pregnancy' (Wellings and Bradshaw, 1994, p. 87). The same process may be afoot in Greece and Portugal. An additional hypothesis is that early initiation implies more risk in countries which do not provide effective sex education in schools and out (Vilar, 1995). This is supported by the fact that the Nordic countries, which have a tradition of school sex education, have no major difficulty with teenage pregnancy, in spite of high proportions of early starters among women.

Within each country, an early or a late sexual debut is the starting point of a specific sexual biography and lifestyle. Early entry to adult sexuality marks the start of a well-identified sexual career characterized by more partners, a more diverse sexual repertoire and some distance from couple and family issues. Late starters have opposite characteristics. In the female population, differences between sexual lifestyles are less pronounced and less connected to age at first intercourse. One may wonder whether early starters are more 'at risk' in terms of HIV contamination. The British survey showed that they used little protection in their youth, but this trend is not so pronounced in other countries (Finland for instance). In their subsequent sex lives, we assume, as was shown in the French survey, that early starters lead 'riskier' lives but are perhaps characterized by greater adaptability to risk, whereas once again the late starters have the opposite characteristics (Bajos *et al.*, 1998).

The second half of the twentieth century, that is from the end of the Second World War onwards, has been characterized by a weakening of religious and moral supervision of young people and the spread of formal education, with the gradual generalization of secondary education and a sharp increase in the number of university students. Whilst religious precepts and influences are known to delay sexual initiation with variable degrees of coercion depending on the religion and society, the effects of education and the school institution on the transition to adult sexuality were not often addressed. Persons who go to secondary school and later to university identify with adult patterns of behaviour less early, as they clearly experience a prolonged teenage role because of their position in the institution and their material dependence. Besides, preoccupation with exams and one's academic career may generate, in some students, an ascetic attitude in which sexual desire, as an element of self-construction, is inhibited. The availability of other- or same-sex partners does not in itself necessarily lead to early intercourse among secondary school students. Conversely, there is no obstacle to social maturation, adult identification and sexual initiation for those who escape school discipline early and enter the labour market. Prolonged studies lead to a more reflective attitude towards sexual initiation; formal teaching may create a mental barrier to the informal teaching of peer groups, which generally promote early initiation. In contrast, those who are no longer receiving formal education are subjected to unrestricted normative peer pressure.

Sex education has been included in the school curricula for teenagers all over Europe, albeit with variable contents and ambitions (Vilar, 1995; Field and Wellings, 1993). According to the few available reports on this subject, it seems that the spread of sex education has had a slight delaying effect on age at first intercourse (Mellanby *et al.*, 1995; Wellings *et al.*, 1995) and increased the rate of contraceptive use at first intercourse markedly (Aggleton, Baldo and Slutkin, 1993; Greydanus, Pratt and Dannison, 1995). Sex education should start early, before students embark on their sexual careers, so as to give them a chance to prepare gradually for this key transition in their lives. Therefore it is necessary to aim at young age groups, 12- or 13-year-olds, rather than 15- or 16-year-olds (Kontula, Rimpelä and Ojanlatva, 1992). Those concerned with the conditions in which young people start their sex lives and with the content of sex education should not necessarily identify an early debut age with a physical or moral danger or consider juvenile abstinence a target. The mutual ignorance of and gap between the representations and expectations of men and women at sexual initiation and the resulting difficulty of interaction are major obstacles to effective prevention among young people. When young men consider their first intercourse to be merely a commitment-free personal experience, they have difficulty understanding young women's aspirations towards responsible relationships and behaviour. When it is not gender-biased, sex education may thus be a great help in promoting the attitudes necessary for concerted prevention by encouraging dialogue between partners.

Notes

1   This chapter deals mainly with first intercourse. It does not of course imply that no sex life or sexual initiation exists before first intercourse.

2   Social reproduction is the process by which social structure is reproduced; spouse and mate choice are a key element in this process (Bozon and Héran, 1989).

3   Our purchase of the British data file enabled us to calculate the indicators needed for this chapter. We should like to thank R. Laurent, S. Deneufchâtel and A. Carré from INED for performing the statistical analysis. Thanks are also in order to M. Meldbye, R. Bigger and J. Jónsdóttir – the investigators who conducted the Danish and Icelandic surveys – for kindly agreeing to provide us with their tables on age at first intercourse, since their questions were comparable to those of the other surveys. Their cooperation is greatly appreciated.

4   The survey was confined to Athens rather than all of Greece. Care must thus be taken not to extrapolate the results to the entire country.
5   This had to be done because of the small sizes of some samples, which would have been an obstacle if we had split the 20- to 49-year-olds into two or three generations.
6   When this chapter was written, an important survey on sexual behaviour in Sweden was being carried out by Bo Lewin.
7   Domination here does not refer to any individual psychological process, but to the gender relations that shape women's spouse and mate preferences (Bozon, 1991).

References

AGGLETON, P., BALDO, M. and SLUTKIN, G. (1993) 'Sex education leads to safer behaviour', *Global AIDS News*, **4**, pp. 1–20.

BAJOS, N., DUCOT, B., SPENCER, B. and SPIRA, A. (1998) 'Trajectoires socio-sexuelles et comportement face au risque de transmission sexuelle du Sida', in BAJOS, N., BOZON, M., FERRAND, A., GIAMI, A. and SPIRA, A. (Eds) *La sexualité aux temps du Sida*, Paris: Presses Universitaires de France.

BARRÈRE-MAURISSON, M.A. and MARCHAND, O. (1990) 'Structures familiales et marchés du travail dans les pays développés. Une nette opposition entre le Nord et le Sud', *Économie et Statistique*, **235**, pp. 19–30.

BOZON, M. (1991) 'Women and the age gap between spouses. An accepted domination?', *Population. An English selection*, **3**, pp. 113–48 (French version: 1990).

BOZON, M. (1996) 'Reaching adult sexuality. First intercourse and its implications', in BOZON, M. and LERIDON, H. (Eds) *Sexuality and the Social Sciences. A French Survey on Sexual Behaviour*, Aldershot: Dartmouth (French version: 1993).

BOZON, M. and HÉRAN, F. (1989) 'Finding a spouse. A survey of how French couples meet', *Population. An English Selection*, **1**, pp. 91–121 (French version: 1987).

BOZON, M. and LERIDON, H. (Eds) (1996) *Sexuality and the Social Sciences. A French Survey on Sexual Behaviour*, Aldershot: Dartmouth (French version: 1993).

CARAËL, M. (1995) 'Sexual behaviour', in CLELAND, J. and FERRY, B. (Eds) *Sexual Behaviour and AIDS in the Developing World*, London: Taylor and Francis.

CAVALLI, A. and GALLAND, O. (Eds) (1993) *L'allongement de la jeunesse*, Le Paradou: Actes Sud.

DUBOIS-ARBER, F., JEANNIN, A., MEYSTRE-AGUSTONI, G., GRUET, F. and PACCAUD, F. (1993) Évaluation de la stratégie de prévention du Sida en Suisse. Quatrième rapport de synthèse 1991–1992, *Cahiers de Recherche et de Documentation*, **82**, Lausanne, Suisse.

EUROSTAT (1993), *Demographic Statistics*, Luxembourg.

FIELD, B. and WELLINGS, K. (1993) *Context of Sexual Behaviour in Europe. Selected Indices*

Relating to Demographic, Social and Cultural Variables, London: St Mary's Hospital Medical School.

GAGNON, J. and SIMON, W. (1973) *Sexual Conduct. The Social Sources of Human Sexuality*, Chicago: Aldine.

GREYDANUS, D., PRATT, H. and DANNISON, L. (1995) 'Sexuality education programs for youth: current state of affairs and strategies for the future', *Journal of Sex Education and Therapy*, **4**, pp. 238–54.

HOEM, J. and RENNERMALM, B. (1985) 'Modern family initiation in Sweden: experience of women born between 1936 and 1960', *European Journal of Population*, **1**, pp. 81–112.

HOFSTEN, E. (1978) 'Consensual unions and their recent increase in Sweden', *Statistical Review*, **1**, pp. 24–32, Stockholm, Sweden.

HUBERT, M. and MARQUET, J. (Eds) (1993) *Comportements sexuels et réactions au risque du sida en Belgique*, Brussels: Centre d'études sociologiques, Facultés universitaires Saint Louis.

JESSOR, R., COSTA, F., JESSOR, L. and DONOVA, J. (1983) 'Time of first intercourse: a prospective study', *Journal of Personality and Social Psychology*, **44**, 3, pp. 608–26.

JOHNSON, A. and WADSWORTH, J. (1994) 'Heterosexual partnerships', in JOHNSON, A., WADSWORTH, J., WELLINGS, K. and FIELD, J., *Sexual Attitudes and Lifestyles*, Oxford: Blackwell Scientific Publications.

JOHNSON, A., WADSWORTH, J., WELLINGS, K. and FIELD, J. (1994) *Sexual Attitudes and Lifestyles*, Oxford: Blackwell Scientific Publications.

JÓNSDOTTIR, J.I. (1996) 'Sexual behaviour among Icelanders: implications for the risk of HIV prevention and planning of AIDS prevention', *Nordisk Sexologi*, **14**, pp. 9–17.

KONTULA, O. (1991) *Cultural terms of sexual initiation* (in Finnish, with English summary, pp. 179–88), Helsinki: Sosiaali-Ja Terveyshallitus.

KONTULA, O. and HAAVIO-MANNILA, E. (1995) *Sexual Pleasures: Enhancement of Sex Life in Finland, 1971–1992*, Dartmouth: Aldershot (see in particular Chapter 5 'The sexual initiation', pp. 46–67).

KONTULA, O. and KOSONEN, K. (1996) 'Sexuality changing from privacy to the open: a study of the Finnish press over the years from 1961 to 1991', *Nordisk Sexologi*, **14**, 3, pp. 34–47.

KONTULA, O., RIMPELÄ, M. and OJANLATVA, A. (1992) 'Sexual knowledge, attitudes, fears and behaviours of adolescents in Finland (the Kiss study)', *Health Education Research*, **7**, 1, pp. 69–77.

LAUMANN, E., GAGNON, J., MICHAEL, R. and MICHAELS, S. (1994) *The Social Organization of Sexuality. Sexual Practices in the United States*, Chicago: University of Chicago Press (see in particular Chapter 9 'Formative sexual experiences', pp. 321–47).

LEWIN, B. and TRAEEN, B. (1993) 'Seeing the real through the eyes of the ideal. Some comments on Traeen *et al.* (1992) account of gender difference in Norwegian young people's sexual behaviour', *Journal of Community and Applied Social Psychology*, **3**, pp. 71–6.

LOYOLA, M.A. (1992) 'Sexualidade e Reprodução' (in Portuguese), *Physis-Revista de Saude Coletiva*, **1**, pp. 93–105, Rio de Janeiro: Rio de Janeiro State University.

MELDBYE, M. and BIGGAR, R. (1992) 'Interactions between persons at risk for AIDS and the general population in Denmark', *American Journal of Epidemiology*, **135**, 6, pp. 593–602.

MELLANBY, A.R., PHELPS, F.A., CRICHTON, N.J. and TRIPP, J.H. (1995) 'School sex education: an experimental programme with educational and medical benefit', *British Medical Journal*, **311**, pp. 414–17.

MESSIAH, A. and MOURET-FOURME, E. (1996) 'Homosexuality, bisexuality: elements of sexual socio-biography', in BOZON, M. and LERIDON, H. (Eds) *Sexuality and the Social Sciences. A French Survey on Sexual Behaviour*, Aldershot: Dartmouth (French version 1993).

PERISTIANY, J.G. (Ed.) (1966) *Honor and Shame: The Value of Mediterranean Society*, Chicago: University of Chicago Press.

POLLAK, M. (1985) 'Male homosexuality or happiness in the ghetto?', in ARIÈS, PH. and BÉJIN, A. (Eds) *Western Sexuality*, Oxford: Blackwell Scientific Publications (French version: 1982).

ROUSSEL, L. (1987) 'Deux décennies de mutations démographiques (1965–1985) dans les pays industrialisés', *Population*, **3**, pp. 429–48.

SANTOS-LUCAS, J. (1993) *Sida. A sexualidade desprevenida dos Portugueses* (in Portuguese), Lisboa: McGraw Hill.

SARDON, J.P. (1993) 'Women's first marriage rates in Europe. Elements for a typology', *Population – An English Selection*, **5**, pp. 119–52 (French version: 1992).

SEGALEN, M. (1981) *Amours et mariages de l'ancienne France*, Paris: Berger-Levrault.

SIMON, W. and GAGNON, J. (1986) 'Sexual scripts: permanence and change', *Archives of Sexual Behaviour*, **15**, 2, pp. 97–120.

SPIRA, A., BAJOS, N. and ACSF GROUP (1994) *Sexual Behaviour and AIDS*, Avebury: Aldershot.

SUNDET, J., MAGNUS, P., KVALEM, I., SAMULSEN, S. and BAKKETEIG, L. (1992) 'Secular trends and sociodemographic regularities of coital debut age in Norway', *Archives of Sexual Behaviour*, pp. 241–52.

TOULEMON, L. and LERIDON, H. (1992) 'Twenty years of contraception in France: 1968–1988', *Population – An English Selection*, **4**, pp. 1–34 (French version: 1991).

TOULEMON, L. and LERIDON, H. (1995) 'La diffusion des préservatifs: contraception et prévention', *Population et Sociétés*, **231**, Paris: INED.

TRAEEN, B., LEWIN, B. and SUNDET, J. (1992) 'The real and the ideal; Gender differences in heterosexual behaviour among Norwegian adolescents', *Journal of Community and Applied Social Psychology*, **2**, pp. 227–37.

TROST, J. (1978) 'A renewed social institution: non-marital cohabitation', *Acta Sociologica. Journal of the Scandinavian Sociological Association*, **4**, pp. 303–15.

TROST, J. (1990) 'La famille : stabilité et changement', in PRIOUX, E. (Ed.) *La famille dans les pays développés: permanences et changements*, Paris: PUF-INED.

VAN DE KAA, D.J. (1987) 'Europe's second demographic transition', *Population Bulletin*, **42**, pp. 1–57.

VAN ZESSEN, G. and SANDFORT, T. (1991) *Seksualiteit in Nederland: seksueel gedrag, risico en preventie van AIDS* (in Dutch), Amsterdam/Lisse: Swets and Zeitlinger.

VILAR, D. (1995) 'School sex education: still a priority in Europe', *Planned Parenthood in Europe*, **23**, 3, pp. 8–11.

WELLINGS, K. and BRADSHAW, S. (1994) 'First intercourse between men and women', in JOHNSON, A., WADSWORTH, J., WELLINGS, K. and FIELD, J. (Eds) *Sexual Attitudes and Lifestyles*, Oxford: Blackwell Scientific Publications, pp. 68–109.

WELLINGS, K., WADSWORTH, J. and JOHNSON, A. (1994) 'Sexual diversity and homosexual behaviour', in JOHNSON, A., WADSWORTH, J., WELLINGS, K. and FIELD, J. (Eds) *Sexual Attitudes and Lifestyles*, Oxford: Blackwell Scientific Publications, pp. 183–224.

WELLINGS, K., WADSWORTH, J., JOHNSON, A., FIELD, J., WHITAKER, L. and FIELD, B. (1995) 'Provision of sex education and early sexual experience: the relation examined', *British Medical Journal*, **311**, pp. 417–20.

Chapter 3

Homosexual and Bisexual Behaviour in European Countries

*Theo Sandfort**

Introduction

The AIDS epidemic has turned male homosexuality into a societal issue that can no longer be marginalized or ignored. In most Western countries, with the exception of southern Europe, the majority of people with AIDS were and still are gay men (*HIV/AIDS Surveillance in Europe*, 1995). Primarily as a consequence of the fear that men who have sexual contacts with men as well as with women might form a bridge between the affected gay community and the heterosexual population, interest in bisexuality has grown as well (Weinberg, Williams and Pryor, 1994).

The AIDS epidemic has stimulated much research into homosexual behaviour, nationally and cross-nationally; money to do so became available in an unprecedented way. For the first time, gay men, as a separate category of people, also became a target of extensive primary prevention. In some European countries, such as the Netherlands and Switzerland, gay men were even integrated into the campaigns directed at the general population. In other countries, such as France, AIDS has reactivated or fostered the growth of the gay and lesbian movements (De Busscher, 1995).

The research about gay men carried out prior to AIDS, as well as that conducted in the context of AIDS, has relied predominantly on convenience samples (Bochow *et al.*, 1994). These studies have answered several important questions about homosexual behaviour. Since it has been shown that convenience samples of gay men tend to be biased (Weinberg, 1970; Harry, 1986 and 1990; Sandfort, 1996), these studies have also generated several other

*The author would like to thank Henny Bos, Stuart Michaels, Ernest de Vroome, Jeffrey Weiss and the group of researchers collaborating in the EU Concerted Action for their support in preparing and writing this chapter.

questions. One might ask, for instance, whether the mean level of education among gay men is indeed higher than among heterosexual men, as most studies in convenience samples seem to suggest. Are urban areas really inhabited by more gay men than rural areas? Are the frequency of casual sex, the degree of behaviour change, and the seroprevalence rate found in gay convenience samples characteristic of the total homosexual population?

Male homosexuality has also been studied in the general population surveys elicited by the AIDS epidemic and carried out to inform general AIDS policy and HIV prevention. Most of these surveys have addressed female homosexuality and bisexuality as well. These surveys have made it possible to assess whether homosexuality is randomly distributed in society, or whether subsamples of homosexual and heterosexual people differ systematically from one another. These surveys also make it possible to assess to what extent the occurrence and expression of homosexuality differ from one country to the next. A major limitation of these surveys is that very large samples are needed to find enough people with homosexual experiences to allow statistical analyses and, consequently, in-depth understanding of homosexuality.

Occurrence and Expression of Homosexuality: Similarities and Differences

To understand similarities and differences between countries in the occurrence and expression of homosexuality, it is important to ponder what homosexuality and bisexuality actually are. In this respect our scientific thinking has changed considerably in the last decades, predominantly as a consequence of historical and cultural-anthropological research.

Homosexuality is usually understood to be a kind of sexual behaviour exhibited by people who have sexual desires for people of their own sex and label themselves homosexual, gay, or lesbian. Here, sexual behaviour is seen as an expression of the person's real self. Implicitly or explicitly, this homosexuality is considered to be a consequence of biological factors and/or a product of family dynamics (see Ellis, 1996 for an overview and discussion of these theories). Homosexual people are seen as the complement to heterosexual people. This conception is part of the common understanding of our socio-erotic world, in which people are either straight or gay, and accordingly have a characteristic, unifying lifestyle. Aside from this 'true' homosexuality, in which desire, behaviour and self-labelling converge, 'situational' homosexuality has been identified as well, especially in circumstances where the opposite sex is not available, such as in prisons and boarding schools.

Bisexuality is usually understood in the context of the heterosexual/ homosexual dichotomy. Quite often it is seen as transitory: uncertain about their real sexual orientation, people experiment with and explore their sexual desires to eventually become either hetero- or homosexual (Troiden, 1989). People who continue to have sex with people of their own as well as the opposite sex are assumed not to be able to choose, to deny their homosexual orientation, or to try to adopt a more accepted, heterosexual lifestyle. Research has shown that for some people, bisexuality is a satisfactory, self-fulfilling condition (Weinberg, Williams and Pryor, 1994).

Although the heterosexual/homosexual dichotomy is experienced as part of a natural order, recent historical, sociological and cultural-anthropological studies have shown that homosexuality is not a one-dimensional, un-equivocal phenomenon, but encompasses a diversity of ways of sexual expression (Plummer, 1975 and 1981; Foucault, 1980; Pollak, 1985; Kitzinger, 1987; Greenberg, 1988; Gagnon, 1990; Herdt, 1990). In general, these studies have shown that the way in which sexuality is expressed and organized is not a 'natural' given, but depends upon a variety of historical, societal and cultural factors. This implies that the social and personal meanings of a behaviour which might appear identical from the outside are in fact divergent. These meanings are dependent upon the way sexuality is organized in a specific culture. It has, for instance, become clear that our current understanding of what a homosexual person is is heavily influenced by late-nineteenth century medical theories (Hekma, 1987).

The variety of ways in which sexuality is organized and expressed is not documented for homosexuality alone. Recently the notion that sexual identities are constructed has also been studied in the field of heterosexuality, showing that sexuality between persons of a different sex has been organized in various ways and has had different meanings for the people involved (Jackson, 1987; Wilkinson and Kitzinger, 1994; Katz, 1995). This constructionist approach has also revealed that even the understanding of ourselves as having a sexual orientation defined by a class of objects (men or women) to whom we feel attracted is a rather recent 'invention' (Halperin *et al.*, 1990).

The fact that even in our contemporary society not all homosexual behaviour is expressed in the form of a homosexual identity has become clear in AIDS studies as well. For instance, Doll *et al.* (1992) showed in a blood donor study that almost a quarter of the men who had had sex with another man in the preceding year did not label themselves as homosexual. This was more often so among Blacks and Hispanics than among Caucasians, indicating that among white men, homosexual self-labelling is a more common practice (compare Seidman, 1993). These findings suggest that labelling oneself as homosexual or lesbian might be dependent upon social and subcultural factors as well. Laumann *et al.* (1994) also showed that there is little overlap between feelings of attraction, actual behaviour and self-labelling, although they examined this over a rather long time frame.

The idea that the kinds of homosexuality we observe are constructed, does not necessarily exclude the roles of biological and interpersonal or developmental factors in the causation of homosexual behaviour. It does, however, imply that these factors in themselves are not sufficient to comprehend all the different forms of homosexual behaviour, as Kinsey (1941) already indicated as early as the 1940s. According to the constructionist approach, a variety of social factors influence the extent to which and way in which homosexual desire is expressed in behaviour and the way this expression is experienced and labelled by the actor and his or her entourage.

As suggested by Laumann *et al.* (1994), cultural and social factors affect not only the expression of homosexuality, but possibly its occurrence as well. According to their recently formulated elicitation/opportunity hypothesis, homosexuality can be promoted by an environment that creates opportunities for and is supportive of this form of behaviour. Conversely, in a negative climate there will be more pressure to conform and a stronger fear of discrimination that inhibits the expression of homosexuality. Laumann *et al.* also present some empirical support for this idea. In their study of a representative sample of US citizens, they found that homosexual people tend to live in urban rather than rural areas. They demonstrate that this is not simply a consequence of gay people's migration to these areas to avoid negative social pressure and to find more opportunities for the expression of their desires, for they found that proportionately more gay than heterosexual men already lived in a city at the age of 16, an age at which they cannot be assumed to have had a major influence on the choice of their family's place of residence. This suggests that the city is a place which offers more opportunities for the development and expression of homosexual behaviour.

Additional support for this elicitation/opportunity hypothesis comes from the finding that fathers of gay men are more highly educated than fathers of heterosexual men (Rogers and Turner, 1991). Neither the homosexual nor the heterosexual offspring can of course be held accountable for this difference, supporting again the idea that environmental factors play a role in the occurrence of homosexual behaviour.

Factors Influencing Occurrence and Expression of Homosexuality

As implied by the elicitation/opportunity hypothesis, the variety in homosexual expression in contemporary Western societies cannot be understood without acknowledging the dominance of heterosexuality. The constant message people receive through a variety of socializing agents is that the proper way for sexuality to be expressed is between a man and a woman. In no European country is homosexuality a legitimate, well-accepted and integrated form of sexual expression valued in the same way as heterosexuality. This has consequences on the occurrence of homosexuality as well as on the way homosexuality is expressed.

The fact that individual constructions of homosexuality are made in a context of condemnation will result in differences between heterosexual and homosexual people. In a society in which homosexual desires are socially unaccepted, whether blatantly or more subtly, men and women who have such desires have to accomplish several tasks to be able to express these desires satisfactorily. They have to integrate this aspect into their understanding of who they are, and in doing so, process the negative stigma related to this form of sexual expression (Shidlo, 1994). They accomplish this more effectively when they are able to make themselves less dependent upon their environment. Since homosexuals, unlike heterosexuals, do not have a 'natural' access to potential partners, they generally have to put more energy into organizing and maintaining a network in order to find partners. Developing economic independence is much more of a necessity for lesbians than for heterosexual women. These processes predict a higher level of social mobility and of migration to urban centres among gay men and lesbians. They also suggest that homosexuals in general are less often religiously inclined and more often opt for progressive political movements. We expect that some of these processes can be observed in the various countries which are included in this overview.

Besides the social pressure to adopt a heterosexual lifestyle, several other factors will influence the kind of homosexuality one may observe. These factors, which will be discussed later, are either expressions or consequences of the dominant heterosexual climate. They are interrelated and will operate on different levels of social organization. As it will become clear, the 'effects' of the differences in social climate will be noticeable in various aspects of homosexuality.

The countries included in this comparison can be distinguished by the legal status of homosexuality (Waaldijk, 1993). The more progressive countries – those that legally acknowledge same-sex relationships or have adopted anti-discrimination legislation – will be more supportive of homosexual expression and gay and lesbian lifestyles than the less progressive countries where specific forms of homosexual expression are still illegal. The latter is, for instance, the case in the UK, where, despite a recent change in the law, the ages of consent for heterosexual and homosexual intercourse still differ. These legal differences between countries will to a certain extent reflect the dominant social values, while changes in these laws will be the result of social pressures from, for instance, the gay and lesbian movement.

Although in general the Church's influence is waning (Halman and De Moor, 1994), the dominant social attitude towards homosexuality will also depend upon the religious situations in the respective countries. Countries like Ireland and Italy, where Roman Catholic doctrine promoting heterosexual monogamy is still dominant, will differ from countries like Sweden and

Germany, where the Church's influence on the organization of social life is practically nil.

The occurrence and expression of homosexuality will also depend upon the general visibility of homosexuality in a given society. This in turn is related to the existence of homosexual subcultures and the strength of a gay and lesbian movement. Subcultures are a crucial factor in the expression of homosexuality, since they offer homosexual men and women opportunities to meet each other, to find potential partners and to develop a shared frame of reference in dealing with an oppressive environment. When a gay and lesbian subculture is strongly developed in a specific country, it will independently support the expression of homosexuality and further the development of various homosexual lifestyles.

This list of societal characteristics influencing the occurrence and expression of homosexuality in a specific country is by no means exhaustive. Countries also vary with regard to socio-geographical factors such as urbanization and population density, which, as has already been indicated, will affect the occurrence and expression of homosexuality as well. On a broader level, countries will differ with respect to their cultural isolation or independence, some being more receptive or vulnerable to cultural influences from other countries.

The social factors discussed thus far will affect the occurrence and expression of homosexuality in the various countries in different ways. Among other things, the process of homosexual identity formation can be expected to be thwarted and delayed in countries with a less tolerant climate towards homosexuality. As a consequence, people will 'come out' at a later stage in life (coming out in this instance refers to the personal acknowledgement and public openness about one's homosexual orientation). In countries with a more negative climate, this will result in a greater discrepancy between the mean age of the people who identify as lesbian or gay and the people who are heterosexual, the latter being relatively younger as a group.

In less supportive social climates, people who eventually 'turn out' to be gay or lesbian may also attempt to ignore their homosexual desires and to adopt a heterosexual lifestyle for a longer period of time. As a consequence one would also expect relatively more homosexuals who are or have been legally married in countries with a less accepting climate. This assumption is supported by the fact that in the Netherlands, which is characterized by a growing acceptance of homosexuality, one finds more men who are or have been married in the older cohorts of men who now identify themselves as homosexuals.

Homosexuality's greater visibility, which will be a consequence but also a cause of a more positive climate in a specific country, will provide homosexual role models. This will make it easier for people to develop homosexual identities. Heterosexual experimentation will no longer be felt to be a personal necessity, which will also contribute to the greater frequency of exclusively homosexual behaviour. In countries where public manifestations of homosexual behaviours and lifestyles are more frequent, specific forms of behaviour will also be identified and labelled as homosexual more readily, not only by society, but also by the people concerned.

Historically, the greater visibility of homosexuality – achieved by, among other things, a strong and successful gay and lesbian movement – may also have resulted in a dichotomous understanding of sexual identity, that is, that people are either straight or gay/lesbian. Bisexuality as an alternative sexual identity will consequently be less viable in countries with a stronger acceptance of homosexuality. At the moment this may, however, be changing as a consequence of the attention paid to bisexuality in recent AIDS research projects, while there is a growing acknowledgement of sexual diversity within the gay and lesbian community itself.

Finally, countries with a more open climate may also counteract the furtive expression of homosexuality and foster finding intimate partners and developing and maintaining gay and lesbian relationships, given that the generally observed shorter duration of gay relationships has been ascribed to the lack of social support and legal recognition of these relationships.

Some of the social factors mentioned here will obviously affect not only the expression of homosexuality, but also people's willingness to report on homosexual experiences in sex surveys. What people have reported about their sexual interactions in the various European general population surveys offers an interesting opportunity to test some of the aspects of the perspective developed above. This opportunity is limited by the way homosexuality has been addressed in the various studies and the other data available. In particular, most studies predominantly focused on behaviour, while only a few studies included questions about aspects such as attraction, identities, and lifestyles.

Cross-nationally we anticipate that people exhibiting homosexual behaviour will have a higher level of education and will more often be found in large towns than rural areas. Between countries we expect differences in the occurrence of (exclusively) homosexual behaviour, with the countries with a generally more positive social climate towards homosexuality showing a higher rate of (exclusively) homosexual behaviour. Furthermore, in countries with a less positive climate, relatively more homosexual behaviour will be exhibited by people who are or have been married. In this chapter we shall also explore the relationship of homosexual behaviour with age and the start of one's sexual career. Differences between men and women will be checked systematically. Finally, the relationship between behaviour and attraction will be described.

Understanding the occurrence and expression of homosexual behaviour, and the factors affecting these, is of great relevance for the prevention of HIV and STD. This information is needed to find out where and how target groups can be reached and which lifestyle and subcultural factors have to be taken into account in order to communicate messages effectively.

Methodological Aspects

To make our comparisons as valid as possible and to understand the limitations of our efforts, it is important to address some methodological issues first. These link to 1) inter-survey comparability, including the way homosexuality has been addressed in the various studies, 2) the way comparisons within and between countries are made statistically, and 3) an *a priori* classification of countries according to their social climates concerning homosexuality.

Variety in Research Designs

As discussed earlier (see Chapter 1), each country had its own approach to designing and conducting its national study. This will have affected the outcomes. To start with, each study used different sampling techniques. Although almost all countries aimed at composing national representative samples (the Greek study, which focused on Athens, was an exception), they did so in various ways, and quite likely with different degrees of success. This may have affected the observed frequencies of specific forms of behaviour. In the Dutch survey, where an extensive follow-up study has been conducted to understand the effects of non-response, it became clear that highly educated women with professional careers were under-represented in the national sample (Van Zessen and Sandfort, 1991). It is quite likely that the sexual lifestyles of these women differ from the lifestyles of monogamously married heterosexual women, who are predominantly homemakers.

Next to the issue of sampling, it should be noted that the national surveys collected data in various ways, ranging from telephone interviews to face-to-face techniques (see Chapter 1). This may have affected the results of the studies, especially those concerning forms of less socially accepted types of behaviour such as homosexuality. Although a French study failed to detect differences between the results of telephone and face-to-face interviews (ACSF Investigators, 1992), it has been documented in the British survey that the more anonymous written questionnaire elicits higher reporting of homosexual behaviour than a personal interview (Johnson *et al.*, 1994). Other methodological studies have shown differences as well (Turner, Miller and Rogers, 1996). People's willingness to answer questions about homosexuality and to disclose a homosexual present or past will also be dependent upon the social climate towards homosexuality within the respective countries, regardless of the quality of the interviewer or the technique applied, with homosexual men and women in less accepting climates being less willing to collaborate.

Assessments of Homosexuality

Aside from the methods of data collection, the national studies also differ in the way homosexuality was surveyed in terms of both the extent to which homosexuality was covered and the specific kinds of questions that were posed.

Some studies applied more than one approach (see also Table 3.1). All countries surveyed male as well as female homosexuality, except for Switzerland, where only male homosexual behaviour was addressed. The following section presents an overview of the diversity of approaches taken in the different studies. Since, except for Switzerland, analogous questions were used to cover male and female homosexuality, only questions addressed to men are presented and discussed here.

Half of the studies focused exclusively on homosexual behaviour (Athens, Belgium, Norway, Portugal, Switzerland), while other studies also asked one or more questions about more internal dimensions like attraction or preferences (Finland, France, Netherlands and Spain). Except for behaviour and attraction, the surveys took different approaches to the time period considered. There are questions dealing with lifetime occurrence ('have you ever . . .') and questions focusing on various specific periods: some questions focused on a recent time period (for example preceding year or preceding five years), whereas others dealt with specific developmental periods (like puberty). In a single instance no time period was specified at all.

With respect to behaviour, three levels of directness were used to elicit responses about possible homosexual experiences, as follows: 1) some studies took a direct approach, asking people specifically whether they had ever had same-sex sexual experiences or with how many women and with how many men they had had sex in their life; 2) others asked about the genders of the people with whom the respondent reported having had sex; and finally

Table 3.1 *Questions and response categories used to address lifetime homosexual behaviour and preference*

BEHAVIOUR

Athens (1990)	'In terms of your sexual activity which of the following statements best describes what you actually do (or did)?' 1: I have had sex only with women – 5: I have had sex only with men
Belgium (1993)	'In the course of your lifetime have you had sex with:' 1: women only – 4: men only, 5: as many women as men
Finland (1992)	'Have you had sexual experiences (arousing fondling or intercourse) with a person of your own sex?' (no/yes once/yes many times)

Table 3.1   *(cont.)*

France (ACSF–1992)	'In the course of your life have you had sexual intercourse with . . .' 1: women only – 5: men only
Germany (West–1990)	'With regard to your sexual activity, which of the following statements best describes what you actually do (or did)?' 1: I have had sex only with women 2: I have had sex mostly with women but occasionally with men 3: I have had sex equally with men and women 4: I have had sex mostly with men but occasionally with women 5: I have had sex with men only
Netherlands (1989)	'Have you ever had sexual contact with a boy or a man? By sexual contact we mean at least masturbation or jacking off.' (yes/no)
Norway (1992)	'Have you ever had sexual partners of your own sex?' (no/yes)
Portugal (1991)	'In terms of your sexual activity which of the following statements best describes what you actually do (or did)?' 1: I have had sex only with women – 5: I have had sex with men only
Spain (1990)	'What is your personal sexual orientation?' 1: I feel attracted or have sexual relations only with the opposite sex (heterosexual) 2: I feel attracted or have sexual relations only with people of my own sex (homosexual) 3: I feel attracted or have sexual relations with people of both sexes (bisexual) 4: I have changed sex (transsexual)
Switzerland (1992)	'Have you engaged in homosexual sex?' (yes/no)
PREFERENCE	
France (ACSF–1992)	'In the course of your life, have you been sexually attracted by . . .' 1: women only – 5: men only
Finland (1992)	'Besides being sexually interested in the opposite sex, people are sometimes also interested in their own sex. Are you at the moment sexually interested in . . .' 1: only the male sex – 5: only the female sex
Netherlands (1989)	'Please give the number which best describes your present sexual preference. Your sexual preference doesn't have to correspond to your sexual behaviour.' 1: exclusively heterosexual – 7: exclusively homosexual

3) in some, respondents were asked to assess their own behaviour on a scale indicating the proportion of male and/or female sexual partners. These approaches will be discussed below.

As can be seen in Table 3.1, same-sex sexual contacts were tackled directly in the Dutch, Finnish, Norwegian and Swiss studies by asking whether or not they had ever occurred. However, different concepts were used to refer to these same-sex experiences. Questions ask about sexual partners of the same sex, sexual contact, and sexual experiences. In the Swiss study, the question put to men reads: 'Have you engaged in homosexual sex?' Men who responded positively to this question were also asked how long it had been since they had last had sex with another man. In the Finnish study, people with same-sex experiences were also asked at which age their first sexual experience with a person of their own sex took place, the kinds of sexual contact they have had, and the number of same-sex partners. They were subsequently asked if they had ever had an orgasm during intercourse with a person of the same sex, an orgasm being described as 'an ending of sexual tension by coming with an intense feeling of pleasure'. In the Dutch survey lifetime occurrence of same-sex sexual contacts was addressed in the section on early sexual experiences, which included various questions assessing first erotic and physical attraction and experiences and actual contacts with persons of the opposite as well as the same sex.

Questions about the occurrence and number of male and/or female sexual partners in different time periods were asked in Belgium, France, Norway, and Portugal.

The gender of specific sexual partners was asked for in Athens (current steady partner), Belgium (first sexual contact, current and previous year partners), France (first relationship, current steady partner, last sexual contact), the Netherlands (steady partner as well as casual partners in different time periods), Norway (current steady partner and casual partners), Portugal (current steady partner) and Switzerland (steady partner and last occasional partner). In a few cases the partner's gender was not asked, although it was sometimes indicated to the respondents, as in the Finnish study, that a partner could be steady or temporary, male or female.

Respondents were asked to assess their sexual behaviour on a scale in the studies carried out in Belgium, France, Greece, Germany, and Portugal. In Spain, one and the same question asked about behaviour as well as sexual preference. In these questions, the period under consideration was specified most of the time.

Questions about sexual preference were included in the French, Finnish and Dutch surveys. The approaches taken in these studies differ completely, however, with respect to the actual words they used to describe attraction (Table 3.1). While the focus in the French study was on lifetime sexual interest, the Finnish study asked about current sexual interest. In the Dutch study people who indicated having had feelings of physical attraction towards people of the same sex at least once were asked whether these feelings were still present and if not, at what age they disappeared. All Dutch respondents were also asked to classify their sexual preference on a seven-point scale ranging from 'exclusively heterosexual' to 'exclusively homosexual'; the categories were shown to the respondent on a response card. The labels 'heterosexual' and 'homosexual' were introduced only after same-sex sexuality had already been discussed extensively in a neutral way.

Consequences of the Variety in Approaches

The way in which homosexuality has been addressed will undoubtedly have affected the various studies' outcomes. It has already been shown that different definitions of sexual contacts have been presented. It is quite likely that a more narrow definition of sexual contact, as used for instance in the Belgian study: 'intimate contact with (vaginal, anal, or oral) penetration', will elicit fewer positive responses than the somewhat broader Dutch and Finnish definitions presented (see Table 3.1). Of course, not just the definition of those crucial terms presented by the interviewer, but also the respondents' understanding of those terms and definitions, will affect their reports. Where no definition of sexual contact was presented it is unclear whether the respondents understood the term as referring specifically to intercourse or as indicating a wider range of sexual techniques.

The surveys also differ with respect to the definition of partner presented to the respondent. Sometimes no specific information was given about this, while at other times a range of partners was described. Indicating that a partner could be male or female quite likely helped people to remember same-sex experiences and consequently led to a higher response rate. It is unclear how respondents interpreted questions in which a time frame was relevant but not specified, as was the case in a few studies, and what kind of effect this had on the responses. It quite likely resulted in under-reporting of the relevant behaviours or experiences. The extensiveness with which homosexual experiences were addressed will also have affected the response rates, for when more questions are asked it becomes more difficult to overlook or 'forget' certain experiences.

Society's negative judgement of homosexuality makes it even more likely that the studies' findings were affected by the approaches taken. Since people may have a tendency not to cover these experiences or just 'forget' them, special care has to be taken to elicit them. It has been shown that the way people are asked about homosexual behaviour influences their answers. An enhanced mode of questioning, that legitimizes a positive response, results in higher rates of reported homosexual behaviour (Catania, 1996). In this context, the fact that almost all the surveys did not literally ask about 'homosexual' behaviour should be seen positively, as the term might elicit negative feelings, inhibiting objective reporting of past experiences. It is also possible, of course, that people who have had same-sex experiences do not label these experiences as homosexual because the term suggests homosexual self-identification, which does not always have to be the case. Despite being direct about homosexuality, most surveys also avoided offending people. They managed this by, for instance, offering the more likely answer categories, referring to heterosexual behaviour, before the answer category indicating homosexual behaviour.

Willingness to report about homosexual experiences will also depend upon the extent to which the naturalness or even superiority of heterosexuality and marriage is implicitly or explicitly communicated to the respondents. A gender-neutral approach with respect to partners and avoiding of the assumption that people usually are married will encourage people to be open about homosexual experiences. It is evident that in this respect it is not just the questionnaire, but also the interviewer's behaviour that matters.

In conclusion, it is difficult to predict how and to what extent the various methodological factors discussed here actually influenced the findings presented in this chapter, because too many variations are possible. Although the consequences of these factors can only be speculated about, it is assumed that these methodological factors will have had an effect. At the same time it is assumed that the inter-country differences presented here cannot be attributed solely to methodological differences.

Comparisons within and between Countries

The data from the various studies allow us to make intra- and inter-country comparisons of lifetime occurrence of homosexuality as well as homosexual behaviour in the preceding year, although the latter could be examined for somewhat fewer countries. Exclusively homosexual behaviour was reported so rarely in most countries, however, that we have had to combine people with both exclusively homosexual experiences and bisexual experiences into one group.

In order to make comparisons between countries, 95 per cent confidence levels were computed for the total samples and subsamples. A difference between countries was considered significant if the two respective confidence levels did not overlap. Within countries, women were compared with men using logistic regression analysis. The same technique was used to test relationships within countries between the occurrence of homosexual contacts on the one hand and age, start of sexual career, level of education, and urbanity on the other hand. These analyses were performed separately for men and women. If other techniques were used they will be specified.

A *Priori* Classification of Countries

The interpretation of potential similarities and differences between countries will be guided by the theoretical perspective developed in the introduction. To make these comparisons meaningful, it is necessary to classify the countries beforehand instead of interpreting empirical differences with hindsight. Various classification criteria, such as the legal situation regarding homosexuality, the presence and strength of a gay and lesbian movement and subculture, and so on, can be used.

In this study I shall classify countries according to the population's acceptance of homosexuality, as described in the European Values Studies (Van den Akker, Halman and De Moor, 1994). As part of this study, people in various countries were asked to indicate on a 10-point scale to what extent they felt that homosexuality could always (10) or never (1) be justified. It is unclear whether respondents in these studies understood the term 'homosexuality' as implying female as well as male homosexuality.

As Table 3.2 shows, people in most countries responded to this question in a significantly different way. According to this classification, the Netherlands has the most positive climate (the difference with regard to all the other countries is significant) and Portugal has the least positive climate. The mean scores for Britain and the USA (not included in the table) were 3.53 and 2.42, respectively.

The resulting hierarchy of countries is almost completely identical to a hierarchy based on answers to the statement 'I would not like to have homosexuals as neighbours' that was included in the same studies.

Finland, Greece (Athens) and Switzerland were not included in the European Values Studies. Being one of the Nordic countries, Finland can be classified in line with Norway, while we assume that Greece will share its value

Table 3.2 *Acceptance of homosexuality in different countries, mean scores (standard deviation)*

	Belgium	France	Germany	Netherlands	Norway	Portugal	Spain
Mean score	3.88	3.92	4.46	7.20	4.14	2.34	3.43
(*sd*)	(3.08)$_c$	(2.95)$_c$	(3.24)$_d$	(3.24)$_c$	(3.49)$_c$	(2.31)$_a$	(2.92)$_b$
N	2594	958	1884	995	1190	1149	2537

Note:
The data are based on the European Values Studies and were collected in 1990 (Van den Akker *et al.*, 1994) and are answers to the question whether homosexuality can 'always be justified, never be justified, or something in between', 1 (never) – 10 (always); means with different subscripts differ significantly from one another (non-overlapping 95% confidence intervals)

patterns with countries like Spain and Portugal. Switzerland, with several discriminatory legal rules concerning homosexuality, can probably be classified somewhere in the middle.

For the purpose of this chapter, the hierarchy based on the European Values Studies is the best available at this moment. For further comparative studies it might be wise to develop more elaborate indices of social climates concerning homosexuality.

In conclusion, the data available from the various European surveys may lend support to the theoretical perspective developed in the introduction. Given all the limitations discussed, by no means do these data constitute a definitive test. Studies with more sophisticated designs will have to be conducted before conclusive evidence in this field can be collected. The theoretical perspective might, however, be useful to elucidate possible empirical differences between countries.

Results

Prevalence of Hetero-, Homo- and Bisexual Behaviour

Different prevalences of both lifetime and one-year hetero-, homo- and bisexual behaviour were observed in the countries studied (Table 3.3). Hetero-, homo- and bisexual behaviour are used here to indicate that people have had sexual contacts with either people of the opposite gender, the person's own gender, or both, in a specific period of time. If 'homosexual experience' is used, it implies at least some level of physical contact.

The percentages presented in Table 3.3 are based on the subgroup of people in each country who were sexually active in the respective period. Since more people are sexually active over their lifetimes than in the preceding year, the sample size for each country is necessarily smaller if the focus is on behaviour in the preceding year.

The table shows some substantial differences between countries with respect to lifetime occurrence of homosexual contacts. Exclusively heterosexual *lifetime* histories were reported by the majority of men and women in each country (Table 3.3). For men this percentage ranged from 86.6 per cent in the Netherlands to 99.1 per cent in Portugal, and for women from 94.2 per cent in Finland to 99.4 per cent in Athens. Complementarily, the percentages of respondents who report having had sex with a person of the same sex at least once in their lifetimes, whether exclusively or in combination with heterosexual experiences, varied from 0.9 per cent in Portugal to 13.4 per cent in the Netherlands for males and from 0.6 per cent in Athens to 5.8 per cent in Finland for females.

Table 3.3 *Proportions of hetero-, bi- and homosexual behaviour during lifetime and in preceding year*

	Athens 1990	Belgium 1993	Finland 1992	France ACSF 1992	Germany West 1990	Netherlands 1989	Norway 1992	Portugal 1991	Spain 1990	Switzerland 1992
LIFETIME										
Men										
Hetero	98.3*	93.9**	95.1	95.7*	95.6	86.6**	94.8*	99.1	92.7	95.3
Homo/bi	1.7_a	6.1_b	4.9_b	4.3_b	4.4_b	13.4_c	5.2_b	0.9_a	7.3_b	4.7_b
Bi	(1.6)	(5.2)		(4.2)	(3.1)	(8.6)		(0.7)	(4.2)	
Homo	(0.1_{ac})	(0.9_{ab})		(0.1_c)	(1.3_{bd})	(4.7_c)		(0.2_{ac})	(3.0_{bde})	
N	774	1222	753	1630	1034	359	1636	1163	427	1266
Women										
Hetero	99.4_a	97.6_b	94.2_c	97.3_{bd}	95.3_{cd}	95.3_{bc}	96.2_{bc}	99.2_a	95.8_{bc}	
Homo/bi	0.6	2.4	5.8	2.7	4.7	4.7	3.8	0.8	4.2	
Bi	(0.6)	(2.1)		(2.6)	(3.9)	(3.9)		(0.4)	(2.9)	
Homo	(0.0_a)	(0.3_{bc})		(0.1_{ac})	(0.8_b)	(0.8_{bc})		(0.5_{bc})	(1.2_{bc})	
N	883	1312	724	1591	1151	509	2135	1065	408	
PRECEDING YEAR										
Men										
Hetero		98.4*		98.7*		93.7**	98.4	99.2		
Homo/bi		1.6_a		1.3_a		6.3_b	1.6_a	0.8_a		
Bi		(0.6)		(0.8)		(1.8)		(0.8)		
Homo		(1.1_a)		(0.5_a)		(4.5_b)		(0.0_c)		
N		1223		1591		332	1479	1099		
Women										
Hetero		99.3		99.6		99.4	98.9	99.5		
Homo/bi		0.7		0.4		0.6	1.1	0.5		
Bi		(0.4)		(0.1)		(0.2)		(0.5)		
Homo		(0.3_a)		(0.3)		(0.4)		(0.0_b)		
N		1312		1534		487	1983	976		

Base: all respondents (18–49 years) who have ever had sex

Note:

Asterisks indicate significant differences between men and women (logistic regression analysis, *p < 0.05, **p < 0.01). Percentages with different subscripts differ significantly from one another (non-overlapping 95% confidence intervals)

With respect to the occurrence of homosexual contacts, some countries differed significantly from others. Men and women in Athens and Portugal reported having had sex with another person of the same sex at least once in their lifetimes significantly less often than all the other countries' respondents. The Netherlands differed significantly from all other countries by having the greatest proportion of men reporting same-sex experiences. Women in Finland reported having had sexual contact with another woman during their lifetimes significantly more often than women in France and Belgium; Germany had more women who reported having had at least one same-sex experience than Belgium.

Within countries, men reported having had at least one sexual contact with a person of the same sex in their lives systematically more often than women did. This difference is significant in five of the seven countries where it could be observed. In the two other cases there seems to be a somewhat greater percentage of women with homosexual experiences, but the difference is not statistically significant.

The number of people reporting homosexual contacts decreases absolutely as well as proportionately when the reference period is shortened. The differences between the *one year period* and lifetime reports of homo- and bisexual behaviour were large in almost all the countries for which this comparison could be made. The greatest decreases were found in the Netherlands, where the percentages of respondents reporting same-sex experiences dropped from 13.4 per cent for lifetime behaviour, to 6.3 per cent for the preceding year for men and from 4.7 per cent to 0.6 per cent for women. Despite the lower frequencies, some countries still differed from others. The Netherlands can be singled out for having the highest proportion of men reporting same-sex sexual contact in the preceding year. None of the country-to-country differences in women's answer rates were significant. In all five countries men reported having had a homosexual experience in the preceding year markedly more often than women; this difference is statistically significant in three of them.

In most countries included in this overview, it is possible to see to which extent the reported homosexual experiences are exclusive or go together with heterosexual experiences. In all countries, with the exception of Portugal, exclusive homosexuality among men and women over their *lifetimes* is less frequently observed than bisexual behaviour (for eight out of the 14 comparisons this difference is significant). Regardless of the systematically larger proportion of people with bisexual histories, countries vary with respect to the degree of difference between bisexual and exclusively homosexual lifetime report rates. For men, Germany, the Netherlands and Spain stand out by having the highest relative reports of exclusively homosexual experiences in their lives. For women the pattern of differences is less clear, although Athens stands out by having no women at all who reported having had exclusively homosexual experiences over their lifetimes. In Germany and the Netherlands – countries which differed from others in the sense that more women reported having had sex with another woman at least once – the proportions of women with exclusively same-sex sexual experiences were relatively high compared with those in other countries.

The relatively lower rate of exclusively homosexual compared with bi-sexual behaviour was seen in some countries for the *preceding year* as well, indicating that relatively more people had sex in the preceding year with both men and women than exclusively with persons of the same sex. For Portugal this difference is significant. More men reported having had exclusively homosexual relations in the preceding year in Belgium and especially the Netherlands than in France, Norway and Portugal.

The data indicate that the majority of people in all the European countries included in this study have exclusively heterosexual sexual histories; exclusively homosexual life histories are relatively rare and even less frequently observed than bisexual life histories. The people with bisexual life histories should by no means be seen as a unified category, as the label 'bisexual' encompasses a variety of histories, including women who feel exclusively attracted to women but have had heterosexual experiences in the past as well, and happily married men who had a homosexual experience during their adolescence, as well as persons who have sex with men and women alternately. Table 3.4 shows the relative occurrences of these different patterns.

In Table 3.4 the data for lifetime sexual experiences and sexual experiences in the preceding year are combined so as to show whether respondents with bisexual lifetime histories had sex in the preceding year with somebody

Table 3.4 *Hetero-, bi- and homosexual behaviour in preceding year for people with a bisexual lifetime history, in percentages of sexually active people*

	Belgium 1993	France–ACSF 1992	Netherlands 1989
MEN			
Hetero	4.6	3.0	7.0
Bi	0.6	0.8	1.7
Homo	0.3	0.3	0.0
N	1223	1572	357
WOMEN			
Hetero	1.8	2.1	3.7
Bi	0.4	0.3	0.2
Homo	0.3	0.1	0.0
N	1312	1524	507

Note:
N includes people with exclusively hetero- and homosexual behaviour during entire life

of their own or the opposite gender or both. The table shows that if people have had sex with both men and women during their life, they will more likely have had sex in the preceding year with only people of the opposite sex than with either exclusively people of their own sex or both men and women. This shows once more that for most people who have had same-sex experiences in their lives, these contacts are incidental. Although the differences in proportions are not significant, a common trend seems to be that people with a bisexual history are more likely to have had sex with both men and women in the preceding year than exclusively with someone of their own sex. The label 'bisexual' could be applied to all people in this table, but is probably more in order for the people with bisexual behaviour throughout their lives as well as in the preceding year. It should be stressed, however, that nothing can be deduced from these data about underlying motives, preferences or self-labelling.

Homosexual Behaviour and Age

The relationship between lifetime homosexual behaviour and current age may also give us some insights as to whether homosexual contacts are related to a specific period in life or occur randomly during a person's sexual career (Table 3.5). In the former case, the percentage of people with homosexual experiences would remain more or less the same after a specific age, in the latter case this percentage would increase continuously with age. This increase can of course also be indicative of a cohort effect, which would imply that younger people would be less likely to engage in or else report homosexual behaviour than older cohorts. Given the small percentages, we shall look at the occurrence of homosexual contacts, regardless of whether the respondent has had heterosexual relationships as well.

In general, the percentages of men who have had sex with another man do not seem to increase substantially in the age brackets above 24. This finding suggests that if a man has had homosexual experiences, the first one is quite likely to have taken place before the age of 25. While some men might continue to have these experiences after this age, others do not. Conversely, first homosexual experiences seem less likely to occur after the age of 25. This seems to apply to all the countries for which data are available. France is an exception, as the proportion of men with homosexual experiences increases steadily with age. The Netherlands shows the opposite trend, that is, older cohorts reporting homosexual experiences significantly less.

For women the patterns are somewhat more varied (Table 3.5). In some countries the percentages of women having had any homosexual experiences are so small that it is impossible to make reliable statements about differences. In other countries, such as Norway, the percentage of women having had

Table 3.5 *Proportions of homosexual behaviour during lifetime and in preceding year by current age*

	Athens	Belgium	Finland	France ACSF	Netherlands	Norway	Portugal	Spain	Switzerland
	1990	1993	1992	1992	1989	1992	1991	1990	1992
LIFETIME									
Men									
18–19	0.0 (47)	1.6 (63)	4.7 (43)	1.1 (91)**	28.6 (14)*	4.9 (82)	0.0 (99)	11.7 (60)	1.1 (88)
20–24	2.4 (123)	6.0 (201)	4.5 (112)	2.6 (270)	18.9 (53)	7.4 (269)	0.5 (219)		6.3 (191)
25–29	2.3 (129)	6.5 (169)	5.0 (121)	3.5 (256)	12.9 (62)	3.1 (294)	1.5 (135)	7.0 (158)	5.6 (232)
30–39	1.2 (246)	6.5 (403)	5.1 (253)	4.7 (533)	13.4 (142)	6.3 (540)	1.3 (400)	7.6 (131)	3.9 (565)
40–49	1.3 (228)	5.8 (411)	4.9 (223)	5.6 (480)	9.6 (83)	4.0 (451)	0.7 (307)	3.8 (78)	4.8 (250)
Women									
18–19	0.0 (29)	0.0 (43)	9.8 (41)*	1.4 (69)	3.8 (26)	4.7 (107)	0.0 (46)	3.6 (84)	
20–24	1.6 (123)	1.7 (181)	4.2 (120)	1.1 (270)	0.0 (79)	2.8 (362)	1.4 (147)		
25–29	0.6 (159)	0.9 (221)	13.6 (110)	3.3 (241)	7.3 (96)	5.0 (362)	0.0 (144)	1.7 (468)	
30–39	0.3 (326)	2.8 (498)	5.3 (243)	3.9 (539)	9.7 (175)	5.1 (721)	1.5 (394)	5.4 (111)	
40–49	0.4 (246)	3.0 (427)	2.4 (210)	2.1 (473)	0.0 (134)	2.0 (559)	0.3 (333)	0.0 (67)	
PRECEDING YEAR									
Men									
18–19		0.0 (62)		0.0 (91)	14.3 (14)*	1.4 (74)	0.0 (89)		
20–24		0.0 (192)		1.5 (262)	9.4 (64)	2.2 (231)	0.5 (207)		
25–29		1.8 (168)		1.6 (248)	9.7 (62)	1.7 (230)	1.6 (129)		
30–39		3.5 (400)		1.5 (528)	4.9 (142)	1.6 (490)	1.3 (385)		
40–49		1.0 (401)		0.6 (462)	2.4 (82)	1.2 (414)	0.5 (205)		
Women									
18–19		0.0 (42)		0.0 (66)	3.8 (26)	0.0 (98)	0.0 (42)		
20–24		1.1 (178)		0.4 (264)	0.0 (79)	0.9 (339)	1.5 (136)		
25–29		0.9 (213)		0.9 (229)	1.1 (95)	1.7 (358)	0.0 (137)		
30–39		0.4 (480)		0.4 (530)	1.7 (176)	1.6 (672)	0.8 (370)		
40–49		0.8 (397)		0.4 (446)	0.0 (134)	0.4 (516)	0.0 (291)		

Notes:
An asterisk indicates a significant relationship between homosexual experience and age (logistic regression analysis, *p < 0.05, **p < 0.01)
The cell sizes are in brackets

homosexual contacts seems to be relatively stable over the different age categories, suggesting that if a woman has homosexual contacts, her first homosexual experience will likely have happened at an early age. In other countries, such as Finland, the percentage fluctuates much more, but the statistical test indicates a decrease with increasing age. It might be that single homosexual experiences are less closely tied to a specific developmental period in the case of women than men.

The finding that, at least for some people, homosexual experiences quite often are bound to a specific age period is, however, supported by related findings from Finland, the Netherlands and Switzerland. Only three of the 37 Finnish men and three of the 41 Finnish women who reported having had sexual experiences with men or women, respectively said that at the present time they were mainly or exclusively interested in same-sex partners. In addition, two-thirds of the Finnish men who reported that they had had at least one homosexual experience said that they had never had an orgasm in these experiences. The figure for women, in contrast, was about 80 per cent, suggesting that these sexual experiences included less extensive ones. Finally, in the Dutch study, fourteen (29.2 per cent) of the 48 men who reported ever having had sex with another man said that they currently considered themselves to be (predominantly) homosexual.

In the Swiss study, men who reported having had at least one sexual experience with another man were also asked how long ago this last experience took place. Sixty per cent of the 55 men reporting such an experience answered that it occurred more than one year ago (all answers of more than one year ago were recorded in one category).

Although 25 seems to be a critical upper age limit, applicable to almost all the countries, the situation differs between countries if we consider the age at which first homosexual contacts are likely to occur. This can be seen by looking at the percentages of men with homosexual experiences in the younger age groups. In some countries, such as Finland and the Netherlands, the percentage of men who have had homosexual experiences does not increase substantially after the age of 19. In Belgium, Greece and Switzerland in particular the percentages in the 20- to 24-year age group are clearly higher than those in the 18- to 19-year age group. This suggests that men who engage in homosexual behaviour in the last three countries 'debut' at a later age.

Examining the start of people's sexual careers gives another perspective on the relationship between homosexuality and age. Do people who engage in homosexual contacts start at the same age or a different age from people who have only heterosexual experiences? Unfortunately, we have no means of determining whether these first experiences were homosexual or heterosexual. Accordingly, we cannot draw any conclusions about possible links between the age of sexual initiation and coming out as gay or lesbian. Furthermore, this analysis disregards potential differences between generations.

Table 3.6 shows no single clear pattern of lifetime behaviour for men across Europe. In Germany there is a significant relationship between having

Table 3.6 *Proportions of people with homosexual experience by age at sexual initiation*

	Athens 1990		France ACSF 1992		Germany West 1990		Netherlands 1989		Norway 1992		Switzerland 1992	
	%	N	%	N	%	N	%	N	%	N	%	N
LIFETIME												
Men												
≤16	1.5	(325)	3.3	(632)	6.8	(352)*	15.3	(111)	6.8	(518)	6.7	(328)
17	1.2	(325)	5.4	(650)	3.0	(394)	10.1	(99)	3.1	(547)	2.4	(466)
≥18	2.5	(121)	4.0	(348)	3.1	(288)	9.3	(140)	6.2	(519)	6.1	(440)
Women												
≤16	0.9	(107)	4.9	(326)*	6.8	(380)*	8.3	(108)	5.7	(761)*		
17	0.5	(379)	2.1	(887)	3.7	(626)	4.8	(250)	3.2	(947)		
≥18	0.5	(392)	1.6	(371)	3.3	(151)	3.4	(148)	2.2	(366)		
PRECEDING YEAR												
Men												
≤16			1.0	(619)			9.0	(111)*	2.1	(476)		
17			0.9	(640)			2.0	(100)	0.6	(504)		
≥18			1.9	(324)			2.1	(140)	2.2	(450)		
Women												
≤16			0.3	(320)			1.9	(108)	1.3	(777)		
17			0.4	(856)			1.2	(250)	0.8	(878)		
≥18			0.3	(357)			0.0	(147)	1.5	(339)		

Notes:
An asterisk indicates a significant relationship between homosexual experience and start of sexual career (logistic regression analysis,
*: p < 0.05, **: p < 0.01)
The cell sizes are in brackets

had homosexual contacts at least once and the start of one's sexual career, to the effect that men who started at an earlier age were more likely to have had sexual contact with the same sex as well. The Netherlands seems to have the same kind of pattern, although the relationship is not significant. For Norway and Switzerland homosexual experiences seem to make it more likely for men to have had either a relatively early or a relatively late start (the differences, however, are not significant). For France and Greece the differences are not substantial enough to make reliable statements.

For women, the relationship between homosexual experiences and age of sexual initiation shows a clearer pattern. It was found in all countries that women who had homosexual experiences were more likely to have started their sexual career at age 16 or earlier. In France, Germany and Norway, this relationship is significant.

The patterns just described can also be seen with regard to homosexual behaviour in the preceding year. Dutch men who had homosexual experiences in the preceding year were more likely to have started their sexual career at an earlier age; for French and Norwegian men it did not seem to matter. For women, differences were absent or not significant.

Educational Level, Place of Residence and Homosexual Experiences

Comparing the level of education versus the occurrence of homosexual experiences in the various countries revealed one pattern to be most common, namely, a higher percentage of people with higher levels of education had homosexual experiences than people with lower levels of education (Table 3.7). This pattern holds true regardless of whether lifetime behaviour or behaviour in the preceding year is considered. The lifetime occurrence of homosexual contacts is significantly related to education for men in France, the Netherlands and Norway. For women this relationship is significant in Athens, West Germany and the Netherlands. This pattern is not, however, found in every country. In Switzerland for instance, there does not seem to be any relationship at all, while in Belgium even the opposite trend can be observed, that is, homosexual experiences occur more often among people with a lower level of education. However, these differences are not statistically significant.

The relationship between homosexual experiences and current place of residence clearly suggests that, in general, homosexuality is much more often an urban than a rural phenomenon (Table 3.8). Regardless of whether one looks at lifetime behaviour or at behaviour in the preceding year, the percentages of people who have had homosexual experiences are higher in large cities or medium-sized towns than in rural areas. In most cases the differences within

Table 3.7 *Proportions of people having had a homosexual experience by education*

	Athens	Belgium	Finland	France ACSF	Germany West	Netherlands	Norway	Portugal	Spain	Switzerland
	1990	1993	1992	1992	1990	1989	1992	1991	1990	1992
LIFETIME										
Men										
Low	0.8 (118)	8.3 (300)	4.0 (551)	2.7 (512)*	5.0 (282)	10.5 (19)*	4.0 (676)*	0.6 (480)	8.0 (163)	6.9 (58)
Medium	1.2 (406)	5.6 (485)	7.8 (77)	4.5 (733)	3.8 (582)	10.6 (227)	4.8 (356)	0.9 (436)	7.1 (99)	4.4 (1036)
High	2.5 (241)	5.2 (461)	7.3 (124)	6.0 (382)	5.4 (168)	20.2 (114)	6.9 (597)	1.2 (245)	6.7 (165)	6.5 (170)
Women										
Low	0.0 (224)*	3.0 (301)	4.6 (478)	2.2 (542)	3.5 (491)*	0.0 (25)**	3.2 (871)	0.6 (509)	2.1 (146)	
Medium	0.2 (456)	3.2 (537)	13.9 (101)	2.2 (650)	5.1 (564)	2.7 (371)	4.2 (455)	1.2 (341)	4.7 (107)	
High	2.0 (196)	1.3 (533)	4.7 (148)	3.8 (398)	8.7 (92)	13.9 (108)	4.3 (793)	0.9 (215)	5.9 (153)	
PRECEDING YEAR										
Men										
Low		2.0 (296)		0.8 (494)*		5.3 (19)*	1.3 (611)	0.7 (456)		
Medium		0.6 (474)		0.8 (719)		4.0 (227)	1.2 (328)	1.0 (411)		
High		2.2 (450)		2.4 (373)		11.4 (114)	2.1 (533)	0.9 (233)		
Women										
Low		0.0 (288)		0.4 (520)		0.0 (25)	1.0 (792)	0.2 (467)		
Medium		1.4 (505)		0.3 (628)		0.8 (372)	1.3 (468)	1.0 (308)		
High		0.4 (515)		0.5 (386)		1.9 (107)	1.1 (72)	1.0 (202)		

Notes:
An asterisk indicates a significant relationship between homosexual experience and age (logistic regression analysis, *p < 0.05,
**p < 0.01)
The cell sizes are in brackets

Table 3.8 *Proportions of homosexual behaviour by place of residence*

	Belgium	Finland	France ACSF	Germany West	Netherlands	Norway	Spain	Switzerland
	1993	1992	1992	1990	1989	1992	1990	1992
LIFETIME								
Men								
Rural	2.6 (38)	4.2 (288)	1.9 (524)**	2.2 (321)**	1.1 (9)**	3.2 (504)**	8.3 (132)	3.6 (505)**
Small towns	5.3 (831)	4.4 (272)	4.5 (379)	2.9 (174)	10.3 (262)	3.9 (761)	5.8 (120)	4.6 (560)
Towns and cities	7.7 (376)	6.9 (189)	5.9 (727)	6.2 (529)	22.6 (93)	10.7 (366)	7.4 (175)	8.7 (195)
Women								
Rural	0.0 (41)	2.8 (251)**	1.8 (457)	3.2 (349)	0.0 (30)*	2.4 (625)**	4.3 (116)	
Small towns	2.3 (903)	6.0 (266)	2.2 (367)	3.8 (184)	3.8 (341)	3.2 (985)	2.7 (111)	
Towns and cities	3.0 (427)	9.1 (209)	3.5 (767)	5.9 (612)	8.6 (139)	6.5 (489)	5.0 (181)	
PRECEDING YEAR								
Men								
Rural	0.0 (38)		0.6 (508)		11.1 (9)*	0.9 (460)**		
Small towns	1.6 (816)		0.8 (370)		4.2 (263)	0.9 (699)		
Towns and cities	2.2 (368)		2.0 (713)		12.0 (92)	4.1 (315)		
Women								
Rural	0.0 (38)		0.2 (445)		0.0 (30)	0.5 (599)**		
Small towns	0.5 (872)		0.3 (352)		0.3 (340)	0.8 (910)		
Towns and cities	1.5 (404)		0.7 (738)		2.9 (140)	2.6 (423)		

Notes:
An asterisk indicates a significant relationship between homosexual experience and place of residence (logistic regression analysis,
* p < 0.05, ** p < 0.01)
The cell sizes are in brackets

each country are statistically significant. The figures for Spain clearly diverge from those of the other countries, showing no relationship between place of residence and the occurrence of homosexuality. The general pattern, however, seems to support the idea that urban life attracts homosexually-inclined people from the countryside and facilitates the expression of homosexuality.

Lifestyle Aspects and Marital Status

Several lifestyle aspects related to homosexuality are examined in other chapters in this volume. Leridon *et al.* (Chapter 5) show that men who have had sex with men, regardless of their current sexual practice, have had more sexual partners in various periods of time. If we look at homosexual behaviour in the preceding year, men with homosexual contacts in Britain and in the Netherlands have had twice as many partners as heterosexual men. For women this relationship is reversed. However, it seems that in the subgroup of people involved in a steady relationship, a systematically higher proportion of gay and lesbian than heterosexual relationships are sexually non-exclusive. Magnus (Chapter 6) shows that both higher proportions of men and women who (also) have had homosexual contacts than people with exclusively heterosexual experiences have had more than five partners in the preceding year. Warszawski (Chapter 7) shows that both men and women who have had homosexual experiences during their life have had a higher frequency of STD than people with exclusively heterosexual experiences. Leridon *et al.* also show that men who have had homosexual relations in their lives as well as during the preceding year have paid for sex more often than men with exclusively heterosexual experiences.

Table 3.9 shows the relationship between the occurrence of homosexuality and marital status. The information depicted allows us to answer several questions. The first question is whether divorced people and singles have a higher rate of homosexual experience in the preceding year, this probably being most indicative of a current homosexual lifestyle. The pattern is clear: people who are currently married have a much lower probability of having had a homosexual experience than people who are separated, divorced, or who have never been married. In most cases these differences are statistically significant. The differences hold not just in the preceding year, but in the lifetime reference period as well: the probability that people who have had same-sex contacts are currently married is smaller than for people with exclusively heterosexual experiences, regardless of when the homosexual experiences occurred. Since we just saw that most lifetime homosexual behaviour takes place at an early age and is not continued, this finding is somewhat surprising. That past-year homosexuality is related to marital status is more self-evident.

Table 3.9 *Proportions of homosexual behaviour (lifetime and preceding year) by civil status*

	France ACSF 1992		Germany West 1990		Netherlands 1989		Norway 1992		Portugal 1991		Switzerland 1992	
	%	N	%	N	%	N	%	N	%	N	%	N
LIFETIME												
Men												
Married	4.0	(858)**	1.8	(445)**	4.3	(187)**	3.0	(757)**	0.2	(651)*	2.7	(594)**
Divorced	4.7	(64)	4.1	(49)	20.0	(15)	8.5	(130)	3.6	(28)	3.6	(56)
Single	4.8	(707)	6.3	(538)	17.6	(216)	6.8	(746)	2.1	(284)	6.9	(613)
Women												
Married	2.0	(929)**	2.4	(657)**	2.8	(352)*	2.2	(1157)**	0.5	(734)		
Divorced	3.3	(120)	5.0	(121)	6.5	(31)	6.8	(177)	0.0	(20)		
Single	3.3	(541)	9.3	(367)	6.9	(189)	5.4	(801)	0.5	(222)		
PRECEDING YEAR												
Men												
Married	0.5	(859)**			0.0	(184)**	0.4	(727)*	0.2	(630)*		
Divorced	0.0	(63)			8.3	(12)	3.7	(109)	4.2	(24)		
Single	2.2	(688)			13.1	(168)	2.5	(640)	1.8	(272)		
Women												
Married	0.2	(921)			0.0	(352)*	0.2	(1118)**	0.3	(707)		
Divorced	0.9	(109)			5.6	(18)	1.4	(148)	0.0	(20)		
Single	0.8	(503)			2.9	(140)	2.5	(717)	0.5	(222)		

Notes:

An asterisk indicates a significant difference between the proportion of married people with homosexual experiences versus divorced and single people with homosexual experiences (logistic regression analysis, *: p < 0.05, **: p < 0.01)

The cell sizes are in brackets

To compare the various countries, we shall now focus on the people with homosexual experiences in the preceding year and compare the proportions of people who are or have been married. Once again, the focus is not on lifetime behaviour, but on behaviour in the preceding year, since the latter is more indicative of a current homosexual orientation. The expectation is that countries with a less positive climate towards homosexuality will have a larger proportion of people with current homosexual behaviour who are or have been married. This percentage ranges from 4.3 to 66.7 per cent. However, these percentages should be interpreted with caution, since the cell sizes on which they are based are very small.

The Netherlands differs from other countries in that only one of 23 men (4.3 per cent) with current homosexual behaviour is or has ever been married. In France, Norway, and Portugal, respectively 4, 7 and 2 out of 19, 23 and 7 men having sexual relations with same-sex partners in the preceding year reported to be or to have been married (respectively 21.1, 30.4 and 28.6 per cent). With regard to women, the first thing that catches the eye is that a larger proportion of women with homosexual experiences in the preceding year are currently or were formerly married. For France, the Netherlands, Norway and Portugal, these percentages are, respectively, 42.9, 20.0, 18.2 and 66.7 per cent (n = 7, 5, 22 and 3, respectively). It is also interesting to look at the subgroup of people reporting homosexual behaviour in the preceding year who are currently married, that is at the time of the survey. None of the Dutch respondents who had same sex contacts in the preceding year are currently married. In France, Norway and Portugal 21.1, 13.0 and 14.3 per cent, respectively, of the men reporting same-sex contacts in the preceding year are currently married. For women these percentages are, respectively, 28.6, 9.1 and 66.7 per cent. Once again, we must stress that the number of people reporting same-sex experiences in the preceding year is small.

Behaviour and Attraction

Although homosexual behaviour is usually assumed to be the expression of a sexual desire for a person of the same sex, the data previously presented do not imply anything about this relationship. Only three out of ten countries asked their respondents about their sexual preference, each using a different approach (see Table 3.1). These questions allow us to explore the relationship between sexual preference or orientation, and behaviour. The term 'preference' will be used here, although, as shown in Table 3.1, it does not exactly match the actual questions posed. People with feelings of attraction for one sex only (in the French and Finnish study) or exclusively or predominantly for one sex (the Dutch study) will be labelled as either heterosexual or

Table 3.10 *Proportions of people with exclusively heterosexual, bisexual and exclusively homosexual experiences by sexual preference*[1]

	Finland 1992			France–ACSF 1992				Netherlands 1989			
	Hetero	Homo/Bi		Hetero	Bi	Homo		Hetero	Bi	Homo	
LIFETIME											
Men											
Hetero	96.4	3.6	(702)	99.0	1.0	0.0	(1539)	92.0	7.7	0.3	(337)
Bi	75.0	25.0	(44)	40.4	58.4	1.1	(89)	12.5	50.0	37.5	(8)
Homo	50.0	50.0	(2)	0.0	66.7	33.3	(3)	0.0	7.1	92.9	(14)
Women											
Hetero	95.8	4.2	(671)	99.5	0.5	0.0	(671)	96.6	3.0	0.4	(495)
Bi	75.0	25.0	(44)	73.8	26.2	0.0	(126)	58.3	41.7	0.0	(12)
Homo	33.3	66.7	(3)	0.0	50.0	50.0	(2)	0.0	0.0	100.0	(2)
PRECEDING YEAR											
Men											
Hetero				99.8	0.2	0.0	(1505)	99.1	0.9	0.0	(337)
Bi				83.1	9.6	7.2	(83)	22.2	44.4	33.3	(9)
Homo				0.0	0.0	100.0	(2)	0.0	7.7	92.3	(13)
Women											
Hetero				99.9	0.1	0.0	(1413)	99.8	0.2	0.0	(494)
Bi				96.6	2.5	0.8	(118)	84.6	15.4	0.0	(13)
Homo				0.0	0.0	100.0	(1)	0.0	0.0	100.0	(2)

Notes:
The cell sizes are in brackets
[1] See Table 3.1 for the various ways in which sexual preference has been measured in the three countries

homosexual. The term 'bisexual preference' is used to classify all other people. This procedure results in a broader category of bisexuality for France and Finland than for the Netherlands.

The distributions of the answers on the original sexual preference scales in Finland, France and the Netherlands are very skewed. In each country, most people reported having an exclusively heterosexual preference (respectively 93.9, 94.4 and 89.4 per cent of the men and 93.5, 92.4 and 92.9 per cent of the women). The proportions decrease rapidly if we move to the homosexual part of the scale. Only for the Dutch men does the declining curve go up again slightly at the (homosexual) end of the scale.

Table 3.10 shows that, regardless of the time period, a larger proportion of people with a bisexual than with a heterosexual preference reported having had sexual contacts with both genders. Although the absolute numbers of people with an exclusively homosexual preference is too small for drawing firm conclusions, it seems that this category has the highest proportion of persons with either bisexual or exclusively homosexual behaviour. Table 3.10 also shows, however, that a stated preference does not exclude sexual contacts that are not in accordance with this preference. Thus, some people stated a homosexual preference but had sexual contacts with persons of the other gender as well, and sometimes even exclusively. This finding might be plausible if one looks at lifetime behaviour, since a current sexual practice does not exclude other past preferences; it is also possible that for some people with a homosexual preference, heterosexual experiences were part of sexual exploration. However, even if one looks at people's sexual behaviour in the more restricted time period of the preceding year, behaviour and preference do not match perfectly. The reverse is true as well: regardless of the time period, some people with exclusively heterosexual or exclusively homosexual experiences reported feeling sexually attracted to both men and women.

Figures 3.1 and 3.2 give an even more detailed picture of the way in which various aspects of homosexuality are interrelated. These figures are based on the Dutch survey, in which same-sex attraction and experiences were covered extensively (Van Zessen and Sandfort, 1991). Since the questions about the occurrence of same-sex love and considerations of being homosexual were put only to people who reported same-sex physical attraction, the true picture will be even more complex.

Of the 385 men and 550 women interviewed, respectively 13.5 per cent and 10.5 per cent said that they had felt *physically attracted* to a person of the same sex at least once in their life. Men reported having experienced these feelings for the first time at a significantly younger age than women (at 14.1 years and 18.1 years, respectively, $p < 0.001$). Two-thirds of these people stated that at the time these feelings were at least somewhat confusing; the same proportion of people, however, said they were pleasurable as well (negative and positive feelings were elicited by independent questions). For over half of these people the feelings of attraction for the same sex disappeared at a later stage in their lives. Not all people who were physically attracted to the

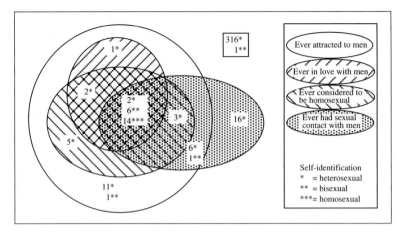

Figure 3.1 *The interrelatedness of various aspects of homosexuality in Dutch men (N = 385)*

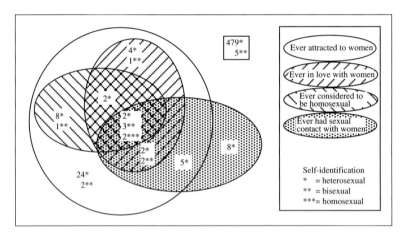

Figure 3.2 *The interrelatedness of various aspects of homosexuality in Dutch women (N = 550)*

same sex had also been in love with someone of the same sex. Physical attraction also does not necessarily coincide with actual sexual experiences, as Figures 3.1 and 3.2 show. The feelings of same-sex attraction preceded the actual sexual contact for almost two-thirds of the people who reported both. For almost all the other people attraction and behaviour occurred in the same year. Only a small group of people reported having had sex first and experiencing same-sex attraction subsequently.

Figures 3.1 and 3.2 suggest that for men it is not so much early sexual attraction or actual homosexual contacts that are predictive of labelling oneself as homosexual at a later stage – having been in love with another man seems to be crucial. For women, labelling oneself as (predominantly) homosexual is much less common than saying that one feels sexual attraction for women.

Although the Dutch data give deeper insights into the relationship between attraction and behaviour, they should be treated with some caution. First of all, the number of cases is generally rather small. Furthermore, the data presented will reflect not only people's actual experiences, but what the person in his current situation is able and willing to remember. This reporting process will of course also be influenced by negative associations, usually attached to homosexuality. Finally, it is not clear whether these findings can be generalized to other Western countries with different attitudes towards homosexuality.

Discussion

This chapter focussed on homo- and bisexual behaviour in ten European countries and the way this behaviour is related to variables such as age and gender, education, urbanity (that is living in an urban environment) and marital status. Both similarities and differences between countries have been identified. These findings are discussed below.

The surveys included in this overview varied substantially in the way data was collected, thereby influencing their outcomes accordingly. The findings presented, however, suggest that the observed differences are not caused by methodological factors alone. This can be demonstrated by looking at the Netherlands, which reported the highest prevalence of male homosexual behaviour in the ten country group. This high prevalence might be attributed to the extensive coverage of homosexuality in the questionnaire, to the relatively wide definition of the term sexual contact, and to the fact that the data were collected in face-to-face interviews. The relatively positive climate in the Netherlands also makes it less necessary to conceal homosexual experiences. These methodological factors will have contributed to the higher rate of homosexual behaviour reported in the Netherlands, but cannot explain why the Netherlands also has the highest rates of *exclusive* homosexuality. More than just methodological factors must play a part as well.

With respect to future research it is important to state that there is not one single, preferred way of addressing homosexuality. The approach taken is heavily dependent on the research questions in the respective studies. In general it seems to be important to promote circumstances in which anxiety is minimized and to eliminate heterosexual bias in the questionnaire, for instance by asking systematically about the partner's gender instead of assuming the opposite gender. The assumption that people are married should also be avoided. Because of its negative connotations, it is better to avoid the label 'homosexual' as much as possible. While this specific study shows the importance of including questions about homosexuality in general population surveys, it also indicates that a more standardized approach would have been helpful.

A general across-the-board finding is that homosexual behaviour quite often seems to be of an incidental, transitional character. If people have homosexual experiences, such experiences are rather more likely to occur before than after the age of 25. A substantial proportion of people with homosexual experiences do not continue to have them as they grow older, but the reason for this is not clear. Regardless of whether or not these homosexual experiences continue to occur in a person's life, having had homosexual contacts seems to be indicative of a somewhat exceptional sexual life style which differs from a more traditional lifestyle characterized by, among others, having had fewer sexual partners and being currently married. Having had homosexual experiences also seems to be related to an early start of one's socio-sexual career.

The findings also show that bisexual behaviour is substantially more frequent if one looks at lifetime data than when a more limited time span is observed, suggesting that 'true' bisexuality occurs rather infrequently. Exclusive homosexuality, however, seems in general to be even more rare than bisexuality.

There seems to be a systematic gender-related difference in the occurrence of homosexual contacts. This difference has already been reported by Kinsey *et al.* (1953) and might be a result of the historically subordinate or repressed status of female sexuality. The finding that women with homosexual experiences in the preceding year are more often married than men with these experiences also seems to reflect women's more economically and socially dependent position in society.

All the surveys revealed systematic differences between people who have had homosexual experiences and people with exclusively heterosexual experiences. Respondents with homosexual experiences tended to be more highly educated and to live in more urban areas. These trends have been observed in other studies as well (Rogers and Turner, 1991; Billy *et al.*, 1993; Johnson *et al.*, 1994; Binson *et al.*, 1995). On the basis of the data reported here, it is not possible to draw any conclusions about the direction of these connections, but both directions are possible. In other words, homosexual experiences may motivate people to become less dependent upon their surroundings. On the other hand, they may also occur more often in surroundings where there is less hostility towards or more support for homosexual experiences. Both explanations, however, testify to the role of social factors in homosexuality. A reporting effect might play a part as well, that is, people with a higher level of education may be less reluctant to report homosexual experiences.

Significant differences between countries have been observed as well. These differences reflect the variety in social climates regarding homosexuality in the various countries. The least homosexual behaviour is observed in countries with the least acceptance of homosexuality. Conversely, homosexual behaviour in general and exclusive homosexuality in particular are reported most frequently in countries with the least negative climate towards homosexuality. First homosexual experiences seem to occur later in life if one lives in a country with a less positive climate towards homosexuality. In such countries people with current homosexual behaviour also seem more frequently to be or to have been married.

This overview included only people who were sexually active in the various periods distinguished. It is quite likely that in countries with less positive attitudes towards homosexuality, people with homosexual preferences refrain from homosexual contacts in general more often than in countries with a more positive climate. Likewise, it is quite possible that in countries with a less positive climate, relatively more people with homosexual preferences avoid homosexual experiences and try to pass as heterosexuals, but such suppositions remain to be verified.

Both the similarities and differences between countries that have been reported here support the idea raised in the introduction that social factors affect the occurrence as well as the expression of homosexuality. Unfortunately, the conclusions which can be drawn for the development of HIV-prevention policies are limited for various reasons. The absolute number of persons with homosexual behaviour in each study is small. Furthermore, very little is known about the respondents who reported homosexual experiences. In most studies it is even unclear in which relational contexts the homosexual experiences occurred and how these people themselves label their experiences. It is also not clear to what extent the people involved actually behave in such a way as to contribute to the spread of HIV, either by catching the virus themselves or by transmitting it to other people. In the latter respect the findings seem to suggest that the chances of 'bisexual' transmission are greater in countries with less exclusive homosexuality, this is, countries with a less accepting climate towards homosexuality.

Although it is not known what actually has been going on sexually in the various homosexual experiences surveyed, it is obvious that the target group for interventions aimed at preventing HIV transmission in sexual relations between men is much bigger than the group of self-identified gay men, for a substantial part of the homosexuality observed here is probably neither experienced nor labelled as such. Obviously, to reach men who have sex with other men but who do not self-identify as gay or homosexual, different communication strategies have to be developed. This finding also underlines the importance of specifically including homosexuality in general prevention campaigns.

Although this overview was unable to assess the merits of convenience samples, other studies have shown that gay men who usually participate in these studies do not resemble the majority of men who have sex with men in a given society (Harry, 1990; Sandfort and De Vroome, 1996). Consequently, studies carried out among gay men in Europe (Bochow *et al.*, 1994; Pollak, 1994) quite probably give a biased picture of the current situation. The general population surveys included in this overview are likely to have reached a different and more representative group of gay men. Given the small numbers of men with recent homosexual contacts, it is unfortunately not possible to say whether these other men, who are usually not recruited for or do not participate in research, have been reached by prevention.

The findings in this overview also suggest that, apart from the gay-identified lifestyle, there may be another specific sexual lifestyle characteristic of a small, albeit not negligible, minority that is associated with a relatively greater risk of transmission of HIV and STD. This lifestyle is characterized by having had not only homosexual experiences but also relatively more sexual partners in one's life. These people apparently start their sexual careers at an earlier age, more frequently have histories of STD and are currently more often in an open relationship. Further identification of this lifestyle might be helpful in designing and targeting specific prevention efforts. Another significant finding is that having had homosexual relations in one's life is a risk indicator for STD for women as well as men.

The kinds of data that were collected in the studies surveyed do not permit any statements about the relationship between self-labelling as homosexual or gay, and health behaviour. In general it is assumed that acceptance of one's homosexual preference and being part of a gay and lesbian community promote healthy lifestyles and general well-being (Pollak, 1985). The data concerning this question are not, however, conclusive (Leserman *et al.*, 1994; Herek, 1995; Sandfort, 1995). This issue seems to involve the interaction of various factors. Being part of a gay subculture also enhances opportunities for meeting (sexual) partners. Furthermore, a specific subculture's dominant social norms about protective behaviour and healthy lifestyles play a substantial role as well. On the other hand, there is at least anecdotal evidence that episodes of depression can be related to unsafe sex and subsequent seroconversion (Sandfort, Hinssen and Bindels, 1991).

It seems obvious that if healthy behaviour is to be promoted, the circumstances in which people live should be supportive of that behaviour. For bisexuals, gay men and lesbians, this means that they should be able to express their sexuality without feelings of guilt and fear of discrimination. This situation is not a reality in any of the European countries, although the social climates may be more positive in some than others. A better understanding of the circumstances in which homosexual contacts occur and in which bisexuals, gay men and lesbians live their lives and the way these circumstances influence their mental as well as physical well-being is relevant for the promotion of healthier lifestyles.

References

ACSF INVESTIGATORS (1992) 'Analysis of sexual behaviour in France (ACSF). A comparison between two modes of investigation: telephone survey and face-to-face survey', *AIDS*, **6**, pp. 315–23.

BILLY, J.O.G., TANFER, K., GRADY, W.R. and KLEPINGER, D.H. (1993) 'The sexual behavior of men in the United States', *Family Planning Perspectives*, **25**, pp. 52–60.

BINSON, D., MICHAELS, S., STALL, R., COATES, T., GAGNON, J. and CATANIA, J. (1995) 'Prevalence and social distribution of men who have sex with men: United States and its urban centers', *Journal of Sex Research*, **32**, 3, pp. 245–54.

BOCHOW, M., CHIAROTTI, F., DAVIES, P., DUBOIS-ARBER, F., DÜR, W., FOUCHARD, F., GRUET, F., MCMANUS, T., MARKERT, S., SANDFORT, T., SASSE, H., SCHILTZ, M.-A., TIELMAN, R. and WASSERFALLEN, F. (1994) 'Sexual behaviour of gay and bisexual men in eight European countries', *AIDS Care*, **6**, 5, pp. 533–49.

CATANIA, J.A. (1996) 'The enhanced mode of questioning in sexual behavior studies', Paper presented at Researching Sexual Behavior: Methodological Issues, The Kinsey Institute, Indiana University, Bloomington, 26–28 April.

DE BUSSCHER, P.O. (1995) 'Relationship between the gay and lesbian movement and the scientific field in France in the time of AIDS', Paper presented at Identity and future of gay and lesbian studies, Zeist, 3–5 July.

DOLL, L.S., PETERSEN, L.R., WHITE, C.R., JOHNSON, E.S., WARD, J.W. and THE BLOOD DONOR STUDY GROUP (1992) 'Homosexually and nonhomosexually identified men who have sex with men: A behavioral comparison', *Journal of Sex Research*, **29**, pp. 1–14.

ELLIS, L. (1996) 'Theories of homosexuality', in SAVIN-WILLIAMS, R.C. and COHEN, K.M. (Eds) *The Lives of Lesbians, Gays, and Bisexuals*, Fort Worth: Harcourt Brace College Publishers, pp. 11–34.

FOUCAULT, M. (1980) *The History of Sexuality*, New York: Pantheon.

GAGNON, J.H. (1990) 'Gender preference in erotic relations: The Kinsey Scale and sexual scripts', in MCWHIRTER, D.P., SANDERS, S.A. and MACHOVER REINISCH, J. (Eds) *Homosexuality/Heterosexuality. Concepts of Sexual Orientation*, New York: Oxford University Press.

GREENBERG, D.F. (1988) *The Construction of Homosexuality*, Chicago: Chicago University Press.

HALMAN, P., and DE MOOR, R. (1994) 'Religion, churches and moral values', in ESTER, P., HALMAN, L. and DE MOOR, R. (Eds) *The Individualizing Society. Value change in Europe and North America*, Tilburg: Tilburg University Press.

HALPERIN, D., WINKLER, J.J. and ZEITLIN, F.I. (1990) *Before Sexuality: The Construction of Erotic Experience in the Ancient Greek World*, Princeton: Princeton University Press.

HARRY, J. (1986) 'Sampling gay men', *Journal of Sex Research*, **22**, 1, pp. 21–34.

HARRY, J. (1990) 'A probability sample of gay males', *Journal of Homosexuality*, **19**, pp. 89–104.

HEKMA, G. (1987) *Homoseksualiteit, een medische reputatie. De uitdoktering van de homoseksuelee in negentiende eeuws Nederland*, Amsterdam: SUA.

HERDT, G. (1990) 'Developmental discontinuities and sexual orientation across cultures', in MCWHIRTER, D.P., SANDERS, S.A. and MACHOVER REINISCH, J.M. (Eds) *Homosexuality/Heterosexuality. Concepts of Sexual Orientation*, New York: Oxford University Press.

HEREK, G.M. (1995) 'Identity and community among gay and bisexual men in the AIDS era', in HEREK, G.M. and GREENE, B. (Eds) *AIDS, psychology, and the lesbian and gay community*, Thousand Oaks: Sage.

HIV/AIDS Surveillance in Europe (1995), Quarterly Report, Saint-Maurice: European Centre of Epidemiological Monitoring of AIDS.

JACKSON, M. (1987) ' "Facts of life" or the eroticization of women's oppression? Sexology and the social construction of heterosexuality', in CAPLAN, P. (Ed.) *The Cultural Construction of Sexuality*, London: Tavistock.

JOHNSON, A.M., WADSWORTH, J., WELLINGS, K. and FIELD, J. (1994) *Sexual Attitudes and Lifestyles*, Oxford: Blackwell.

KATZ, J.N. (1995) *The Invention of Heterosexuality*, New York: Dutton.

KINSEY, A.C. (1941) 'Criteria for a hormonal explanation of the homosexual', *Journal of Clinical Endocrinology*, **1**, pp. 424–8.

KINSEY, A.C., POMEROY, W.P., MARTIN, C.E. and GEBHARD, P.H. (1953) *Sexual Behavior in the Human Female*, Philadelphia: W.B. Saunders.

KITZINGER, C. (1987) *The Social Construction of Lesbianism*, London: Sage.

LAUMANN, E.O., GAGNON, J.H., MICHAEL, R.T. and MICHAELS, S. (1994) *The Social Organization of Sexuality. Sexual Practices in the United States*, Chicago: The University of Chicago Press.

LESERMAN, J., DISANTOSTEFANO, R., PERKINS, D.O. and EVANS, D.L. (1994) 'Gay identification and psychological health in HIV-positive and HIV-negative gay men', *Journal of Applied Social Psychology*, **24**, 24, pp. 2193–208.

PLUMMER, K. (1975) *Sexual Stigma: An Interactionist Account*, London: Routledge and Kegan Paul.

PLUMMER, K. (Ed.) (1981) *The Making of the Modern Homosexual*, London: Hutchinson.

POLLAK, M. (1985) 'Male homosexuality – or happiness in the ghetto', in ARIÈS, P. and BÉJIN, A. (Eds) *Western Sexuality: Practice and Precept in Past and Present Times*, Oxford: Basil Blackwell.

POLLAK, M. (1994) *The Second Plague of Europe. AIDS Prevention and Sexual Transmission among Men in Western Europe*, Binghamton, New York: Haworth.

ROGERS, S.M. and TURNER, C.F. (1991) 'Male–male sexual contact in the U.S.A.: findings from five sample surveys, 1970–1990', *Journal of Sex Research*, **28**, pp. 491–519.

SANDFORT, T.G.M. (1995) 'HIV/AIDS prevention and the impact of attitudes towards homosexuality and bisexuality', in HEREK, G.M. and GREENE, B. (Eds) *AIDS, Psychology, and the Lesbian and Gay Community*, Thousand Oaks: Sage.

SANDFORT, T.G.M. (1996) 'Sampling male homosexuality', Paper presented at Researching Sexual Behavior: Methodological Issues, The Kinsey Institute, Indiana University, Bloomington, 26–28 April.

SANDFORT, T.G.M. and DE VROOME, E.E.M. (1996) 'Homoseksualiteit in Nederland:

een vergelijking tussen aselecte groepen homoseksuele en heteroseksuele mannen', *Tijdschrift voor Seksuologie*, **20**, 3, pp. 232–45.

SANDFORT, T.G.M., HINSSEN, H. and BINDELS, P. (1991) 'Backgrounds of recent seroconversions among gay men', Paper presented at Biopsychosocial aspects of HIV infection, First International Conference, Amsterdam, 22–25 September 1991.

SEIDMAN, S. (1993) 'Identity and politics in a "Postmodern" gay culture: some historical and conceptual notes', in WARREN, M. (Ed.) *Fear of a Queer Planet. Queer Politics and Social Theory*, Minneapolis: University of Minnesota Press, pp. 105–42.

SELL, R.L. and PETRULIO, C. (1996) 'Sampling homosexuals, bisexuals, gays, and lesbians for public health research: a review of the literature from 1990 to 1992', *Journal of Homosexuality*, **30**, 4, pp. 31–47.

SHIDLO, A. (1994) 'Internalized homophobia: conceptual and empirical issues in measurement', in GREENE, B. and HEREK, G.M. (Eds) *Lesbian and Gay Psychology: Theory, Research and Clinical Applications*, Thousand Oaks: Sage.

TROIDEN, R.R. (1989) 'The formation of homosexual identities', *Journal of Homosexuality*, **17**, 1/2, pp. 43–73.

TURNER, C.F., MILLER, H.G. and ROGERS, S.M. (1996) 'Survey measurement of sexual behaviors. Problems and progress', Paper presented at Researching Sexual Behavior: Methodological Issues, The Kinsey Institute, Indiana University, Bloomington, 26–28 April.

VAN DEN AKKER, P., HALMAN, L. and DE MOOR, R. (1994) 'Primary relations in Western societies', in ESTER, P., HALMAN, L. and DE MOOR, R. (Eds) *The Individualizing Society. Value Change in Europe and North America*, Tilburg: Tilburg University Press.

VAN ZESSEN, G. and SANDFORT, T.G.M. (1991) *Seksualiteit in Nederland. Seksueel gedrag, risico en preventie van AIDS*, Amsterdam: Swets and Zeitlinger.

WAALDIJK, K. (1993) 'The legal situation in the Member States' in WAALDIJK, K. and CLAPHAM, A. (Eds) *Homosexuality: A European Community Issue*, Dordrecht: Martinus Nijhoff.

WEINBERG, M.S. (1970) 'Homosexual samples: Differences and similarities', *Journal of Sex Research*, **6**, 4, pp. 312–25.

WEINBERG, M.S., WILLIAMS, C.J. and PRYOR, D.W. (1994) *Dual Attraction. Understanding Bisexuality*, New York: Oxford University Press.

WILKINSON, S. and KITZINGER, C. (1994) 'The social construction of heterosexuality', *Journal of Gender Studies*, **3**, 3, pp. 307–16.

Chapter 4

Sexual Practices and Their Social Profiles

*Theo Sandfort, Henny Bos, Elina Haavio-Mannila and Jon Martin Sundet**

Introduction

How often do people have sex and what do they actually do when they have sex? In the context of AIDS and STD, these issues are of great importance, since people's sexual behaviour is one of the most important determinants of the AIDS epidemic's further development. In this chapter we shall answer these questions as they pertain to people in various countries in Europe and explore differences between countries as well as identify patterns these countries have in common. The focus of this chapter is not on risk behaviour, but on the way sexuality in general is structured by social and demographic factors such as gender, age, and educational level. These insights are essential if one wants to promote the adoption of safer sexual practices effectively.

The emergence of AIDS is not the first time that interest arose as to how people behave sexually. People's sexual practices have been of interest for ages, for a variety of reasons and from different perspectives, such as art and literature, religion, scientific disciplines such as anthropology and psychoanalysis, and sexual education. Before presenting the results of our analyses, we shall sketch some of these perspectives to put our topic in a broader context. In doing so we do not claim to present an exhaustive overview of each perspective. From the perspectives of religion and psychoanalysis, for instance, a lot more has been written about people's sexual practices than can be presented here.

*The authors would like to thank Ernest de Vroome, Jeffrey Weiss and the group of researchers collaborating in the EU Concerted Action for their support in preparing and writing this chapter.

Art and Literature

Human sexual practices have been depicted in paintings, sculptures, literature, and other means of artistic expression (Kronhausen and Kronhausen, 1978; Kearny, 1982; Bullough, 1994). Depicting sexual acts is not a recent phenomenon. These depictions can be observed in almost any civilization. This does not, however, imply that these expressions were not considered to be objectionable in certain times or societies. They can be seen on Greek vases from the fifth century BC, on the wall paintings in Pompeii, and on eleventh- and thirteenth-century Japanese bridal scrolls. Sexual practices have been expressed in the drawings and etchings of artists such as Picasso (1881–1973) and Schiele (1890–1918). Some artists – Rowlandson (1756–1827) in England and Sergel (1740–1814) in Sweden – are known nowadays primarily for their erotic works. Extensive descriptions of sexual acts are part of the literary works of authors such as De Sade (1740–1814).

The motive for including sexual practices in artistic expressions is not necessarily to make an erotic or sexual appeal to the viewer. Some depictions have clear religious or magical meanings; examples include the stone carvings in the Indian 'love-temples' and primitive wood sculpture and pottery from Africa and South America. Other depictions are primarily instructive, or constitute a celebration of sexual pleasure and, related to this, of fertility and procreation. Sexual acts have also been depicted as part of ordinary life, as in Rembrandt's (1606–69) 'The Monk in the Cornfield'; these 'erotic' depictions should not be considered as predecessors of our current pornography. Sometimes sexual acts are depicted for humorous purposes, as in the so-called dirty comic strips published in the US in the 1930s, in which figures such as Popeye, Dick Tracy, and Betty Boop drift into various erotic adventures (Dirty Comics, n.d.), or to express opinions about society, as in the satirical works of the German artist George Grosz (1893–1959). Other depictions of sexual acts were meant to entertain or to stimulate people sexually. There is of course a blurred overlap between erotic art and pornography, the latter representing depictions of sexual acts with the intent to elicit sexual arousal in the viewer (although the pretence of art can be used to conceal pornographic intentions).

The various motives behind depictions of sexual practices do not, of course, exclude each other. Besides, artists' intentions do not dictate how people 'consume' their products; the latter will be largely dependent on both the cultural context and personal background of the person involved. As Reinisch, Ziemba-Davis and Sanders (1990) argue, the expression of erotic images in art and literature shows 'the universality of various sexual activities, including AIDS risk-related behaviours, throughout nearly all of history and in nearly every culture. Although some of these behaviours might have been stigmatized or disapproved of at various points in time or in various cultures, few would deny that their depiction in art indicates that they were at least known, if not widely practiced' (p. 46).

Religion

Sexual acts have also been considered from a religious perspective (Brundage, 1994). Canon law (the legal system of the Catholic Church) specified how, when, and with whom sexual intercourse should be performed and which practices were unacceptable. The latter included sodomy, which was a collective term for a variety of practices like fellatio, cunnilingus and anal intercourse. Procreation was the only legitimate aim of sexual interactions. Although canon law affected sexual behaviour in other eras more strongly then in our times, it has not fully disappeared from our contemporary attitudes towards specific sexual practices. Other religions also set rules for sexual behaviour. Classical Hinduism considers oral–genital sex to be impure. The opposite is true for another Eastern religious and philosophical system, Taoism. This tradition includes teachings on mastering the differences in male and female sexual arousal, with cunnilingus presented as one of the sexual techniques to liberate and activate the female.

Sex Manuals

The advice given in (Western) sex manuals, predominantly in those published in the first half of the twentieth century, centres on genital intercourse which, as we shall later see, is also a cornerstone of traditional psychoanalysis. One of these books, which constituted the basis for various others, is Van de Velde's *Ideal Marriage* (1930), translated from the Dutch into various languages and published all over the world. According to Van de Velde (1873–1937), sexual intercourse should be the highlight of a range of episodes that includes the prelude, love play, afterplay and afterglow. Omitting love play in sexual interactions is foolish, according to Van de Velde, and although oral sex ('the genital kiss') is considered as part of sexual foreplay, he avoids discussing it: 'It may be constructed from what has already been said in detail, about the kiss in general, and about the special structure of the feminine organs' (1930, p. 170). He does, however, offer an elaborate scheme of positions in which people can have intercourse that he calls a systematic 'synousiology' after the Greek term for coitus. Much later, as part of the so-called sexual revolution, came books with photographs of people having sex together in various positions. Most popular were Toft and Fowlie's (1969) 'Variations' series, originally published in Denmark. Such books had large sales in various countries. The pictures were helpful on a practical level and a welcome addition to Van de Velde's more cognitive guidelines.

How to perform oral sex and how to improve related technical skills have become an integral part of many contemporary sex education books. Elaborate instructions on how to perform specific sexual acts are not a recent phenomenon, though. Some of the most well-known examples are the Eastern love books, such as the Kama Sutra, dating from the second century BC. These books provide endless descriptions of sexual techniques, each one with its particular name, complete with tips on how best to give the partner full enjoyment, all in order to promote spiritual perfection.

Psychoanalysis and the Social Sciences

The interest that the social sciences have shown in sexuality is quite recent (Bozon and Leridon, 1996), anthropology being an exception. Although anthropology's interest in sexuality goes far beyond specific sexual practices, these practices – especially as they occurred in 'other' cultures (Frazer, 1994) – have been described extensively and discussed in early anthropological works. These practices were predominantly studied as expressions of less controlled and therefore 'less civilized' cultures. Collections of these descriptions can, for example, be found in Iwan Bloch's *Strange Sexual Practices* (*c.* 1933). Given the many printings of these kinds of books, such expressions of more unbridled sexuality probably spoke not only to the imaginations of anthropologists, but to those of lay people as well, and probably still do!

Another scholarly discipline with a strong interest in sexuality is of course psychoanalysis. In the traditional psychoanalytic approach the focus is not so much on specific practices as on the erogenous zones associated with anal, oral, and genital sex. In fact, these zones even gave their names to specific stages in the development – not just sexual, but general development – of the personality. Genital sexuality is considered the final stage of healthy development. According to psychoanalysis, mature sexuality is expressed in genital intercourse. Other pleasures, such as oral and anal sex, may be experienced as part of sexual foreplay, but can never be the ultimate aim of a sexual interaction (Person, 1987). In fact, when oral sex becomes the main mode of sexual expression, this is considered a perversion, resulting from a fixation at the oral level or castration fear. Fellatio then becomes the denial of the penis or the equivalent of biting off the penis (Kline, 1987).

One of the pioneers of the empirical description of sexual practices in Western societies was Alfred Kinsey. Although he is usually considered to have blazed this trail, several researchers went before him. Davis (1929), for example, studied extensively the sex lives of 2200 married and unmarried women. Kinsey and co-workers (Kinsey *et al.*, 1948, 1953) applied a very elaborate and ingenious interviewing and coding system (Pomeroy, Flax and Wheeler, 1982) to document the diversity of human sexual practices and impact of social factors. Their findings demonstrated the gap between official norms and what people did. These findings, extensively disputed at the time, had a major impact on social life (Gagnon, 1988).

Since Kinsey's landmark study, other investigations have been carried out to explore the correlates of specific sexual practices, predominantly among specific groups such as students and young people. To give a few examples, Hart *et al.* (1991) studied the relation between sexual practices and pregnancy. They showed that although there was a general decline in libido, coital frequency, and orgasm during pregnancy, there were no changes in the frequencies of oral and anal sex and masturbation. Reinholtz and Muehlenhard (1995) demonstrated that people's perceptions of their genitals are related to sexual activity. Simply put, more positive and fewer negative genital perceptions are associated with more frequent participation in and enjoyment of oral–genital behaviour. Gagnon and Simon (1987) demonstrated a cohort effect on the occurrence of oral practices, from which they concluded that oral sex has become part of the sexual scripts of many young people over the last 50 years and is now a common component of sexual relations in contemporary marriage.

The wealth of data on sexual practices which became available because of AIDS-related research has made it possible to explore further questions. From an epidemiological perspective Messiah and Pelletier (1996), for example, studied whether people's sexual practices are dependent on whether they have sex with a casual or regular partner. One of their findings was that non-penetrative and oral practices were more frequent with occasional partners. The data on sexual practices presented in this chapter also come from surveys triggered by AIDS.

Frequency of Sex: Instruction Books and Clinical Sexology

The frequency with which people should make love has also been addressed in sexual instruction books (Rusbridger, 1986). Recommendations about the frequency of sex often proceeded from considerations about health – and control over sexual impulses has long been considered a necessity for healthy men – as well as bridging the gap, or finding the right compromise, between the strengths of female and male desires. Advice given differed from once a month to several times a week. This was dependent on the kind of work people ('men') were involved in, that is, men who did little creative work were 'allowed' a greater frequency than men who unconsciously used their 'sexual energy' in other ways. Nowadays, instruction books acknowledge the wide range in the frequency of sexual behaviour between people and within a given individual's sexual history. As with other aspects of sexual life, the major tone of most sex education books is now one of reassurance ('You are not abnormal') and offers an acknowledgement of diversity. In instruction books from the 1970s and 1980s a minimum level of sexual involvement is, however, also suggested. Alex Comfort (1972) advises in his *Joy of Sex* that a frequency much under twice a week suggests that one could be getting much more out of sex.

Too little and too much interest in sex have been the subjects of clinical sexology as well. Excessive sexual activity used to be known as 'nymphomania' in the female and 'satyriasis' in the male (Allgeier, 1994); 'sexual compulsive behaviour' is the more current term (Coleman, 1991). Usually, excessive sexual behaviour refers to having many partners. Coleman, however, also distinguishes compulsive sexuality in a relationship and compulsive auto-eroticism. Excessive sexuality is considered to be the result of a variety of causes, such as emotional tension, low self-esteem, and early childhood trauma or abuse. It can also be the result of an inordinate need to be accepted by the other sex, an attempt to deny homosexual feelings, or frequent sexual contacts without gratification or orgasm.

It is unclear when sexual behaviour should be considered to be excessive. According to Coleman (1991), this should be defined in terms of the outcomes of the behaviour: for example when a person engaging in this form of behaviour puts him- or herself and other people at risk for STD, illnesses, and injuries, he or she endures great emotional suffering and often experiences moral, social and legal sanctions. It should be realized that the definition of 'excessive' is not based on objective criteria alone; a normative dimension quite often seems to be involved as well. Groneman (1995) has demonstrated that the concept of nymphomania has a function in the construction and regulation of female sexual desire as well as in women's societal position in general (see also Levine and Troiden, 1988; and Irvine, 1995).

At the other end of the scale, little or no sexual interest or activity or 'hyposexuality', is classified as a specific mental disorder (American Psychiatric Association, 1994). Since there is also no objective measure of what constitutes too little interest, a subjective criterion has to be fulfilled, namely, that it should cause the person distress.

The AIDS Perspective

Although interest in what people do sexually and how often they do it is not new, AIDS has put this interest in a completely new light. Some sexual practices play a major role in transmitting the virus that causes this disease. 'Unprotected' anal sex and vaginal intercourse have turned out to be the major vectors, while the role of other techniques, such as oral sex, is still debated (Lane, Holmberg and Jaffe, 1991).

Prior to AIDS, many people were used to being considerate in their (hetero)sexual behaviour in order to prevent new life, at least if they did not want to conceive a baby. AIDS made it necessary to adjust one's sexual behaviour in order to prevent death. Although other STDs threatened people long before AIDS and various interventions have been carried out to prevent the transmission of traditional STDs (Brandt, 1987), the threat of AIDS and worldwide efforts to prevent HIV transmission are unprecedented. AIDS also caused the printing and dissemination of numerous safer sex leaflets and brochures. Instructions about practising safer sex have also been spread through videos ranging from the humorous to the dramatic. Because of AIDS, numerous sex education books have had to be revised. 'Safer sex' is probably the most generally and rapidly spread concept of health behaviour ever, and although it has been used in connection with contraception, safer sex is much more strongly associated with HIV transmission.

AIDS has made it necessary to monitor risky sexual behaviour and to improve our understanding of why some people engage in certain behaviours and others do not. However, the sexual techniques through which HIV can be transmitted are not the only ones of interest; looking at other sexual techniques as well might help us to understand how people cope with the risk of AIDS. Do people continue to perform the same sexual techniques? Do they take the right precautions and start to use condoms? Or do they switch to sexual practices with no or smaller risks of HIV transmission? If one is to attempt to change people's sexual behaviours, understanding the factors that structure sexuality is a prerequisite.

The Organization of Sexual Practices

Recent general population sex surveys initiated in response to AIDS give us the opportunity to explore three distinct aspects of people's sexual practices. The first one is the frequency with which people currently involved in steady heterosexual relationships have sexual contact. The second is how many people in various countries have ever in their life practised various sexual techniques. The third issue is masturbation as a solitary practice. We shall explore whether the various countries for which data on these three practices are available differ from one another. This exploration is not guided by a theory about differences in sexuality between countries, since such a theory is lacking. We shall then investigate possible connections between these three aspects of sexuality and various background factors, namely, gender, age, onset of sexual career, and various socio-demographic factors.

Differences between men and women might be the result of differences in their respective sexual scripts. According to Gagnon and Simon (1973), these scripts are a set of learned rules which help people to interpret a situation as sexual and instruct them what to do and why. The male script for sexual encounters prescribes an active role for men, while the dominant role for women is that they should be passive, although there are indications that these differences are declining as well (Oliver and Hyde, 1993). This difference between the scripts might affect sexuality itself, as well as the reporting of certain behaviours, in the sense that men inflate and women play down their sexual activity.

Given the cross-sectional design of the surveys, age can be indicative of two different processes: psychosexual maturation within the individual, and cultural changes over time which have affected cohorts of people differently. Within the individual, ageing will be related to an increase in experience of various sexual techniques. On the other hand, specific sexual practices, such as masturbation, might be more often practised in specific developmental periods. One might also expect that as a consequence of ageing, there is a decline in the frequency with which people have sex, increasing age being an indicator of not necessarily a less satisfying, but in general a less active sexual life. Looking at age cohorts may reveal that sexual behaviour patterns have changed over time in the various countries. Younger cohorts may have been affected more by the liberal changes that took place in their country's sexual climates in the various countries, which took place in the 1970s. As a consequence, they are more likely to have engaged in relatively less common sexual practices compared with older cohorts. Changes in sexual climate may also have influenced differently people's willingness to report about these practices.

People's sexual practices may also be affected by the time of onset of their sexual careers and the numbers of partners they have had in specific periods, both of which can be considered indicators of the strength of people's *sexual interest*. As a consequence, people who start their sexual careers relatively early in life will have sex with their steady partner more frequently when they get older; the same appears to apply to people with higher numbers of sexual partners. An early start of one's sexual career and more sexual partners will probably also induce higher masturbation frequencies. A stronger interest in sexuality will also increase the likelihood that people engage in less common sexual practices. We cannot rule out the reverse effects as well, in the sense that being sexually active increases one's interest in sex.

Socio-demographic factors of interest include level of education, religious involvement, occupational status, and degree of urbanization.

By creating broader normative perspectives, *education* is usually assumed to be positively related to sexual permissiveness. As such, education may induce a greater willingness to engage in more intimate or less common sexual practices. For women, higher levels of education may also induce a relatively stronger sense of autonomy in their relationship with men, giving them more control over their sexuality.

With respect to *religious involvement*, we assessed the effect of degree of importance attributed to religion and church attendance. In general, religious involvement seems to have the opposite effect, deterring people from sexual exploration. The causal relation between attitudes and behaviour will probably be bi-directional. Not only will lower levels of sexual restrictiveness promote an openness for new experiences. It is, however, also possible that practising specific techniques, especially the less common ones, might induce less restrictive attitudes in people. A more direct assessment of normative aspects on people's sexuality was possible for the Netherlands.

Especially for women, *employment status* might affect sexuality as well. We shall compare homemakers with those who are in paid jobs or the smaller group of women who are currently unemployed. Since women who are part of the paid labour force may have a more independent social position than homemakers, they may also be more permissive, resulting in a higher level of experience of less common sexual practices.

People's sexuality might differ in relation to where they live: compared with people living in *rural areas*, people in *cities* may have more social space and more opportunities for (sexual) exploration. As a consequence, these people may be more permissive and have more positive attitudes towards less common sexual practices.

We shall also assess whether two aspects of the *relationship status* are related to sexuality, namely, whether partners live together or separately, and the length of relationship. Given relatively more opportunities, one might expect partners who share a household to have sex more frequently than partners who live separately. It is quite possible that people who do not live with their partners differ from people who do in several other respects that are stronger determinants of the occurrence of various sexual practices. Not living with the steady partner could, for example, also reflect a specific lifestyle characterized by less restrictive sexual norms. It is commonly assumed that the longer a relationship lasts, the less frequent sexual intercourse becomes. It should, however, be realized that people in longer-lasting relationships are also more likely to belong to the older age cohorts, and, as has been suggested before, may have been less affected by the general changes in sexual climate.

Subsequent to these factors affecting sexual behaviour, we were interested in seeing how lifetime experience of specific practices is related to more recent sexual activities: does one continue to practise specific techniques if one has done them once, or are techniques bound to specific phases in one's sexual career? We shall also explore whether the different sexual practices are related to one another. For example, does having experience of one sexual technique increase the likelihood of having experience of other techniques as well?

Methods

Making comparisons between countries and identifying common trends regarding the sexual practices reported by their inhabitants are complicated tasks. The main reason for this is that the various surveys applied quite divergent approaches in addressing this subject. This variety is possible because the approaches vary with respect to five distinct aspects, namely,

- the specific sexual practices addressed and the ways they were defined in the questionnaires;
- the subsamples for which data about practices were obtained;
- the specificity of the partner with whom practices have occurred;
- the time periods considered in which the occurrence of specific practices were assessed; and
- the ways in which the frequencies of the practices were measured.

These five aspects varied independently not only between the studies, but also in relation to one another within the various surveys, further complicating the possibility of making cross-national comparisons. The only form of behaviour where comparing countries is somewhat less problematic is masturbation, since no other party is involved and there is only variation between approaches on the four remaining dimensions. But, as will be shown, the possibility of making valid comparisons is slight, even with respect to masturbation. We shall now describe the variety of approaches used in the surveys and show some of their consequences, the way in which data have been adjusted to allow for comparisons, and the statistical analyses performed to make comparisons between countries and to identify common trends.

The Variety of Approaches in Studying Sexual
Practices

To make valid comparisons between countries, it is important to understand how the data were collected in the specific surveys. It would also have been interesting to see why specific choices were made in the separate surveys. For example, it is not unlikely that researchers with an epidemiological perspective will have been interested in different aspects of sexual behaviour than sexologists, resulting in different topics and question formats. Since the task of comparing surveys is already complex enough, we decided, however, not to pursue this point. We shall also refrain from in-depth discussion of how the data were collected and how that might have affected the final results. One of the possible variations has to do with the way the respondent's answers were coded: Did an interviewer code the respondent's answers using pre-existing categories or did the respondent do that him/herself? If general response categories were presented to the respondent, either on an answer card or in a written questionnaire, it is unclear how the respondent interpreted the labels presented; it is very likely that the respondents did not interpret the labels the same way and different response sets might be related to the respondent's gender.

Specific Sexual Practices

The most general 'practice' addressed in most surveys is just *sex* or *making love*. Most of the time this term was not specified.[1] It is unclear how respondents interpreted these general concepts and whether their interpretations within a survey varied. Did all respondents equate 'sex' with intercourse or did they understand it much more broadly? It seems, however, that at least for hetero-sexual people, these general terms can be equated with (vaginal) sexual intercourse. The reported frequencies of making love are almost completely identical to the frequencies of intercourse in the three countries where we were able to check this; furthermore, in the French study 98 per cent of the respondents stated that they had engaged in intercourse the last time they had 'had sex'.

The specific sexual practices studied were vaginal intercourse, anal inter-course, oral–genital sex (usually split into active and passive), oral–anal con-tact (subdivided into being anally stimulated by the partner and orally stimulating the partner's anus), hand–genital contact (fondling; active and passive; the Finnish study more restrictively asked about stimulation of one's partner's genitals and giving satisfaction without sexual intercourse), and hand–anal contact (active and passive). None of the studies addressed all these sexual techniques. In the French study male and female respondents involved in same-sex sexual relationships were asked about the occurrence of 'fist-fucking'. Finally, the occurrence of masturbation was assessed in the Dutch, Finnish and French survey.

Subsamples Concerned

The surveys differ with respect to the parts of the sample to which questions about specific practices were addressed. In some surveys, questions about the occurrence of sexual practices were put indiscriminately to all respondents in the survey, in others only to those who had ever been sexually active or who had been active in the past month or year, and in still others only to those who reported having a steady partner.

Partner Specificity

The surveys discussed the occurrence of sexual practices with respect to specific persons or in more general ways (see Table 4.1). Some surveys asked questions about contacts with partners with whom the respondent was currently living; other studies discussed practices with steady partners in general, regardless of whether the respondent lived with this person. Sexual practices with casual partners were explored as well in several studies, either in a general way or for different casual partners specifically. In a few cases practices were discussed in general, without specifying any partner.

Frequencies and Time Periods

Basically five different approaches were used to assess the frequencies of specific sexual practices in combination with the specific time periods considered, as follows (see Table 4.1):

1) whether a specific practice ever occurred in a respondent's life or another specified period.
2) the exact number of times a specific behaviour occurred in a specific period of time (for example, the past seven days, a fortnight, the preceding four weeks, or a month).[2]
3) an estimation by the respondent of how often a specific practice had occurred over a specific period of time ranging from the last seven days to one's whole life and expressed in either a precise or a more general statement. An example of the latter would be 'never, rarely, occasionally, often, nearly always'. A variation on this way of assessing frequencies was to contextualize the specific practices by asking how often a person does specific things 'when he/she is making love with his/her partner'.[3]
4) whether a specific practice occurred in the last sexual encounter a person had.
5) how long ago a specific practice was performed.

In some of the cases where general frequency categories were used, these categories were non-contiguous. Examples can be found in the Belgian and Finnish surveys, where respectively 'practically every day' and 'several times a week', and 'once a week' and 'two or three times a month' were offered as adjacent categories. It is not known what happened to answers falling between

Table 4.1 *Questions about frequency of sex and (sub-) samples addressed in various surveys, with original (•) and constructed categories*

	Athens 1990	Belgium 1993	Finland 1992	France 1990	Germany West 1990	Netherlands[1] 1989	Norway 1992	Spain 1990	Switzerland 1992
Sample addressed	People in steady relationship	People in steady relationship	All respondents	All respondents	People in steady relationship	People in steady relationship	People who are married or cohabiting[1]	All respondents	All respondents
Question	In the *last 4 weeks* have you had sex with your husband/regular partner? How many times have you had sex in the *last 4 weeks?*	On average how many times do you have sex (= intimate contact with vaginal, anal or oral penetration)?	How often have you had sexual intercourse (= a man's penis entering a woman's vagina) during the *last month?*	In all, how many times have you had sex over the *past 4 weeks?*	In the *last 4 weeks* have you had sex with your husband/regular partner? How many times in the *last 4 weeks?*	The frequency of having sex varies greatly among *relationships*. Please indicate how often you made love to each other over the *past 3 months?*	How often have you and your *spouse/cohabitant* had sexual intercourse during the *last month?*	How often do you have sexual action?	How many times have you had sex in the *last 7 days?*
Constructed frequency categories:	**Original frequency categories:**								
Less than once a week	• 1–3 times a month	• sporadically, with periods of intense activity • occasionally • several times a month	• once a month • 2–3 times a month	• 1–3 times a month	• 1–3 times a month	• < every 2 months • around once a month • around 2–3 times a month	• less frequently • once a fortnight	• several times a year • 2–3 times a month	• < once a week
1 to 4 times a week	• 4–16 times a month	• at least once a week • several times a week	• once a week • 2–3 times a week • 3–4 times a week	• 4–15 times a month	• 4–16 times a month	• around once a week • around twice a week • around 3–4 times a week	• 1–2 times a week • 3–4 times a week	• 2–3 times a week	• 1–4 times a week
5 times or more per week	• 17+ times a month	• practically every day	• 5–6 times a week • every day or more often	• 16+ times a month	• 17+ times a month	• 5+ times a week	• 5–6 times a week • daily • several times a day	• once a day • 2–4 times a day • 5+ times a day	• 5+ times a week

[1] Non-cohabiting respondents were asked: How many times have you had sexual intercourse in the *last month?*: • once, • twice, • 3–4 times (less than once a week); • 5–10 times, • 11–20 times (1–4 times a week); • 21–30 times (5 or more times a week)

these response categories. What actually happened probably depended on whether the respondent or the interviewer had to classify the answer. It is also likely that within a specific study interviewers solved this problem differently, unless they had been specifically instructed how to handle this matter, which seems unlikely. This obviously affects the reliability of the data. Finally, the validity of the data may have been affected by the range of frequency categories provided by communicating to the respondents the range in which an answer had to fall in order to be acceptable.

Interactions between Dimensions within Studies

As said before, the various factors discussed above varied independently not only between studies but within studies as well, further complicating the possibility of making valid comparisons between countries. For example, the frequency labels and time periods specified within surveys were not necessarily consistent for either the sexual practices surveyed or the various (categories of) partners distinguished. In the Belgian survey the respondent was asked if he/she had ever performed specific sexual practices with his/her current sexual partner. So, performance of that practice with another person would not have been recorded. The resulting data are of course of limited value if one wants to look at lifetime behaviour, since the majority of respondents in all countries seem to have had more than one partner in their lives, with a consistently higher percentage of men with more than one partner than women. In the Greek study all respondents were asked how often they had sexual intercourse, while the frequency of sex in general was asked only of people involved in a steady relationship. In the Norwegian survey the occurrence of anal intercourse was asked only with respect to people who were not current sexual partners. Another feature of this study was that the occurrence of intercourse was assessed differently for relationships with a spouse or a person one was living with than for relationships with other sexual partners.

Selection and Adjustments

As a consequence of the large variety in approaches taken in the various studies, valid comparisons between countries could be made only for the three topics presented in the introduction. The respective choices made, necessary adjustments and unavoidable exceptions will be discussed here. In a few cases we had to accept an indicator that was not completely equivalent in order to include as many countries as possible in each comparison. These exceptions will also be indicated at the bottom of each of the subsequent tables and are included in the interpretations of the findings. For countries which are not included in specific comparisons, specific data were not available or it was impossible to derive information that could be compared validly with data from other studies.

Frequency of Sex in Ongoing Relationships

Since 'having sex' and 'making love' were the practices assessed in almost all the surveys and could be considered to be identical to intercourse, we selected 'having sex/making love' as the first practice to explore,[4] paying particular attention to the frequency of sex with the steady partner. Nine countries could be compared with respect to this question.

There are practical and conceptual reasons for focusing on steady relationships. First, in most studies, data about sexual practices are available only for people who had steady sexual partners at that time. To make valid country-to-country comparisons the samples should be as identical as possible. Consequently, people with no current partners had to be excluded. Not excluding people without a steady relationship in the other studies would have invalidated the comparisons, since men and women without steady partners reported significantly and substantively lower frequencies of sex than men and women with steady partners. Second, it is unclear on which basis people who were not involved in an ongoing sexual relationship answered questions about current sexual practices; their reports might limit the validity of the data.[5] Furthermore, we decided to look at heterosexual contacts only, as the number of people having had same-sex sexual contacts was almost systematically too small to be treated independently and including data about homosexual practices might have confounded the results.[6]

It was not possible for all surveys to look at all people involved in steady relationships. In a few cases (France, Norway and Spain) data were collected only from respondents who were currently *living with* a sexual partner. Other studies also had data from respondents who currently *had* a sexual partner, regardless of whether the person was living with that partner. Since substantial numbers of the people involved in a sexual relationship do not seem to live with their partners and, as we shall see later, there are differences between people who do and do not live with their current sexual partners, this further limits the validity of our comparisons.

In the studies that assessed the frequency of sex in general, without referring to a specific partner, we were able to sample the necessary data, since in these cases the relationship status was asked independently at another moment in the interview. It is not clear how valid the resulting data are, since the reported frequencies might include sex with people other than the steady partner as well.

Finally, we looked only at people in steady relationships who reported having had sex in a specific recent period and excluded the ones who reported a zero frequency. This was done because in most surveys the frequency of sex was asked only of people who reported having sex with their steady partners. In a few other studies, however, the question about frequencies was put to all respondents. These studies revealed that in most countries from 0.2 per cent to 6.8 per cent of the respondents involved in steady relationships had not had sex in a recent period. The much higher percentages in Switzerland were due to the fact that the respondents were asked to state the exact frequency of sexual contacts in the preceding week. Since this is a very short time interval, it is more likely that a larger number of people had to report 'none'. Including the respondents in a steady relationship who reported a zero frequency of having sex would thus have invalidated the comparisons.

To make comparisons between countries meaningful we had to create new, comparable frequency categories in which the frequency formats used in the various surveys could be reliably captured. We started with the surveys where no exact frequencies were asked, as they presented the biggest problems of comparability. We grouped the various response categories in such a way that the ones that were truly comparable or even identical would end up in a single category (see Table 4.1). The only possible way to do this seemed to be to construct the following three common frequency categories: less than once a week, one to four times a week, and five or more times a week. More categories would have required too many arbitrary decisions and thus reduced the validity of the comparisons. This procedure means that some of the new answer categories contain two, even three original answer categories from a specific survey. A clear example of this is Spain, where the frequencies of the response categories 'more than five times a day', 'two to four times a day', and 'once a day', were lumped together in the response category *five or more times a week*. As a consequence, actual differences between countries may have become less detectable, even disappeared.

The data from countries where exact frequencies were elicited were categorized on the basis of the calculated number of times per week. The only problem here was where to include people who reported having sex or making love more often than 16 times and fewer than 20 times per four weeks, since they would fall between the second and third categories. Since the data available for France were such that people who reported having had sex 16 or more times in the preceding four weeks were grouped in one category, a somewhat arbitrary decision was made to include 17 times, 18 times and 19 times per four weeks in the third category for the countries where this was possible. For the French data, people who reported having had sex 16 or more times a week were placed in the third category (five or more times a week).

The results of these decisions can be seen in Table 4.1. The table also shows to which respondents the reported data apply and whether a general or more specific definition of having sex or making love was applied.

Lifetime Occurrence of Various Sexual Practices

Next we looked at lifetime data about all other sexual practices with other persons, that is how many people had ever practised a specific sexual technique. Lifetime experience of vaginal intercourse was included as well. It was virtually impossible to establish common frequency categories for these sexual practices. The most informative and valid approach here was thus to look at whether people ever performed these practices or not. For a few countries it was also possible to check what percentages of people performed these techniques recently.

Although the topic does not suggest the exclusion of people who are currently not involved in a steady relationship, selection was necessary here as well, as in some studies data about sexual practices were available only for people currently involved in steady relationships. We chose to make the samples for all studies comparable by excluding people who were not involved in a steady relationship. A somewhat odd consequence of this decision was that somebody categorized as ever having practised a specific technique did not necessarily practise the technique with the current steady partner.[7]

Masturbation Frequency

The Dutch, Finnish and French surveys were the only ones in which data on *masturbation* were available. However, each of these surveys handled masturbation using completely different formats (see Table 4.9), making it impossible to create comparative response categories. The Dutch survey asked for a more or less exact frequency, while the French survey offered more abstract frequency categories. The Finnish respondents were asked how long ago they had last masturbated. In line with the first two, the latter can be viewed as an indicator of masturbation frequency, that is, the longer ago a person masturbated, the less often he or she might be assumed to masturbate in general. We consequently did not compare countries but looked for common trends only.

Analyses for Assessing Common Trends and Differences

We used the following statistical techniques to make comparisons between countries and to identify common trends within countries:

- To compare the frequencies with which people have sex in the various countries we first calculated mean frequencies, based on the three newly constructed frequency categories. Confidence intervals were then calculated and inspected for overlap. Confidence intervals were also computed for the numbers of people (percentages) who reported ever having practised specific sexual techniques and subsequently inspected for overlap. Countries were assumed to differ significantly if confidence intervals did not overlap.
- To identify common trends within countries with respect to the frequency of sex in steady relationships we inspected whether the distributions of the newly created frequency categories and the respective common factors were independent by computing Chi^2.
- To see whether various common factors were related linearly to lifetime occurrence of specific sexual techniques and to masturbation frequency we calculated Spearman rho coefficients. Since these relationships do not necessarily have to be linear, we calculated Chi^2 as well.
- To see whether the lifetime occurrences of the various techniques are related to one another we calculated Chi^2. The relationship between the occurrence of various techniques and masturbation frequency was studied by calculating Spearman rho coefficients.

The only way to identify common trends within countries was to use bivariate analysis techniques. This made it difficult to interpret the findings, since we could not control for confounding variables and assess the roles of various factors independently. Multivariate analyses would have yielded more in-depth insights, but were impossible to carry out for practical reasons.

The Frequency of Sex in Steady Relationships

The frequency with which people report having sex with their current steady partners differs significantly between the various countries, for men and women alike (Table 4.2). The lowest frequencies for men and women were reported in Belgium and the highest frequencies for men and women in France. Both Belgium and France differ significantly from each other as well as from almost all of the other countries included in this comparison. Spain, on the other hand, differs significantly from only two countries, Belgium and France. This may partly be attributed to the relatively wide confidence interval. Ranking the countries by the mean frequencies for men and women taken separately yields an almost completely identical order (see Figure 4.1).

Although methodological factors will certainly have affected the outcomes, it is unlikely that the differences between the countries can be

Table 4.2 *Frequency of sex per week*

	Athens	Belgium[1]	Finland[2]	France[3]	Germany West	Netherlands	Norway[2,3]	Spain[3]	Switzerland
	1990	1993	1992	1990	1990	1989	1992	1990	1992
MEN									
Less than once a week	−11.6	29.9	22.3	−8.9	18.8	22.3	23.0	21.1	24.4
One to four times a week	74.6	66.1	72.0	+76.5	68.8	75.0	67.3	+64.3	59.7
Five or more times a week	+13.8	3.9	5.7	14.5	12.5	2.7	+9.7	14.6	15.9
Mean	2.02	1.74	1.83	2.06	1.94	1.80	1.87	1.94	1.92
N	571**	558	579	1077**	634	296	808*	185	935
WOMEN									
Less than once a week	+16.6	34.4	27.4	+13.0	17.0	19.3	23.1	23.8	26.3
One to four times a week	73.9	66.2	68.6	−72.9	72.0	78.5	70.6	64.3	59.8
Five or more times a week	−9.5	2.4	4.0	14.1	11.0	2.1	−6.3	11.9	13.8
Mean	1.93	1.71	1.77	2.01	1.94	1.83	1.83	1.88	1.87
N	736	636	577	1069	800	466	1310	168	983

Base: Men and women in current steady heterosexual relationships

Notes:

An asterisk indicates a significant difference between men and women (X^2, *p < 0.05, **p < 0.01). Proportions with a + or − indicate relatively bigger or smaller proportions than expected

[1] Belgium: Frequencies of penetrative sex, not of making love in general

[2] Finland, Norway: Frequencies of vaginal intercourse, not of making love in general

[3] France, Norway, Spain: Only for people who have a steady partner and live with that partner as well

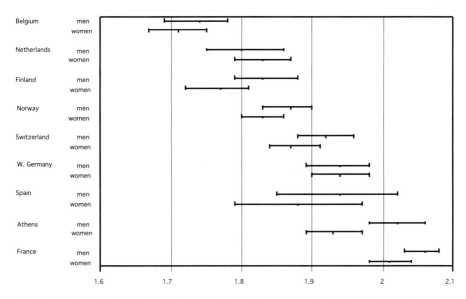

Figure 4.1   *Mean frequencies and confidence intervals (95%) of sexual intercourse per week*

attributed to them exclusively.[8] However, it is hard to interpret the observed differences between countries in general. One distinction seems to be evident, though, namely, the fact that the southern European countries are in the top of the hierarchy, for men as well as for women, while almost all of the northern European countries have lower average frequencies. This finding seems to support the cultural stereotype that people in relatively warmer climates are more passionate and have sex more often. The geographical proximity of Belgium and the Netherlands and Norway and Finland also seems to be reflected in the ranking by average frequency. It is quite possible that these countries have common geographical and cultural climates. More background information and more precise measurements are needed to be able to make more definitive statements.

Tables 4.3 and 4.4 show that the frequency with which people in ongoing steady relationships report having sex varies in relation to several background factors, as discussed below.

Gender and Age

Men reported having sex with their steady partners more frequently than women in seven of the nine surveys; this difference is statistically significant in three countries (see Table 4.2). In Germany men and women reported the same mean frequency, while in the Netherlands women reported a somewhat

Table 4.3 Frequency of sex per week for men (percentages)

	Athens 1990				Belgium[1] 1993				Finland[2] 1992				France[3] 1990			
	<1	1-4	5+	N	<1	1-4	5+	N	<1	1-4	5+	N	<1	1-4	5+	N
Age																
18–19	+46.2	-46.2	7.7	(13)	7.7	65.4	26.9	(26)	8.3	41.7	50.0	(12)	+41.7	58.3	0.0	(12)
20–24	14.1	-56.3	+29.7	(64)	28.4	66.2	5.4	(74)	19.0	76.2	4.8	(63)	-1.5	70.1	+28.4	(67)
25–29	9.6	67.5	+22.9	(83)	27.4	67.1	5.5	(73)	18.2	71.7	10.1	(99)	7.9	76.8	15.2	(164)
30–39	8.1	77.5	14.4	(209)	27.5	69.4	3.1	(193)	19.3	75.4	5.3	(207)	7.3	78.4	14.2	(422)
40–49	12.9	+82.2	-5.0	(202)	35.2	61.7	3.1	(193)	26.8	69.2	4.0	(198)	10.7	77.2	12.1	(429)
Start sexual career																
Early	10.2	73.7	16.1	(236)					-15.5	76.3	+8.2	(207)	-5.3	75.1	+19.6	(398)
Intermediate	12.5	74.2	13.3	(248)					25.5	69.7	4.8	(208)	8.3	77.1	14.7	(436)
Late	12.6	78.2	9.2	(87)					26.7	70.2	3.1	(161)	+15.8	78.3	-5.8	(240)
No. of partners last 12 months																
1					29.5	67.2	3.3	(478)	24.0	72.6	-3.5	(430)	9.0	+78.0	-13.0	(991)
2					28.9	65.8	5.3	(38)	24.1	67.2	8.6	(58)	9.1	-63.6	+27.3	(55)
3–4					43.3	53.3	3.3	(30)	-10.6	76.6	12.8	(47)	8.7	-56.5	34.8	(23)
5+					9.1	63.6	+27.3	(11)	11.4	71.4	+17.1	(35)	0.0	50.0	+50.0	(8)
No. of partners last 5 years																
1					29.3	67.4	3.3	(368)					9.7	+78.8	-11.6	(699)
2					30.5	61.0	8.5	(59)					11.0	79.4	9.6	(136)
3–4					32.8	67.2	0.0	(58)					7.0	70.5	+22.5	(129)
5+					31.0	63.4	5.6	(71)					-3.2	+63.8	+33.0	(94)

No. of partners whole life

	A	A	A	A (n)	B	B	B	B (n)	C	C	C	C (n)	D	D	D	D (n)
1									**+32.9**	**65.7**	**1.4**	**(70)**	12.6	**+83.2**	**–4.2**	(143)
2									**21.4**	**76.2**	**2.4**	**(42)**	**+17.5**	72.2	10.3	(97)
3–4									**28.6**	**68.8**	**2.6**	**(77)**	**+13.7**	76.3	10.0	(190)
5–9									**25.3**	**70.7**	**4.0**	**(99)**	5.4	76.2	18.4	(147)
10+									**–16.4**	**74.8**	**+8.8**	**(274)**	**–5.8**	75.9	**+18.3**	(486)
Education																
Low	13.0	80.0	7.0	(100)	30.5	65.6	3.9	(12)	21.3	72.3	6.4	(422)	6.6	75.1	**+18.4**	(381)
Medium	12.2	73.8	13.9	(237)	27.2	68.5	4.3	(232)	20.8	75.0	4.2	(48)	8.6	79.2	12.2	(475)
High	10.1	72.7	17.2	(227)	32.7	63.8	3.6	(196)	26.6	69.7	3.7	(109)	**+13.1**	74.3	12.6	(222)
Urbanization																
Low					50.0	44.4	5.6	(18)	21.0	73.4	5.6	(214)	10.6	74.4	15.0	(360)
Medium					30.9	65.5	3.6	(391)	23.3	70.2	6.5	(215)	6.8	81.7	11.6	(251)
High					26.2	69.1	4.7	(149)	22.4	72.8	4.8	(147)	9.0	75.3	15.7	(465)
Cohabitation																
Not cohabiting	12.9	68.2	18.9	(132)	35.8	61.3	2.9	(137)	27.4	66.7	6.0	(84)				
Cohabiting	11.2	76.5	12.3	(439)	28.3	67.5	4.3	(421)	21.4	72.9	5.7	(495)				
Duration																
<1 year	**10.0**	**65.0**	**+25.0**	**(40)**	40.8	53.1	6.1	(49)	25.0	66.7	8.3	(24)				
1–4 years	**12.9**	**–64.7**	**+22.3**	**(139)**	23.4	72.1	4.5	(111)	18.6	74.4	7.0	(129)				
>5 years	**11.3**	**+79.0**	**–9.7**	**(391)**	30.2	66.3	3.5	(398)	22.9	72.5	4.6	(414)				

Base: Men in current steady heterosexual relationships

Notes:

Percentages in bold type indicate dependent distributions (X^2, $p < 0.05$). Proportions with a + or – indicate relatively bigger or smaller proportions than expected

[1] Belgium: Frequencies of penetrative sex, not of making love in general

[2] Finland, Norway: Frequencies of vaginal intercourse, not of making love in general

[3] France, Norway, Spain: Only for people who have a steady partner and live with that partner as well

Table 4.3 *(cont.)*

	Germany West 1990				Netherlands 1989				Norway[2,3] 1992				Switzerland 1992			
	<1	1–4	5+	N	<1	1–4	5+	N	<1	1–4	5+	N	<1	1–4	5+	N
Age																
18–19	18.2	54.5	27.3	(220)	0.0	100.0	0.0	(7)	0.0	25.0	+75.0	(4)	+43.2	−32.4	24.2	(37)
20–24	13.6	65.4	+21.0	(81)	16.3	83.7	0.0	(49)	−13.5	70.3	+16.2	(74)	29.4	51.4	19.3	(109)
25–29	15.7	65.7	+18.7	(134)	19.0	76.2	4.8	(42)	20.3	69.9	9.8	(143)	27.3	−50.3	+22.4	(165)
30–39	17.0	71.4	11.6	(224)	26.6	70.2	3.2	(124)	26.2	64.8	9.0	(344)	20.8	+63.6	15.6	(409)
40–49	+24.9	71.1	−4.0	(173)	23.0	74.3	2.7	(74)	23.5	69.1	7.4	(243)	22.5	+69.6	−7.8	(204)
Start sexual career																
Early	16.7	67.2	+16.2	(204)	14.3	82.4	3.3	(91)	18.6	65.4	+16.0	(237)	23.6	−52.0	+24.4	(254)
Intermediate	−14.6	+73.5	11.9	(260)	25.3	69.9	4.8	(83)	22.0	70.1	7.8	(268)	25.0	60.7	14.3	(336)
Late	+28.0	63.4	8.5	(164)	26.7	72.5	0.8	(120)	+27.2	67.1	−5.7	(283)	24.4	+64.5	−11.1	(332)
No. of partners last 12 months																
1					22.5	75.3	2.2	(267)					24.8	60.5	14.7	(850)
2					21.4	78.6	0.0	(14)					20.0	53.3	26.7	(45)
3–4					27.3	63.6	9.1	(11)					26.7	46.7	26.7	(30)
5+					75.0	25.0	0.0	(4)					66.7	33.3	0.0	(9)
No. of partners last 5 years																
1					24.4	74.2	−1.4	(213)								
2					15.8	84.2	0.0	(19)								
3–4					29.0	64.5	6.5	(31)								
5+					−6.1	84.8	+9.1	(33)								

	I				II				III				IV			
No. of partners whole life																
1	+23.0	67.9	-9.1	(187)	28.8	71.2	0.0	(59)	24.2	70.4	-5.4	(186)	29.8	60.9	-9.3	(161)
2	19.8	71.9	8.3	(121)	21.9	78.1	0.0	(32)	31.1	65.6	3.3	(61)	24.6	63.8	11.6	(69)
3-4	-10.7	66.9	+22.3	(121)	20.3	78.0	1.7	(59)	25.0	69.7	5.3	(132)	28.4	62.7	-9.0	(134)
5-9	16.0	62.0	22.0	(50)	+33.3	64.8	1.9	(54)	25.5	64.1	10.3	(145)	20.3	63.2	16.5	(182)
10+	16.7	72.2	11.1	(18)	-13.6	79.5	+6.8	(88)	-17.4	67.4	+15.3	(236)	23.4	56.4	+20.2	(337)
Education																
Low	18.8	70.0	11.2	(250)	33.3	53.3	+13.3	(15)	22.3	65.7	12.0	(359)	29.8	51.1	19.1	(47)
Medium	15.9	69.0	15.2	(277)	-19.5	+77.9	2.6	(195)	23.5	67.5	9.0	(166)	24.6	59.3	16.2	(749)
High	25.5	66.0	8.5	(106)	29.7	68.9	1.4	(74)	23.7	69.1	7.2	(278)	22.1	65.4	12.5	(136)
Urbanization																
Low	20.1	69.1	10.8	(314)	28.6	57.1	14.3	(7)	20.1	70.0	9.9	(283)	21.9	62.3	15.8	(379)
Medium	12.4	72.9	14.7	(129)	23.3	74.4	2.2	(227)	24.4	65.3	10.3	(360)	27.7	58.1	14.2	(430)
High	19.4	66.7	14.0	(186)	17.7	79.0	3.2	(62)	24.1	67.9	8.0	(162)	20.2	57.1	22.7	(119)
Cohabitation																
Not cohabiting	14.9	64.4	+20.7	(174)	14.8	78.7	+6.6	(61)					+32.8	-51.3	15.9	(232)
Cohabiting	20.4	70.2	-9.4	(457)	24.3	73.9	-1.7	(230)					-21.7	+62.4	15.9	(704)
Duration																
<1 year	15.9	60.2	+23.9	(88)	5.6	83.3	+11.1	(18)	-9.6	57.8	+32.5	(83)				
1-4 years	15.3	67.1	+17.6	(170)	14.9	81.1	4.1	(74)	17.4	71.1	11.6	(242)				
>5 years	21.5	72.1	-6.4	(376)	+27.6	71.4	-1.1	(185)	+28.3	67.1	-4.6	(477)				

Base: Men in current steady heterosexual relationships

Notes:

Percentages in bold type indicate dependent distributions (X², p < 0.05). Proportions with a + or − indicate relatively bigger or smaller proportions than expected

[1] Frequencies of penetrative sex, not of making love in general

[2] Frequencies of vaginal intercourse, not of making love in general

[3] France, Norway, Spain: Only for people who have a steady partner and live with that partner as well

Belgium: Frequencies of penetrative sex, not of making love in general

Finland, Norway: Frequencies of vaginal intercourse, not of making love in general

Table 4.4 Frequency of sex per week for women (percentages)

	Athens 1990				Belgium[1] 1993				Finland[2] 1992				France[3] 1990			
	<1	1–4	5+	N	<1	1–4	5+	N	<1	1–4	5+	N	<1	1–4	5+	N
Age																
18–19	8.7	82.6	8.7	(23)	39.1	52.2	8.7	(23)	31.8	59.1	9.1	(22)	0.0	–0.0	+100.0	(3)
20–24	16.9	–62.7	+20.5	(83)	27.8	68.4	3.8	(79)	27.1	63.5	+9.4	(85)	8.6	71.4	20.0	(105)
25–29	–8.1	78.7	13.2	(136)	22.4	76.6	0.9	(107)	33.0	60.4	6.6	(91)	+20.4	–66.0	13.6	(162)
30–39	13.6	+78.4	8.0	(287)	35.6	62.3	2.1	(236)	24.6	+73.9	–1.5	(203)	–9.5	+79.2	–11.3	(432)
40–49	+27.1	–68.1	–4.8	(207)	32.1	65.8	2.1	(190)	27.3	70.5	2.3	(176)	15.3	69.3	15.3	(365)
Start sexual career																
Early	14.9	71.3	13.8	(94)					29.1	65.9	5.0	(179)	16.2	–64.4	+19.4	(216)
Intermediate	17.1	74.6	8.3	(205)					27.3	70.0	2.6	(227)	–9.2	+75.7	15.1	(597)
Late	16.7	74.1	9.2	(436)					25.7	69.6	4.7	(171)	+19.9	72.7	–7.4	(256)
No. of partners last 12 months																
1					30.6	67.4	2.0	(598)	26.3	+70.5	–3.3	(491)	12.9	73.3	13.9	(1025)
2					42.9	46.4	10.7	(28)	38.5	56.4	5.1	(39)	13.5	64.9	21.6	(37)
3–4					71.4	28.6	0.0	(7)	37.5	54.2	8.3	(24)	20.0	60.0	20.0	(5)
5+					0.0	100.0	0.0	(4)	17.6	64.7	+17.6	(17)	0.0	0.0	0.0	(0)
No. of partners last 5 years																
1					29.6	68.8	1.6	(493)					13.6	74.1	–12.3	(803)
2					35.4	59.5	5.1	(79)					10.9	67.9	+21.2	(156)
3–4					32.4	64.7	2.9	(34)					16.7	63.6	19.7	(66)
5+					42.3	50.0	7.7	(26)					2.9	77.1	20.0	(35)
No. of partners whole life																
1									26.6	71.2	2.2	(139)	13.3	74.5	2.2	(376)
2									26.8	71.8	1.4	(71)	12.7	+78.4	–8.9	(213)
3–4									25.6	70.2	4.1	(121)	12.6	73.1	14.3	(182)
5–9									30.5	63.3	6.3	(128)	8.8	70.3	+20.9	(148)
10+									25.5	68.4	6.1	(98)	16.9	–63.4	+19.7	(142)

Education																
Low	20.5	70.3	9.2	(195)	**32.1**	**64.2**	**3.7**	**(134)**	28.8	68.2	3.1	(393)	15.1	71.5	13.4	(411)
Medium	15.4	73.4	11.3	(364)	**27.4**	**+71.8**	**-0.8**	**(259)**	27.5	65.2	7.2	(69)	12.0	72.2	15.9	(435)
High	15.1	78.5	6.4	(172)	**35.8**	**-60.8**	**3.3**	**(240)**	22.6	72.2	5.2	(115)	11.6	75.9	12.5	(224)
Occupation																
Paid work and unemployed	16.5	73.4	10.1	(417)	26.4	71.2	2.4	(455)	27.4	68.8	3.8	(471)	11.9	73.6	14.5	(754)
Looking after home	16.5	73.9	9.5	(284)	31.3	67.7	1.0	(99)	30.8	66.7	2.6	(39)	17.0	69.9	13.1	(282)
Urbanization																
Low					38.5	61.5	0.0	(13)	26.6	70.6	2.8	(214)	**15.6**	**72.5**	**12.0**	**(334)**
Medium					32.2	65.5	2.3	(438)	25.5	70.2	4.3	(208)	**+17.5**	**68.3**	**14.2**	**(240)**
High					29.7	67.6	2.7	(185)	31.0	63.9	5.2	(155)	**-9.7**	**74.8**	**15.5**	**(496)**
Cohabitation																
Not cohabiting	13.8	76.1	10.1	(109)	**+44.8**	**-53.6**	**1.6**	**(125)**	28.3	64.6	7.1	(99)				
Cohabiting	17.1	73.5	9.4	(626)	**-28.1**	**+69.5**	**2.4**	**(509)**	27.2	69.5	3.3	(478)				
Duration																
<1 year	**13.8**	**69.0**	**17.2**	**(290)**	40.0	52.5	7.5	(40)	**25.8**	**61.3**	**+12.9**	**(31)**				
1–4 years	**-9.6**	**72.6**	**+17.8**	**(135)**	35.2	62.0	2.8	(108)	**27.1**	**64.3**	**+8.6**	**(140)**				
>5 years	**+18.2**	**74.6**	**-7.2**	**(571)**	30.1	68.3	1.6	(489)	**28.3**	**70.2**	**-1.5**	**(392)**				

Base: Women in current steady heterosexual relationships

Notes:

Percentages in bold type indicate dependent distributions (X^2, $p < 0.05$). Proportions with a + or − indicate relatively bigger or smaller proportions than expected

[1] Belgium: Frequencies of penetrative sex, not of making love in general

[2] Finland, Norway: Frequencies of vaginal intercourse, not of making love in general

[3] France, Norway, Spain: Only for people who have a steady partner and live with that partner as well

Table 4.4 (cont.)

	Germany West 1990				Netherlands 1989				Norway[1,2] 1992				Switzerland 1992			
	<1	1–4	5+	N	<1	1–4	5+	N	<1	1–4	5+	N	<1	1–4	5+	N
Age																
18–19	14.3	66.7	19.0	(21)	11.8	82.4	5.9	(17)	6.3	56.3	+37.5	(16)	30.6	59.2	10.2	(49)
20–24	12.7	67.6	+19.7	(142)	19.4	76.1	4.5	(67)	-15.8	68.4	+15.8	(177)	30.9	-46.9	+22.2	(162)
25–29	14.8	72.5	12.7	(142)	19.8	78.0	2.2	(91)	23.8	69.7	6.5	(261)	27.4	61.1	11.4	(175)
30–39	14.6	75.6	9.7	(308)	20.5	78.3	1.2	(161)	23.4	73.5	-3.0	(499)	23.7	61.8	14.5	(393)
40–49	+26.2	69.5	-4.3	(187)	18.5	80.0	1.5	(130)	26.6	68.9	4.5	(357)	23.7	+67.2	-9.1	(186)
Start sexual career																
Early	13.8	71.2	+15.0	(260)	14.4	82.5	3.1	(97)	21.1	72.3	6.6	(441)	20.5	63.2	16.2	(185)
Intermediate	16.1	73.1	10.8	(342)	18.1	80.5	1.3	(226)	23.5	69.4	7.1	(591)	29.6	56.4	14.0	(541)
Late	+21.7	72.3	-6.0	(184)	23.7	73.4	2.9	(139)	24.6	71.4	4.0	(248)	23.8	64.3	11.9	(252)
No. of partners last 12 months																
1					19.4	78.8	1.8	(443)					26.0	60.6	13.4	(938)
2					23.5	64.7	11.8	(17)					40.0	40.0	20.0	(35)
3–4					0.0	100.0	0.0	(3)					12.5	12.5	25.0	(8)
5+					0.0	100.0	0.0	(3)					50.0	50.0	0.0	(2)
No. of partners last 5 years																
1					19.4	79.1	1.5	(402)								
2					24.0	72.0	4.0	(25)								
3–4					17.9	75.0	7.1	(28)								
5+					11.1	77.8	11.1	(9)								
No. of partners whole life																
1	16.9	74.8	8.3	(278)	20.4	77.9	1.7	(181)	21.5	72.9	5.6	(447)	28.6	61.0	-10.5	(287)
2	19.4	72.7	7.9	(165)	11.8	84.9	3.2	(93)	27.7	67.9	4.4	(159)	24.3	64.0	11.8	(136)
3–4	15.9	66.9	+17.2	(151)	22.0	76.1	1.8	(109)	21.8	71.2	7.0	(243)	-19.9	63.7	16.4	(226)
5–9	12.1	72.7	15.2	(33)	20.0	78.0	2.0	(50)	25.8	66.9	7.3	(260)	27.0	55.2	17.8	(174)
10+	0.0	60.0	+40.0	(5)	24.2	72.7	3.0	(33)	19.7	71.8	8.5	(142)	+33.1	52.1	14.8	(142)

				(N)				(N)				(N)				(N)
Education																
Low	14.9	73.7	11.4	(350)	13.0	82.6	4.3	(23)	24.7	69.3	6.0	(567)	25.7	60.2	14.2	(113)
Medium	17.2	71.0	11.7	(383)	19.3	79.3	1.4	(348)	22.6	71.4	6.0	(318)	25.8	60.8	13.3	(802)
High	28.1	67.2	4.7	(64)	20.2	75.3	4.5	(89)	21.3	71.8	6.9	(422)	35.4	49.2	15.4	(65)
Occupation																
Paid work and unemployed	16.5	71.6	11.9	(461)	19.2	78.6	2.1	(234)	24.5	70.1	5.4	(971)				
Looking after home	19.5	72.9	7.6	(262)	20.3	78.7	1.0	(207)	21.9	72.7	5.5	(183)				
Urbanization																
Low	17.1	72.5	10.4	(375)	17.2	79.3	3.4	(29)	23.6	71.0	5.4	(441)	26.8	61.2	12.0	(433)
Medium	17.2	71.4	11.5	(192)	18.5	79.0	2.5	(319)	23.4	71.1	5.5	(595)	26.8	59.3	13.9	(440)
High	15.8	72.4	11.8	(228)	22.0	77.1	0.8	(118)	21.1	69.3	9.6	(251)	22.9	57.1	20.0	(105)
Cohabitation																
Not cohabiting	**11.6**	**72.7**	**15.7**	**(172)**	21.5	75.4	3.1	(65)					32.8	53.9	13.2	(204)
Cohabiting	**18.6**	**71.6**	**9.8**	**(624)**	19.0	79.2	1.8	(390)					24.6	61.4	14.0	(779)
Duration																
<1 year	**−8.4**	**63.9**	**+27.7**	**(83)**	**9.1**	**77.3**	**+13.6**	**(22)**	**−12.2**	**69.1**	**+18.7**	**(123)**				
1–4 years	**+12.8**	**68.1**	**+19.1**	**(188)**	**18.8**	**80.0**	**1.2**	**(85)**	**+20.1**	**70.7**	**+9.3**	**(334)**				
>5 years	**+19.3**	**75.0**	**−5.7**	**(523)**	**20.2**	**78.3**	**1.5**	**(337)**	**+26.1**	**70.9**	**−3.1**	**(844)**				

Base: Women in current steady heterosexual relationships

Notes:

Percentages in bold type indicate dependent distributions (X^2, $p < 0.05$). Proportions with a + or – indicate relatively bigger or smaller proportions than expected

[1] Belgium: Frequencies of penetrative sex, not of making love in general

[2] Finland, Norway: Frequencies of vaginal intercourse, not of making love in general

[3] France, Norway, Spain: Only for people who have a steady partner and live with that partner as well

higher mean frequency than men. This general difference between men and women is in line with predictions derived from their respective sexual scripts. It is interesting to see, however, that two of the three countries where men reported significantly higher frequencies of sexual contact, that is, France and Greece (Athens), are both countries where sex-role stereotypes are still more vigorously endorsed (Hofstede, 1991). This suggests that the reporting of sexual behaviour is affected differently by sex-role stereotypes.

An inspection of Table 4.3 and 4.4 also shows that, as expected, the frequency with which people have sex declines over the years. These tables also illustrate that for at least a few countries this is only part of the story, however. For men and women in Norway and former West Germany and women in Finland, younger age cohorts reported higher frequencies of having sex proportionately more often than the older age groups. For men and women in Athens and Switzerland, and for men in France, however, the situation is different, for relatively larger percentages of the people in the youngest age groups reported having sex infrequently. It seems that for persons with steady partners in these countries, the frequency of having sex first increases with age, then diminishes. It should be noted that this pattern cannot be attributed to not yet being involved in a relationship, since all people included in Table 4.3 were currently involved in a steady relationship.

Level of Sexual Interest

As expected, people who started their sexual careers earlier in life were found to have sex with their steady partners more frequently when they got older than 'late starters' did. This trend is found in seven out of the nine countries. The effect of early sexual initiation may be stronger for men than women, since the correlation is significant in five countries for men but in only two countries for women. Interestingly, we found that in most countries, regardless of the time period concerned (whole life, preceding last five years or preceding year), both male and female respondents who reported having had more sex partners also said they had sex more frequently with their current steady partners. These trends were significant in several countries, especially if one looks at a longer time period, and once again more often for men than for women.

Socio-demographic Factors

For women, there seems to be no relationship between the level of *education* and the frequency of sexual contact with the current sexual partner (the

significant differences in Belgium are difficult to interpret). For men, however, the following trend was observed in several countries: men with a lower
level of education more often reported higher frequencies of sex than men
with higher levels of education. This trend is significant for men in France and
the Netherlands.

The role of *religion* could be assessed for Athens, West Germany and the
Netherlands (not in table). Only for Dutch males did we see a significant
inverse relationship between church attendance and frequency of sex, that is,
the more often people attend services, the less often they have sex. This
relationship was not found for Dutch women or West German men and
women. The importance people in Athens and West Germany attached to
religion in their lives was also not related to the frequency of having sex.

Whether people live in *urban centres* or *rural areas* does not seem to affect
the frequency with which people have sex with their partner. Except for
women in France there are no significant differences. The significant findings
for France are difficult to interpret.

Relationship Status

The expectation that, given relatively more opportunities, partners who share
a household have more frequent sex than partners who live separately is
supported by the data for Belgian women and Swiss men only. Dutch men who
live separately, however, reported higher frequencies of having sex than men
who live together with their steady partner. It is quite likely that these significant relationships are confounded by other common variables such as age.

The suspected inverse correlation between the frequency of having sex
and length of the relationships is clearly supported by the findings in the
various countries. These differences are significant in nine of the 12 possible
comparisons.

**The Lifetime Prevalence of Various Sexual
Techniques**

Do people in the various countries differ with respect to the specific sexual
techniques they have ever practised with other persons? Here our concern
is not the frequency with which people do certain things but lifetime experience. Table 4.5 shows the percentages of the respondents in the various
countries who reported having ever practised specific sexual techniques.
As mentioned earlier, only people who are currently involved in a steady

Table 4.5 *Lifetime occurrence of sexual practices*

	Lifetime in general				Current partner	
	Athens 1990	Finland 1992	France ACSF 1990	Germany West 1990	Belgium[1] 1993	Netherlands[2] 1989
MEN						
Fondling, passive	96.3 (94.8–97.8)			95.5 (94.0–97.0)		94.9 (92.4–97.4)
Fondling, active	98.0** (96.8–99.2)	93.7** (91.7–95.7)		97.8* (96.7–98.9)		97.3 (95.4–99.2)
Vaginal intercourse	99.5 (98.8–100.0)			98.7** (97.9–99.5)		95.2 (92.7–97.7)
Oral sex, passive	44.7** (40.6–48.8)	87.3 (84.5–90.1)	82.7 (79.6–85.8)	66.8** (63.3–70.3)		72.3 (67.2–77.4)
Oral sex, active	40.4** (36.4–44.4)	90.3*** (87.8–92.8)	87.9*** (85.2–90.6)	76.6*** (73.5–79.7)	78.53[3] (75.1–81.9)	81.4*** (76.9–85.9)
Mouth–anus, passive	5.3 (3.4–7.2)			9.2 (7.0–11.4)		
Mouth–anus, active	8.3*** (6.0–10.6)			12.2* (9.2–14.6)		
Anal intercourse	15.3** (12.3–18.3)	26.0 (22.5–29.5)		19.8* (16.8–22.8)	17.5 (14.3–20.7)	5.8** (3.1–8.5)
N (min.–max.)	562–574	551–596	1107–1110	688–774	555–557	291–292

WOMEN

Fondling, passive	95.6 (94.1–97.1)			96.6 (95.4–97.8)		94.6 (92.5–96.7)
Fondling, active	94.6 (93.0–96.2)	91.0 (88.7–93.3)		96.0 (94.7–97.3)		95.9 (94.1–97.7)
Vaginal intercourse	98.9 (98.1–99.7)			99.8 (99.5–100.0)		96.3 (94.6–98.0)
Oral sex, passive	35.8 (32.3–39.3)	85.2 (82.3–88.1)	85.1 (82.1–88.1)	60.3 (57.0–63.6)		74.2 (70.2–78.2)
Oral sex, active	31.9 (28.5–35.3)	82.8 (79.7–85.9)	77.2 (73.7–80.7)	68.4 (65.3–71.5)	74.33[3] (70.9–77.7)	67.0 (62.7–71.3)
Mouth–anus, passive	5.3 (3.7–6.9)			11.7 (9.5–13.9)		
Mouth–anus, active	2.5 (1.4–3.6)			9.1 (7.2–11.0)		
Anal intercourse	10.1 (7.9–12.3)	23.0 (19.6–26.4)		15.5 (13.1–17.9)		11.6 (8.7–14.5)
N (min–max)	721–731	570–599	1113	856–1001		461–464

Base: Men and women in current steady heterosexual relationships

Notes: An asterisk indicates a significant difference between men and women (X^2, *p < 0.05, **p < 0.01, ***p < 0.001)

[1] Belgium: Percentage of people who ever practised a technique with current partner

[2] Netherlands: Percentage of people who recently practised a technique with current partner

[3] Frequency of oral sex in general

relationship are included in this table, in order to promote comparability between countries. If a person reported having practised a specific sexual technique, this does not, however, mean that he/she performed it with his/her current partner. For Belgium and the Netherlands, however, only data about experiences with the current steady partner (concerning the whole duration of the relationship and a recent unspecified period, respectively) were available.

As Table 4.5 shows, the relative numbers of people who have ever fondled or had sexual intercourse do not differ significantly in the countries included in this comparison.[9] We do, however, find significant differences for some other practices.

For active as well as passive oral sex, and for men as well as for women, we find the same differences between countries. In Athens and West Germany, the proportions of people reporting experience of this technique are lower than in other countries, whilst the two countries differ from each other as well. Given the fact that in Belgium and the Netherlands we are looking at experiences with the current partner only, the percentages of people reporting experience of oral sex seem to be relatively high. The Dutch percentages are significantly higher than those reported for Athens; a higher percentage of Dutch than German women likewise reported having experience of passive oral sex.

The people in the various countries show different levels of experience of anal sex. Compared with women in Athens, relatively more women in Germany reported having ever practised this sexual technique (the same questionnaire was used in both countries), while in Finland an even higher percentage of women reported having experience of this technique than in Germany. The percentage of Belgian women is also greater than the percentage of women in Athens. Finally, significantly more women in Germany than Athens reported ever having had sexual contacts in which they stimulated their partners' anuses with their mouths or were themselves stimulated this way.

If we look at the overall differences between the countries, people in Athens seem to be the least experienced; within steady relationships they make love relatively frequently, but with a more one-sided repertory. The Finns, and to a somewhat lesser extent the French, show up as the relatively most experienced people sexually.

The hierarchies of sexual techniques based on the proportions of people who report having ever practised them do not differ between countries. The techniques that are less common in one country are less common in other countries, too. Fondling and intercourse are the most common – almost all people in all countries for which data are available have fondled or had intercourse at least once. Oral sex is clearly less common, and anal sex even less. Mouth–anus contacts seem to have been experienced by the smallest number of people in each country.

One might expect people who have practised a specific, less common sexual technique to have used other less common techniques as well. Table 4.6

Table 4.6 *Correlations between lifetime occurrence of various practices*

| | Lifetime | | | | | | | | Current partner | |
| | Athens 1990 | | Finland 1992 | | France ACSF 1990 | | Germany West 1990 | | Netherlands[1] 1989 | |
	never	ever	never	ever	never	ever	never	ever	never	ever
MEN										
Oral sex passive										
oral active	7.0 (314)	81.8 (253)***	7.7 (52)	97.4 (456)***	22.0 (132)	90.9 (963)***	7.4 (163)	85.0 (535)***	13.0 (54)	85.7 (237)***
mouth–anus passive	0.3 (312)	11.6 (250)***					1.8 (228)	12.9 (456)***		
mouth–anus active	1.0 (312)	17.5 (251)***					2.6 (231)	17.1 (461)***		
anal	3.2 (314)	30.4 (253)***	1.5 (66)	30.4 (474)***			3.0 (232)	28.4 (461)***	4.9 (81)	6.2 (211)
Oral sex active										
mouth–anus passive	0.0 (336)	13.3 (226)***					1.2 (162)	11.7 (523)***		
mouth–anus active	0.0 (336)	20.7 (227)***					2.4 (165)	15.3 (528)***		
anal	3.3 (338)	33.2 (229)***	2.4 (83)	27.0 (134)***			1.8 (165)	25.5 (529)***	5.6 (54)	5.9 (237)
Mouth–anus passive										
mouth–anus active	0.8 (516)	56.5 (46)***					4.0 (624)	92.1 (63)***		
anal	11.7 (532)	73.3 (30)***					14.0 (623)	79.4 (63)***		
Mouth–anus active										
anal	10.5 (516)	66.0 (47)***					11.8 (609)	77.4 (84)***		

139

Table 4.6 *(cont.)*

| | Lifetime | | | | | | | | Current partner | |
| | Athens 1990 | | Finland 1992 | | France ACSF 1990 | | Germany West 1990 | | Netherlands[1] 1989 | |
	never	ever	never	ever	never	ever	never	ever	never	ever
WOMEN										
Oral sex passive										
oral active	4.1 (465)	82.1 (257)***	32.0 (97)	98.7 (451)***	10.3 (165)	88.8 (947)***	7.2 (274)	85.4 (584)***	34.9 (152)	93.8 (307)***
mouth–anus passive	0.9 (464)	13.3 (255)***					5.0 (343)	16.5 (504)***		
mouth–anus active	0.2 (465)	6.6 (256)***					1.8 (340)	14.2 (506)***		
anal	2.6 (465)	23.7 (257)***	3.9 (51)	29.3 (495)***			3.8 (340)	23.1 (507)***	14.3 (119)	10.9 (341)
Oral sex active										
mouth–anus passive	0.6 (491)	16.5 (231)***					2.9 (275)	16.1 (573)***		
mouth–anus active	0.0 (492)	7.9 (229)***					0.4 (273)	13.4 (574)***		
anal	2.6 (492)	26.1 (230)***	6.3 (95)	27.9 (463)***			2.6 (274)	21.6 (574)***	12.5 (152)	11.3 (310)
Mouth–anus passive										
mouth–anus active	3.4 (702)	82.4 (17)***					0.7 (755)	73.5 (98)***		
anal	7.2 (681)	57.9 (38)***					8.6 (752)	66.7 (99)***		
Mouth–anus active										
anal	8.7 (703)	61.1 (18)***					9.3 (773)	74.4 (78)***		

Notes:
Percentages presented in table are of people who have ever practised a sexual technique for subsamples that have or have never practised another technique with corresponding cell sizes
An asterisk indicates a significant difference between people who have ever practised a sexual technique for subsamples that have or have never practised another technique with corresponding cell sizes (X^2, *p < 0.05, **p < 0.01, ***p < 0.001)
[1] Netherlands: Percentage of people who recently practised a technique with current partner

140

shows that this is generally the case. It would be interesting to know what the determining factors are in this respect.

For Athens and West Germany we were able to explore whether people continue to practise specific sexual techniques if they have used them once or whether techniques are bound to specific phases in one's sexual career. We did this by checking how many of the people who had ever practised a specific sexual technique reported using the same technique in the past four weeks as well. The resulting pattern is the same for men and for women in both countries. With respect to the generally most frequently observed sexual techniques, such as fondling (active and passive) and vaginal intercourse, around 95 per cent of the people who said they ever did this had performed the technique in the previous four weeks. To the extent that other specific practices are generally practised less often, smaller percentages of the people who ever used these techniques used them in the past four weeks. The percentages range from 74 per cent to 82 per cent for active and passive oral sex; 47 per cent to 66 per cent for active and passive mouth–anus contacts; and 39 per cent to 57 per cent for anal intercourse. These findings underline the popularity or higher acceptability of techniques such as fondling and inter- course. Some people continue to practise other techniques once they have experienced them, while others seem to stop practising them. The dynamics behind these processes still have to be explored.

Gender Differences

There are several differences in male and female report rates. These differ- ences are generally in line with the discussed differences in men's and wom- en's sexual scripts. With respect to the active and passive variants of some sexual techniques there are consistent differences between men and women. For example, more men have ever practised active oral sex than passive oral sex, while the reverse is true for women (the exceptions are men in Athens and women in West Germany). With respect to mouth–anus contacts we observe the same difference in the two countries for which data are available: Athenian and West German men more often reported having practised mouth–anus contacts actively than passively, while for women the reverse relationship applies. Even for active and passive fondling we find the same trends. Here men's and women's reports of both their own and their partners' behaviour seem to be congruent.

If we look across countries at the percentages of people who have ever practised one specific sexual technique, we see even more gender-related differences. For one thing, when these percentages differ significantly, the male rate is consistently higher. The emerging pattern is more intriguing, however. Men and women do not differ with respect to passive fondling,[10] but do with respect to active fondling (more men than women report active fondling). The same pattern is found for oral sex in Finland, France and the Netherlands, that is, there are no gender-specific differences with regard to passive oral sex but there are significant differences regarding active oral sex (more men than women report having experience of this technique). In Athens and West Germany more men than women reported having had experience of both active and passive oral sex. Anal sex and the active role in mouth–anus contacts is reported by more men than women in both Athens and West Germany.

Experience versus No Experience of Specific Techniques

Several cross-national factors seem to differentiate people who have ever or never practised a specific sexual technique. This is especially true for the less commonly reported sexual techniques such as oral and anal sex. When a factor is related to a sexual technique in one country, it almost always has the same effect in other countries. The common factors rarely distinguished between people who have engaged in fondling and intercourse and those who have never tried them. The predominant reason for this is that almost everybody in each country has practised these techniques at least once, resulting in

Table 4.7 *Lifetime occurrence of sexual practices by various common factors for men*

	Lifetime				Current partner	
	Athens	Finland	France ACSF	Germany West	Belgium[1]	Netherlands[2]
	1990	1992	1990	1990	1993	1989
Age						
fondling passive	ns	–	–	ns	–	ns
fondling active	ns	–	–	ns	–	ns
intercourse	ns	ns	–	0.14***	–	ns
oral sex passive	−0.31***	−0.09*	−0.09**	−0.10*	–	−0.13*
oral sex active	−0.32***	−0.14**	ns	ns°	ns°	−0.14*
mouth–anus passive	−0.09*	–	–	–	ns	–
mouth–anus active	−0.14***	–	–	–	ns°	–
anal intercourse	ns	ns°°	–	ns	ns	ns
Start sexual career						
fondling passive	ns	–	–	ns	–	ns
fondling active	ns	–	–	ns	–	ns
vaginal intercourse	−0.09*	ns	–	ns	–	ns
oral sex passive	−0.11*	−0.16***	−0.12***	−0.10**	–	−0.19**
oral sex active	ns	−0.15***	−0.06*	ns	ns	−0.18**
mouth–anus passive	ns	–	–	−0.12**	–	–
mouth–anus active	ns	–	–	−0.14***	–	–
anal intercourse	ns	−0.13**	–	−0.09*	ns	ns

Table 4.7 *(cont.)*

	Lifetime				Current partner	
	Athens	Finland	France ACSF	Germany West	Belgium[1]	Netherlands[2]
	1990	1992	1990	1990	1993	1989
No. of partners last 12 months						
fondling passive	–	–	–	–	–	ns
fondling active	–	–	–	–	–	ns
vaginal intercourse	–	ns	–	–	–	ns
oral sex passive	–	0.14***	0.10**	–	–	ns
oral sex active	–	0.10*	0.06*	–	ns	ns
mouth–anus passive	–	–	–	–	–	–
mouth–anus active	–	–	–	–	–	–
anal intercourse	–	0.18***	–	–	ns	0.12*
No. of partners last 5 years						
fondling passive	–	–	–	–	–	ns
fondling active	–	–	–	–	–	ns
vaginal intercourse	–	–	–	–	–	ns
oral sex passive	–	–	0.22***	–	–	0.16**
oral sex active	–	–	0.47***	–	ns	0.13*
mouth–anus passive	–	–	–	–	–	–
mouth–anus active	–	–	–	–	–	–
anal intercourse	–	–	–	–	ns	ns
No. of partners lifetime						
fondling passive	–	–	–	ns	ns	ns
fondling active	–	–	–	0.09*	–	ns
vaginal intercourse	–	ns	–	ns	–	ns
oral sex passive	–	0.21***	0.23***	0.10*	–	0.28***
oral sex active	–	0.17***	0.17***	0.12**	–	0.25***
mouth–anus passive	–	–	–	0.10*	–	–
mouth–anus active	–	–	–	0.12**	–	–
anal intercourse	–	0.17***	–	0.12**	–	ns
Education						
fondling passive	ns	–	–	0.12**	–	ns
fondling active	ns	–	–	0.11**	–	ns
vaginal intercourse	ns	ns	–	ns°	–	ns
oral sex passive	0.13*	ns	ns	0.13***	–	ns
oral sex active	0.18***	−0.09*	ns	0.23***	ns	ns
mouth–anus passive	0.11**	–	–	ns	–	–
mouth–anus active	0.14***	–	–	ns	–	–
anal intercourse	0.12**	ns	–	ns	ns	ns
Urbanization						
fondling passive	–	–	–	ns	–	ns
fondling active	–	–	–	ns	–	ns
vaginal intercourse	–	−0.09*	–	ns	–	ns
oral sex passive	–	ns	ns	0.12**	–	ns
oral sex active	–	ns	ns	0.10*	ns	ns
mouth–anus passive	–	–	–	ns	–	–
mouth–anus active	–	–	–	ns	–	–
anal intercourse	–	ns	–	0.11**	ns	ns
Cohabitation						
fondling passive	ns	–	–	ns	–	ns
fondling active	ns	–	–	ns	–	ns
vaginal intercourse	ns	ns	–	ns	–	ns
oral sex passive	−0.28***	ns	–	−0.11**	–	ns
oral sex active	−0.27***	ns	–	−0.08*	ns	ns
mouth–anus passive	−0.09*	–	–	ns	–	–
mouth–anus active	−0.12**	–	–	ns	–	–
anal intercourse	0.10*	ns	–	ns	ns	ns

Table 4.7 *(cont.)*

	Lifetime				Current partner	
	Athens	Finland	France ACSF	Germany West	Belgium[1]	Netherlands[2]
	1990	1992	1990	1990	1993	1989
Duration						
fondling passive	ns	–	–	ns	–	ns
fondling active	ns	–	–	ns	–	ns
vaginal intercourse	ns	ns	–	0.12**	–	ns
oral sex passive	−0.25***	ns	–	−0.24***	–	ns°°
oral sex active	−0.27***	ns	–	ns°°°	ns°°	ns
mouth–anus passive	−0.09*	–	–	−0.09*	–	–
mouth–anus active	−0.12**	–	–	−0.08*	–	–
anal intercourse	−0.11*	ns	–	ns	ns	ns

Base: Men in current steady heterosexual relationships
Notes:
Percentages presented in table are of people who have ever practised a sexual technique
An * and a ° indicate a significant difference between the sexual practice and the common variables
(Spearman R: *p < 0.05, **p < 0.01, ***p < 0.001, and for X^2, °p < 0.05, °°p < 0.01, °°°p < 0.001)
[1] Belgium: Percentage of people who have ever practised a technique with current partner; frequencies of oral sex active are frequencies of oral sex in general
[2] Netherlands: Percentage of people who recently practised a technique with current partner

a small variance. Tables 4.7 and 4.8 show for which countries and combinations of factors and sexual techniques it was possible to explore the relations. These tables also present an overview of all the significant linear and non-linear relationships that could be identified. In this section we shall present general trends rather than discussing each significant relationship independently. We shall illustrate these trends with specific examples to give an idea of the size of the effects. Our observations are based not just on the correlation coefficients in the tables, but also on inspection of the raw frequency tables, for we found that trends that were significant in some countries could quite often be observed in other countries as well, without being statistically significant. We considered this procedure to be valid, especially since the recoding resulted in a sizeable loss of variance, thereby limiting the possibility for effects to be significant. Given space limitations, however, we could not include all the relevant frequency tables in this book.

Age

The assumption that because of increasing opportunities more people in the older age groups have experience of specific techniques than in the younger age group is only partly supported by the data. It seems to apply to active and passive fondling and intercourse only, not to the other techniques. An

Table 4.8 *Lifetime occurrence of sexual practices by various common factors for women*

	Lifetime				Current partner	
	Athens	Finland	France ACSF	Germany West	Belgium[1]	Netherlands[2]
	1990	1992	1990	1990	1993	1989
Age						
fondling passive	ns	–	–	ns	–	ns
fondling active	−0.09*	–	–	ns	–	ns
vaginal intercourse	ns	ns	–	0.08*	–	ns°
oral sex passive	−0.26***	−0.22***	−0.07*	ns	–	−0.18***
oral sex active	−0.24***	−0.23***	−0.07*	ns	ns	−0.19***
mouth–anus passive	ns	–	–	ns	–	–
mouth–anus active	ns	–	–	ns	–	–
anal intercourse	ns	−0.13***	–	ns	−0.09*	0.11*
Start sexual career						
fondling passive	ns	–	–	−0.07*	–	ns
fondling active	ns	–	–	−0.07*	–	ns
vaginal intercourse	ns	ns	–	ns	–	ns
oral sex passive	−0.11**	−0.11*	ns	−0.12***	–	−0.14*
oral sex active	−0.10**	−0.16***	−0.09**	−0.09*	ns	−0.12*
mouth–anus passive	ns	–	–	−0.09*	–	–
mouth–anus active	ns	–	–	−0.10**	–	–
anal intercourse	ns	−0.21***	–	−0.08*	ns	ns
No. of partners last 12 months						
fondling passive	–	–	–	–	–	ns
fondling active	–	–	–	–	–	ns
vaginal intercourse	–	ns	–	–	–	ns
oral sex passive	–	ns	ns	–	–	0.14**
oral sex active	–	ns	0.08**	–	ns	0.10*
mouth–anus passive	–	–	–	–	–	–
mouth–anus active	–	–	–	–	–	–
anal intercourse	–	0.14***	–	–	ns	ns
No. of partners last 5 years						
fondling passive	–	–	–	–	–	ns
fondling active	–	–	–	–	–	ns
vaginal intercourse	–	–	–	–	–	ns
oral sex passive	–	–	0.08**	–	–	0.17***
oral sex active	–	–	0.17***	–	0.14***	0.17***
mouth–anus passive	–	–	–	–	–	–
mouth–anus active	–	–	–	–	–	–
anal intercourse	–	–	–	–	ns	ns
No. of partners lifetime						
fondling passive	–	–	–	ns	–	ns
fondling active	–	–	–	ns	–	ns
vaginal intercourse	–	ns	–	ns	–	0.10*
oral sex passive	–	0.08*	0.18***	0.10*	–	0.19***
oral sex active	–	0.13**	0.27***	0.10**	–	0.19***
mouth–anus passive	–	–	–	ns	–	–
mouth–anus active	–	–	–	0.10**	–	–
anal intercourse	–	0.25***	–	0.12**	–	ns
Education						
fondling passive	0.13***	–	–	0.10**	–	ns
fondling active	0.10**	–	–	ns	–	ns
vaginal intercourse	ns	ns	–	ns	–	ns
oral sex passive	0.21***	0.15***	0.20***	0.12***	–	0.16***
oral sex active	0.28***	0.11**	0.14***	0.16***	0.12**	0.15*
mouth–anus passive	0.13***	–	–	ns	–	–
mouth–anus active	ns	–	–	ns	ns	–
anal intercourse	0.15***	0.08*	–	ns	ns	ns

Table 4.8 *(cont.)*

	Lifetime				Current partner	
	Athens	Finland	France ACSF	Germany West	Belgium[1]	Netherlands[2]
	1990	1992	1990	1990	1993	1989
Occupation						
fondling passive	−0.10**	–	–	ns	–	−0.11*
fondling active	−0.10**	–	–	ns	–	−0.10*
vaginal intercourse	ns	ns	–	ns	–	ns
oral sex passive	−0.60***	ns	−0.08**	ns	–	−0.11*
oral sex active	−0.15***	ns	−0.13***	ns	−0.12**	−0.14**
mouth–anus passive	−0.11**	–	–	ns	–	–
mouth–anus active	ns	–	–	ns	–	–
anal intercourse	ns	ns	–	ns	ns	ns
Urbanization						
fondling passive	–	–	–	0.08*	–	ns
fondling active	–	–	–	ns	–	ns
vaginal intercourse	–	ns	–	ns	–	ns
oral sex passive	–	ns	0.11***	0.10*	–	ns
oral sex active	–	ns	0.06*	0.08*	ns	ns
mouth–anus passive	–	–	–	ns	–	–
mouth–anus active	–	–	–	ns	–	–
anal intercourse	–	0.11**	–	0.09*	ns	ns
Cohabitation						
fondling passive	ns	–	–	ns	–	ns
fondling active	ns	–	–	ns	–	ns
vaginal intercourse	0.07*	ns	–	ns	–	ns
oral sex passive	−0.14***	ns	–	−0.07*	–	−0.09*
oral sex active	−0.14***	ns	–	−0.11***	ns	ns
mouth–anus passive	ns	–	–	ns	–	–
mouth–anus active	ns	–	–	ns	–	–
anal intercourse	ns	ns	–	−0.07*	ns	ns
Duration						
fondling passive	−0.18***	–	–	ns	–	ns
fondling active	ns	–	–	ns	–	ns
vaginal intercourse	ns	ns	–	ns	–	ns
oral sex passive	−0.14***	−0.15***	–	−0.08*	–	0.15**
oral sex active	−0.15***	−0.13**	–	−0.09*	ns	0.11*
mouth–anus passive	−0.08*	–	–	ns	–	–
mouth–anus active	ns	–	–	−0.14***	–	–
anal intercourse	−0.08*	−0.10*	–	ns	ns	ns

Base: Women in current steady heterosexual relationships
Notes:
Percentages presented in table are of people who have ever practised a sexual technique
An * and a ° indicate a significant difference between the sexual practice and the common variables
(Spearman R: *p < 0.05, **p < 0.01, ***p < 0.001, and for X², °p < 0.05, °°p < 0.01, °°°p < 0.001)
[1] Belgium: Percentage of people who have ever practised a technique with current partner; frequencies of oral sex active are frequencies of oral sex in general
[2] Netherlands: Percentage of people who recently practised a technique with current partner

example is the occurrence of intercourse in West German men and women: whereas 85.3 per cent of the 34 male and 92.9 per cent of the 28 female 18–19-year-olds had ever practised vaginal intercourse, the percentages jumped to 99.4 per cent of the 163 25–29-year-old male and 100 per cent of the 164

20–24-year-old female respondents in this survey. All the other significant correlations between age and the various techniques were negative, however, suggesting that people in the oldest age cohorts are less likely to have ever practised the more specific sexual techniques.

Closer inspection of the breakdown of people with experience of specific techniques by age reveals a more complicated picture. In the oldest age group (40–49 years) we consistently find a significantly smaller proportion of both men and women who report having ever practised oral sex (active and passive) than in the one or two preceding age categories (respectively 30–39 years and 25–29 years). In some cases the proportion in the oldest age category is even smaller than that in the youngest age category (18–19 years). An example of a significant non-linear relation between age and oral sex is found in the Netherlands, where 83.3 per cent, 85.1 per cent, 83.7 per cent, 87.1 per cent and 67.6 per cent of the men and 61.1 per cent, 81.5 per cent, 78.9 per cent, 65.0 per cent and 54.6 per cent of the women in the 18–19, 20–24, 25–29, 30–39 and 40–49 age categories, respectively, said that they had ever practised active oral sex. The same trend is found for active and passive mouth–anus contacts and anal sex, that is rising percentages of experienced people in the higher age categories, except for the last age category, where in several cases a significantly smaller percentage stated having been involved in anal sex.[11] A clear example of this is given by Finland. In this survey, the number of men who said they ever practised anal sex peaks at 32.3 per cent in the 30–39 age category, then falls to 19 per cent in the 40–49 age category. In contrast, the highest percentage of women reporting ever having practised anal sex is in the 25–29 age category (29.5 per cent), after which the percentage declines to 14.2 per cent in the 40–49 age category.

The findings support the idea that both individual maturation and cultural changes are at work, affecting the age cohorts differently. First, people become more experienced in the course of their sexual careers (this applies especially to the most common sexual practices like fondling and intercourse), although after a specific age (around 35) people no longer engage in new practices. Second, sexual behaviour patterns have changed over time in the various countries, since people in younger age cohorts are more likely to have engaged in relatively less common sexual practices than the respondents in the oldest cohorts included in this overview.

Level of Sexual Interest

As expected, the start of one's sexual career and number of sexual partners are related to a broader range of sexual experience. In the Netherlands relatively more early than late starters have ever performed oral sex on their partner (89.8 per cent of 88 men and 75.3 per cent of 97 women for the former versus 73.5 per cent of 117 men and 59.7 per cent of 134 women for the latter). In the case of passive oral sex these figures are respectively 84.1 per cent of the male and 84.4 per cent of the female early starters versus 63.6 per cent of the male and 67.2 per cent of the female late starters. The more sexual partners French men and women have had in their lives, the more often they have experience of both passive and active oral sex (for active oral sex: 76.4 per cent of 144 men with one partner compared with 94.4 per cent of 497 men who claim to have had 10 or more sexual partners in their lives; for women the percentages are 64.3 per cent of 387 persons and 92.2 per cent of 154 persons).

We also find differences, albeit somewhat smaller ones, in relation to the number of partners in the preceding year. In Finland, for instance, we see that 21.9 per cent of 443 men and 20.8 per cent of 510 women with one sexual partner in the preceding year had ever practised anal sex versus 50.0 per cent of 36 men and 66.7 per cent of 18 women with five or more partners in the preceding year.

Socio-demographic Factors

As expected, people with higher levels of education engaged in specific sexual practices more often than people with lower levels of education. This trend can be observed and is significant for several countries and for various techniques. A clear example is Athens: 15.6 per cent of the men with the lowest level of education (n = 96) and 46.7 per cent of the men with the highest level of education (n = 229) reported having ever practised active oral sex; for passive oral sex these percentages were respectively 25.0 per cent and 49.1 per cent. For women in Athens these percentages were respectively 10.2 per cent versus 46.1 per cent and 16.7 per cent versus 44.9 per cent (for respectively 186 less educated and 178 highly educated women). Interestingly, the trend of increasing experience with higher levels of education was also found for active and passive fondling. For example, 96.6 per cent of the women with a higher level of education in Athens reported having ever fondled their partners' genitals compared with 90.3 per cent of the women with the lowest level of education.

Anal sex seems to be the only practice that does not show this trend. For men in Finland and women in the Netherlands the reverse trend is observed, and for Belgian men this reverse trend is even significant: 24.0 per cent of the men with the lowest level of education (n = 129) compared with 17.9 per cent of the men with the highest level of education (n = 195) reported having engaged in anal sex with the current sexual partner. It is quite possible that a permissive attitude does not promote engaging in anal sex. The reason for this could be that anal sex, unlike oral sex, may be less intimate emotionally, since it does not require contact between mouth and genital parts or anus. Furthermore, anal sex may also be an adequate substitute for vaginal intercourse. Practising anal sex preserves the woman's 'virginity' and was also a relatively safe (before the AIDS pandemic) and effective means of contraception. The negative correlation between level of education and the occurrence of anal sex might be related to different attitudes towards anal functions.

For Athens, West Germany and the Netherlands it was possible to explore the effect of *religious involvement* on the occurrence of sexual practices. Regardless of which indicator we look at, for example the importance attached to religion or church attendance, the pattern is clear: greater religious involvement is related to less experience of almost all sexual techniques (vaginal intercourse excepted) for both men and women. What is more, this finding applies to three different religions: Greek Orthodox, Roman Catholic and Protestant. The effect seems to be stronger in Athens than in West Germany. In the Netherlands, there are no differences related to religious faith. With respect to actual church attendance we find small, significant differences for men, in that men who attend religious services reported less experience of fondling their partners' genitals (93.8 per cent of 80 men versus 98.6 per cent of 212 men), passive oral sex (61.3 per cent versus 76.4 per cent), and active oral sex (68.8 per cent versus 86.3 per cent). It is quite likely that the church's impact on daily life in the Netherlands has become less strong. This does not mean that differences in people's attitudes towards sexuality have disappeared as well. When these attitudes are correlated with sexual practices, it seems that men and women who hold more permissive attitudes also more often reported having practised specific techniques. These relations are significant with respect to passive and active oral sex. Women who reported ever having fondled a partner's genitals also reported significantly higher levels of permissiveness than women who had never engaged in such fondling.

We also observed a general trend with respect to the current *place of residence*. In general, people who live in bigger cities more often reported having ever practised the less common sexual techniques. This trend is seen in all the countries included in the overview except for men in France. In Germany the differences between the three levels of urbanization are significant for passive and active oral sex and for anal sex, both for men and for women. To give an example, 16.5 per cent of the 351 German men living in rural areas compared with 28.2 per cent of the 195 men living in cities reported having had anal sex; for German women these percentages are respectively 12.3 per cent (of 416 women) and 20.1 per cent (of 239 women).

Looking at the *employment status*, we expected that women who have (or are looking for) paid work have more sexual experience, especially with regard to the less common sexual practices. This does indeed seem to be the general trend for almost all combinations of countries and sexual techniques, the exception being oral sex in Finland, where relatively few women identified themselves as homemakers. An example of this trend is oral sex in French women: 80.2 per cent and 86.7 per cent of the women with paid work (n = 788) reported experience of respectively active and passive oral sex, compared with 68.4 per cent and 80.2 per cent of homemakers (n = 294). A more extreme example is passive oral sex in Athenian women: 85.0 per cent of 207 women with paid work reported ever having had this experience compared with 24.8 per cent of the 270 homemakers.

Relationship Status

Since cohabitation and the relationship's length are reflections of the current situation, it would be somewhat surprising if they were related to lifetime experience of certain sexual practices. There are, however, systematic correlations for some countries and techniques. There is a general trend for people who do not live with their steady partners to have proportionately more experience of specific sexual practices than people who do. A significant difference is, for example, found for Dutch women: 72.5 per cent of the 386 women who live with their steady partners have had passive oral sex compared with 84.4 per cent of the 64 women who do not.

There is also a trend related to the duration of the person's ongoing relationship. As a rule, respondents who were involved in relationships that had already lasted five or more years reported proportionately less experience of the less common sexual techniques than respondents involved in shorter relationships. This trend is seen in several countries and for several techniques. There are no situations in which the reverse was detected. An example of the differences is provided by Finland, where 20.4 per cent of the women involved in relationships lasting five or more years (n = 407) said they had practised anal sex, while 28.1 per cent and 30.6 per cent of the women involved in relationships lasting respectively up to one year or between one and five years said they had ever practised anal sex (n = 407, 32, and 144, respectively). Relationship duration is also related to passive fondling in women from Athens, for all 34 women involved in a relationship lasting up to one year reported ever having had their genitals fondled by a partner, compared with 96.3 per cent of the 135 women involved in relationships lasting one to five years, and 80.4 per cent of the women involved in longer-lasting relationships (n = 648). People with broader sexual interests may have more problems staying in a relationship and favour variety, although this is unlikely. It should, however, also be realized that people in longer-lasting relationships are more likely to belong to the older age cohorts, and, as has been suggested before, may have been less affected by the general changes in the sexual climate.

Frequency of Masturbation

The questions asked about masturbation and answer formats used in the various studies are too divergent to allow cross-national comparison of the frequency of masturbation. Table 4.9, which presents the available data, suggests that fewer Finnish men and women than Dutch and French people say they have never masturbated. This is not actually true, but a consequence of the fact that in the Finnish survey respondents were asked about lifetime behaviour, while in the Dutch and the French survey the question focused on current masturbation frequency. Despite these disparities, it is possible to identify a pattern common to all three countries, namely, systematically more women than men said that they never masturbated, while among those who did, women likewise reported masturbating significantly less often than men. The actual gender difference might be smaller, since it is quite likely less acceptable for women to report this kind of behaviour than it is for men.

Ever having practised a specific sexual technique that might be seen as an indication of a more open sexual attitude is also related to masturbation frequency, at least for people in the Netherlands. Thus, in the Dutch survey, respondents who had practised passive oral sex masturbated more often than those who had never done so (80 per cent of the men and 59.3 per cent of the women who had ever practised passive oral sex reported masturbating at least once a month compared with 62.1 per cent of the men and 30.1 per cent of the women who never practised oral sex.) We find the identical relationships for women who have practised active oral sex and both men and women who have practised anal sex.

We explored other relationships between background factors and frequency of masturbation, checking for linear as well as curvilinear trends.[12] The results are presented in Tables 4.9 and 4.10. Table 4.10 shows the percentages of respondents in various subcategories who reported masturbating frequently. Almost all factors seem to be related to the frequency of masturbation in each of the three countries.

Age

Masturbation frequency is related to age, albeit with a gender-specific difference. Overall, younger men masturbate more frequently then older men; there seems to be a steady decline from age 18 onwards. It seems that for women, masturbation frequency first goes up with age, then decreases. This is most visible in the French data, where the curvilinear trend is significant for women. The curvilinear trend can be observed also in the Netherlands and

Table 4.9 *Frequency of masturbation and its relation to common factors and other sexual techniques*

	Finland 1992		France 1990		Netherlands 1989	
	Men	Women	Men	Women	Men	Women
When did you last masturbate?						
I have never masturbated	9.2	20.2				
over 10 years ago	13.8	17.2				
1–10 years ago	16.8	18.5				
in the past year	20.8	21.7				
in the past month	18.5	14.1				
in the past week	17.5	7.5				
in the past 24 hours	3.5	0.8				
You have masturbated …						
never			15.7	49.7		
rarely			20.9	16.9		
sometimes			49.2	26.5		
often			14.2	7.0		
On average how often do you masturbate?						
I never masturbate					18.1	44.5
less than once a month					19.0	28.4
one to several times a month					30.1	19.3
one to several times a week					28.2	7.2
every day					3.9	0.5
several times a day					0.7	0.0
N[1] / N[2]	601	604	1686	1663	415	566
Gender	−0.22***		−0.35***		0.39***	
Age	−0.25***	−0.23***	−0.10***	0.07**	−0.30***	−0.11**
Start of sexual career	−0.02	−0.18***	−0.08**	−0.05	−0.07	−0.17***
No. of partners last 12 months[3]	0.16***	0.17***	0.12***	0.14***	0.26***	0.13*[1]
No. of partners last 5 years[4]	0.07	0.27***	0.16***	0.19***	0.36***	0.32***[1]
No. of partners lifetime[5]	0.22***	0.22***	0.19***	0.32***	0.15**	0.30***[1]
Education	0.10**	0.11*	0.17***	0.29***	0.23***	0.25***
Urbanization					0.16***	0.06
Relation					0.33***	0.21***
Cohabitation	−0.19***	−0.10*	−0.11***	+0.06*	−0.27***	−0.09*
Duration	−0.16***	−0.17***			−0.27***	−0.14**
Different sexual practices[2]						
Making love			ns	ns		
Fondling passive					ns	0.13**
Fondling active					ns	0.09*
Intercourse					ns	ns
Oral sex passive					0.23***	0.23***
Oral sex active					ns	0.24***
Anal					13*	ns

Notes:

An asterisk indicates a significant difference between men and women (X[2]; *p < 0.05, **p < 0.01, ***p < 0.001)

[1] Percentage of people who recently practised a technique with current partner

[2] Only for people currently involved in a steady relationship

[3] For Netherlands: People who have had more than 1 partner in the last 12 months

[4] For Netherlands and France: People who have had more than 1 partner in the last 5 years

[5] For Netherlands and France: People who have had more than 1 partner in their lifetimes

Table 4.10 *Proportions of people who frequently masturbate*[1]

	Finland 1992				France 1990				Netherlands 1989			
	Men		Women		Men		Women		Men		Women	
	%	N	%	N	%	N	%	N	%	N	%	N
Age												
18–19	41.2	(17)	4.2	(24)	25.7	(105)	2.9	(102)	51.6	(33)	11.6	(43)
20–24	31.3	(66)	16.3	(86)	13.1	(289)	4.0	(297)	46.1	(76)	9.9	(91)
25–29	28.6	(98)	14.7	(95)	20.4	(269)	8.7	(253)	41.8	(67)	13.5	(104)
30–39	21.3	(220)	6.6	(214)	14.5	(539)	10.3	(543)	28.7	(150)	6.7	(181)
40–49	11.5	(200)	3.7	(185)	8.7	(484)	4.9	(468)	14.6	(89)	2.7	(147)
Start of sexual career												
Early	19.6	(210)	13.3	(187)	15.0	(640)	10.6	(330)	33.0	(115)	11.4	(114)
Intermediate	23.5	(213)	5.2	(229)	14.9	(657)	6.1	(884)	29.9	(107)	7.1	(267)
Late	18.2	(165)	6.7	(180)	11.7	(351)	7.2	(376)	25.4	(150)	5.1	(155)
No. of partners in last 12 months												
0									41.3	(29)	7.3	(41)
1	17.8	(438)	6.9	(507)	11.9	(1357)	6.2	(1423)	20.5	(287)	5.6	(463)
2	28.3	(60)	12.5	(40)	23.7	(139)	17.1	(82)	64.7	(34)	25.9	(27)
3–4	30.5	(46)	12.5	(24)	23.5	(68)	30.0	(20)	66.7	(21)	40.0	(10)
5+	36.1	(36)	27.8	(18)	35.3	(34)	28.6	(7)	83.3	(18)	25.0	(4)
No. of partners in whole life												
0					0.0	(6)	0.0	(3)	53.8	(26)	14.3	(21)
1	20.3	(74)	5.1	(138)	5.2	(172)	1.3	(468)	19.1	(68)	3.5	(199)
2	20.9	(43)	2.7	(75)	9.2	(141)	8.4	(296)	23.7	(38)	4.6	(107)
3–4	20.1	(80)	5.5	(128)	11.6	(293)	8.3	(303)	25.3	(75)	4.9	(123)
5–9	21.2	(92)	9.8	(132)	15.0	(266)	9.2	(260)	35.5	(76)	16.9	(71)
10+	21.6	(277)	17.5	(103)	18.4	(734)	14.6	(247)	41.6	(125)	25.0	(44)
No. of partners in last five years												
0					100.0	(2)			38.5	(13)	5.6	(18)
1					9.8	(779)	5.8	(970)	18.3	(228)	4.5	(422)
2					13.7	(233)	7.0	(270)	42.9	(28)	2.5	(40)
3–4					21.3	(272)	11.9	(201)	45.5	(55)	29.3	(41)
5+					21.2	(312)	13.5	(111)	58.5	(65)	34.8	(23)

Table 4.10 *(cont.)*

| | Finland 1992 | | | | France 1990 | | | | Netherlands 1989 | | | |
| | Men | | Women | | Men | | Women | | Men | | Women | |
	%	N	%	N	%	N	%	N	%	N	%	N
Education												
Low	17.5	(436)	5.9	(406)	9.7	(527)	3.2	(554)	19.1	(21)	4.0	(25)
Medium	39.2	(51)	19.2	(73)	12.5	(768)	7.6	(687)	26.6	(248)	5.5	(400)
High	26.3	(114)	9.6	(125)	23.9	(389)	11.1	(425)	46.4	(142)	14.9	(134)
Occupation												
Paid work	38.6	(488)	21.8	(495)	13.0	(1364)	7.2	(1141)	27.6	(301)	8.4	(285)
Unemployed	34.8	(66)			14.6	(103)						
Looking after home			14.6	(41)			7.6	(315)	28.6	(42)	4.0	(223)
Urbanization												
Low	17.7	(221)	7.8	(218)	10.7	(540)	5.4	(464)	33.3	(9)	6.9	(29)
Medium	23.2	(228)	6.8	(220)	14.1	(389)	5.4	(392)	28.6	(304)	6.7	(390)
High	21.5	(149)	10.8	(166)	17.0	(753)	8.7	(809)	45.2	(102)	10.9	(147)
Relationship												
No									57.9	(107)	18.2	(99)
Yes									24.0	(308)	5.5	(467)
Cohabitation												
Not cohabiting	38.0	(92)	14.9	(108)	20.8	(571)	6.5	(537)	47.1	(68)	18.2	(66)
Cohabiting	17.8	(509)	6.9	(496)	10.9	(1114)	7.2	(1128)	18.0	(234)	3.6	(390)
Duration												
<1 year	33.3	(27)	12.5	(32)					55.0	(20)	14.3	(21)
1–4 years	29.4	(136)	14.4	(145)					31.7	(79)	10.5	(193)
<5 years	17.0	(424)	5.8	(411)					16.4	(188)	3.0	(338)

Note:
[1] Finland: 'last time in past week or past 24 hours'; France: 'often'; Netherlands: 'once a week or more often'

Finland. It should be noted, however, that in the Netherlands and Finland, the relation is linearly significant. This suggests that although (more frequent) masturbation starts later in women, women in the oldest age category masturbate the least often. Thus, 39.5 per cent, 42.9 per cent, 39.4 per cent, 45.3 per cent and 49.7 per cent of the Dutch women aged 18–19, 20–24, 25–29, 30–39 and 40–49 years, respectively, said that they had never masturbated. There might be a cohort effect for women as well, as suggested by the Finnish data, where 27.6 per cent of the women in the oldest age category said that they had never masturbated in their lives, compared with 16.2 per cent of the women between 20 and 39 years of age.

Level of Sexual Interest

As expected, masturbation frequency is also related to when people started their sexual careers. Late starters generally reported masturbating less frequently than early starters. The number of sexual partners – the second indicator of level of sexual interest – is also positively correlated with masturbation frequency, regardless of the period considered (whole life, past five years or preceding year). However, these trends are not significant in all cases. The pattern is somewhat disrupted by the relatively high masturbation frequencies of respondents who reported no sexual partners. In such cases, masturbation should quite likely be seen as a substitute for sexual intercourse; not having had sexual partners clearly does not imply a lack of sexual interest.

Socio-demographic Factors

As expected, people with higher levels of education reported masturbating more often than people with lower levels of education. This statistically significant trend is seen for men and women in all countries, although upon closer inspection the trend seems to be more curvilinear for the Finns. According to the Finnish data, men and women with a medium level of education tend to masturbate more frequently than men and women with higher or lower levels of education; it is unclear how this should be interpreted.

In the Netherlands it was possible to explore the connections between religiousness and attitudes towards sexuality and masturbation frequency. Both parameters are clearly related to masturbation frequency. Dutch women who belonged to a religious faith and men and women who attended religious services reported masturbating less often than other people, while the highest percentages of both men and women who said that they never masturbated were in the group that attended religious services (25.9 per cent of 81 male 'worshippers' versus 20.4 per cent of 216 male 'non-worshippers', and 54.7 per cent of 159 female 'worshippers' versus 44.3 per cent of 307 female 'non-worshippers'). Restrictive sexual attitudes, which are probably linked closely to being religious, also correlate with lower masturbation frequencies (Spearman rho = 0.33, $p < 0.001$ and 0.37, $p < 0.001$ for men and women, respectively).

Overall, urbanization has a noticeable effect on masturbation frequency, although the percentages do not increase steadily with increasing urbanization in all countries. People who live in rural areas tend to report masturbating less often than people in urban areas across Europe.

Relationship Status

Being in a relationship clearly seems to affect the frequency with which people masturbate. Unfortunately, data on this are available for the Netherlands only. Being in a steady relationship generally seems to prompt people to stop masturbating. For example, 21.1 per cent of the 308 Dutch men and 47.8 per cent of the 467 Dutch women involved in a steady relationship said that they never masturbated, compared with 9.3 per cent of the men and 29.3 per cent of the women without a steady relationship. If being in a relationship does not stop people from masturbating, it will generally decrease the frequency with which people masturbate. The possibility that the opportunity of having sexual contact influences masturbation frequency negatively is suggested by the fact that Dutch respondents living with their steady partners reported masturbating less frequently than those who were not. The same is found for Finnish men and women and French men, although in these cases the groups of people classified as non-cohabiting also included people who were not involved in a steady relationship, thereby increasing the discrepancies between these groups and people living with a steady partner.

Being in a steady relationship also seems to affect masturbation frequency in a different way, for the longer the respondents' steady relationships, the less frequently they masturbated. This can be attributed partly to age, since the longer-lasting the relationship, the higher the mean age of the people involved. The frequency with which people have sex within a steady relationship is statistically related to masturbation frequency. This relationship is clear in the case of French men and Dutch women: if they make love to their partners frequently, they also tend to masturbate more often. This shows that having frequent sex with a steady partner does not 'eliminate' the desire or urge to masturbate. Both behaviours are probably consequences of a stronger sexual desire.

Limitations, Major Findings and Unresolved Issues

It has been possible to identify several common trends as well as a few differences between countries regarding people's sexual practices. Our undertaking was seriously hindered, however, by the diversity of approaches taken in the various studies. Having to adjust the data may have concealed some of the real differences between countries. The fact that it was practically impossible to apply multivariate analyses further limited the possibility of disentangling the various patterns of relations between variables.

Documenting the ways in which researchers have surveyed the topic of sexual practices has been quite instructive. We came across a few interview questions in specific surveys that we thought were somewhat inadequate. In one of the surveys, respondents were asked whether they had *already* engaged in a specific sexual practice. We do not know how respondents interpreted the question. We can imagine, though, that some of them wanted to avoid giving the impression that they were sexually behind the times and answered 'yes' without actually having engaged in the specific practice. In other studies we thought the answer formats were inadequate. This was, for instance, the case where people were asked to report lifetime frequency of masturbation. Usually it will be impossible to express this on a unipolar scale, ranging from never to very often. Some other studies failed to indicate the period about which the respondents had to report the frequency of a specific practice. In general we found that a few questions were too general, resulting in very broad answers and giving the respondent a lot of room for projection. At the other end of the scale, researchers should not expect respondents to be able to answer questions that ask for more details than the person can remember or reconstruct.

It was unclear what prompted the various researchers to adopt specific approaches and time frames. These choices should of course be based on both content and methodological factors. The variety of approaches indicated, however, that some haphazard factors played a role in their decisions as well. We think that these choices have to be made more explicit: Why do we want to know something, and why do we use a specific format?

A major limitation of the data presented here is that they represent reported rather than actual behaviour. Since reporting about sexual behaviour is not a neutral activity, the outcomes were definitely affected. This effect does not necessarily have to be the same for all respondents. The findings themselves – for instance, the observed gap in the frequencies with which men and women in relationships report having sex – suggest that reported behaviour is not identical to actual behaviour. The exact magnitude of the effect, however, is hard to assess. In sexological studies this difficulty is practically impossible to overcome, since observation is not a viable alternative. To improve the validity of sexological studies, it would be worthwhile to get a better understanding of how various factors influence the reporting of sexual behaviours and to find ways to diminish the gap between actual behaviour and reporting about it. Still, we think that it is unlikely that all the observed differences can be attributed exclusively to different reporting biases.

Major Findings

There are several differences between the sexual practices of people in the various countries. Within steady relationships, people in northern European countries report having sex less often than people in southern European countries. It is interesting to see, however, that in southern European countries, where sex-role stereotypes are more vigorously endorsed, men report higher frequencies than women.

While some sexual techniques, such as genital fondling and intercourse, seem to be practised by almost everybody who engages in sex, other techniques, such as oral sex and especially anal sex, are fairly rare. The hierarchies based on the percentages of the population who engage in specific sexual practices do not differ between countries. There are, however, differences between countries in the actual proportions. In general, people in Athens turn out to have a somewhat restricted repertory, while inhabitants of Finland and, to a lesser extent, France seem to have the most diversified experiences.

A more important conclusion seems to be that, although countries do differ in some respects, they have much more in common. The various factors explored in this chapter seem to structure people's sexual practices in identical ways, regardless of the country of residence.

The data show a clear sexual career effect. Although there are differences with respect to the age at which people start to have frequent sex, this frequency subsequently declines as people get older. Part of the sexual career involves gradually acquiring experience in various techniques, although this process seems to stop for most people around the age of 35. Furthermore, some people have a wider range of experiences than others. In general, people who start their sexual careers earlier have a higher frequency of sex with their partners, and end up with a broader range of sexual experiences, than late starters. Earlier starters seem to masturbate more often, too. The relatively high frequency of masturbation reported by people currently without partners suggests that not having a sexual partner should not necessarily be interpreted as a lack of sexual desire.

People's sexual practices also seem to depend upon gender. Men report higher frequencies of sexual contact with their steady partners, are more likely to have ever practised specific sexual techniques, and report having practised the active forms more often than the passive forms. Fewer men than women report that they have never masturbated, while the masturbation frequencies are higher in the case of men than women. Basically, there are three perspectives from which these differences can be explained. First of all, these differences may not necessarily be real but result from differences in reporting behaviour. For men it is more desirable to boast about their sexual accomplishments, while women are expected to be sexually modest. There are indications that this difference in reporting did affect the outcomes. The other two perspectives both assume that the differences are real, but offer completely opposite explanations. The evolutionary approach (Buss, 1994) assumes that men and women have faced different problems of reproduction for millions of years. As a consequence, men and women are psychologically not the same in the realm of sexuality and stronger sex 'drives' and a greater interest in sexual variety are assumed to be typically male. The other approach puts the stress on learning, that is, based on their biological gender, people learn to perform the behaviours that are expected to characterize males and females within a society (Howells, 1986). These sex-role expectations affect sexual behaviour itself, for proponents of this approach claim that people learn that 'sex [is] for men, and women ha[ve] to bear it because they [need] men' (Safilios-Rothschild, 1977, p. 107). According to this learning perspective, sex-role stereotypes have defined men's and womens interest and involvement in love and sex in diametrically opposed directions.

It would be interesting to see to what extent differences in both women's and men's sexual behaviours can be explained by their level of sex-role identification. The finding that the sexuality of women who are involved in paid work does differ from homemakers supports the learning perspective, although the evolutionary approach has never claimed that gender-related behaviours are completely immutable. Both perspectives may contribute to a full understanding of what people do sexually. Given the diversity between countries regarding the social distance between masculine and feminine roles, this topic could be studied very fruitfully from a cross-national perspective.

Next to developmental and gender differences, people's sexual practices seem to be affected by normative factors. At least that is how we interpret the differences related to level of education, religion and place of residence. A larger percentage of people with higher levels of education have practised less common sexual techniques. They also report masturbating more frequently, which might be the result of fewer normative inhibitions to do so. Religious involvement seems to correlate with less sexual variety. This is quite likely the consequence of higher levels of sexual restrictiveness, which are characteristic of almost all Western religious systems. When it comes to place of residence, cities may offer a greater variety of sexual models and more practical opportunities to explore different behaviours than rural habitats. The fact that 'opportunity' plays a role is evident, since living with a partner generally results in more frequent sexual activity than living alone. Finally, whether people are sexually permissive or restrictive will quite likely be both a consequence and a cause of engaging in specific behaviours.

Like others (Laumann *et al.*, 1994), we found differences that should be interpreted as a consequence of changes in the sexual climate over time. The younger age cohorts in the various studies more often reported having ever engaged in several less common sexual practices than the older cohorts.

The import of the various findings for HIV prevention is not obvious. In designing prevention policies one should take into account the various factors that shape human sexuality, for instance, by including them in the targeting of campaigns. Furthermore, this review has revealed the supremacy of vaginal intercourse in the sexual interactions of both men and women. From the perspective of HIV and STD prevention it might be desirable to have people practise a broader range of less risky sexual techniques than vaginal and anal intercourse. Our findings make us wonder, however, how malleable sexual behaviour is. For prevention purposes, encouraging people to make sexual intercourse as safe as possible will probably be the most productive course.

Unresolved Issues

Several issues could not be addressed in this cross-national exploration of people's sexual practices. Although not stated explicitly, the various surveys seemed to be built on the assumption that sexuality is something either two persons do together or people do on their own. Sexual interactions in which three or more persons are involved were addressed in the Finnish and French surveys only. The use of accessories during sex was not addressed at all. Furthermore, sexual practices in interactions of people of the same sex could not be compared.

Another limitation of this exploration is that the prevalence of sexual practices was addressed independently and from a lifetime perspective only. It would be interesting to know whether the various techniques are practised independently or whether the less common ones are always practised as foreplay prior to vaginal intercourse. How are the various techniques combined in a sexual encounter? How do people move from kissing to oral sex? Which 'path' do they take? Furthermore, it is unclear how the less commonly practised techniques come about: Why do people engage in new experiences? Are they introduced to them by a steady or casual partner? Why do people try, stick with, or drop specific practices, and why do some people never engage in specific practices? How do preferences for specific techniques come about? If we assume that several techniques are not appealing by nature, how do people come to appreciate some and reject others?

The labels used for the various techniques might suggest that we were talking about identical behaviours. Even from a physical perspective this does not have to be the case. The issue of who is in which position has not been addressed. With respect to vaginal intercourse, for instance, it would be interesting to know whether positions are fixed or whether people alternate. It is quite possible that people's preferences regarding specific positions might differ as well from one country to the next.

Several studies have looked for correlations between attitudes and specific sexual behaviours. The reasons for engaging in specific activities, which will differ between individuals as well as within individuals, have seldom been addressed. Oral sex, for instance, may be practised as a form of contraception, to express deep intimate feelings or as an alternative for intercourse during pregnancy or when intercourse is painful. Sexual techniques may also be practised out of curiosity or as an experiment. How is the meaning people give to vaginal intercourse related to the meaning of other sexual practices? Are there heterosexual people for whom vaginal intercourse is not indispensable? What is exciting about oral sex, the reward of your partner's pleasure and excitement or something else? How do practices contribute to sexual satisfaction in particular and to well-being in general?

The results of this study make clear that the explanation for sexual variety between people should not be sought on an individual level only. Various social factors contribute to this variety as well. How these factors actually influence sexual behaviour should be studied more extensively. For instance, the precise role of urban life might become clearer if we studied how migration between rural and urban areas affects people's sexual values and behaviours. These questions, whether studied nationally or cross-nationally, seem less relevant from the HIV and STD prevention standpoint. However, prevention in this field can be effective only if the factors constituting sexuality are understood and taken into account.

Notes

1 In the Belgian survey the concept of 'sex' was specified by indicating that it referred to penetrative sex (vaginal, oral, or anal). In the Spanish survey the frequency of the *sex act* was assessed. In Finland and Norway the occurrence of 'sex' in general or 'making love' was not addressed.

2 It is not clear in these cases whether the researchers took exact numbers for specific recent time periods to be averages for longer time periods or were not interested in this, or whether the researchers expected that these deviations would level out for the total group.

3 Two idiosyncratic frequency categories were used in the Belgian and Spanish surveys. In the Belgian study the response category 'sporadically, with periods of

intense activity' was available in the questionnaire as well. The Spanish self-administered questionnaire included the category 'I cannot (impotence)'. The Spanish response categories were exceptional not only because of the inclusion of this category, but also because of the many categories for comparatively rather high frequencies ('5 times a day or more', '2 to 4 times a day' and 'once a day'). One might wonder whether the high frequency categories are indicative of a social norm and whether the presence of the impotence category is related to this.

4   For Finland and Norway only intercourse frequencies were given; no general frequencies of having sex or making love were available.

5   The decision to focus on steady relationships is of course somewhat arbitrary, too, since it is not always clear how long they have already lasted or how 'serious' they are and whether they will continue to exist. Besides this, the operational definitions of steady relationship vary from one study to the next.

6   Due to practical circumstances, the French love-making frequency data for respondents with same-sex partners could not be extracted from the sample.

7   Except for Belgium, since in the Belgian survey people were asked whether they had ever practised a specific technique with their current sexual partners (lifetime occurrence in general was not tackled). For the Dutch sample lifetime occurrence is based on information about current sexual behaviour within the ongoing steady relationship; lifetime data as such were not collected in this survey. Using less comparable indicators was preferred to having fewer countries to compare.

8   The higher frequencies for France and Spain could be a consequence of the fact that for these countries (as well as for Norway) we had data only for people who lived together. People in a relationship who live together might have sex more frequently and consequently increase the average frequency compared with countries where people who do not live together were also included. However, this seems not to be the case. When we compare the average frequencies only for people who live together in the various countries, we get almost exactly the same results. This is in line with the finding that living situation (apart or together) does not have an unequivocal effect on the frequency of having sex in the various countries, as we shall see later.

9   The smaller proportion of people in the Netherlands (compared with Athens and West Germany) who reported ever having had intercourse is explained by the fact that in the Netherlands only data about recent intercourse with the current partner were included.

10 The only exception is West Germany, where women reported having experienced this significantly more often than men.

11 Dutch women are an exception: for them, greater age is predictive of having practised anal sex.

12 The latter was done by inspecting adjusted residuals in rows and in columns in cases where the overall distribution of the variables was not independent (and Chi^2 was significant); we looked for –, +, – and +, –, + patterns in particular.

References

ALLGEIER, A.R. (1994) 'Nymphomania', in BULLOUGH, V.L. and BULLOUGH, B. (Eds) *Human Sexuality: An Encyclopedia*, New York: Garland.

AMERICAN PSYCHIATRIC ASSOCIATION (1994) *Diagnostic and Statistical Manual of Mental Disorders*, 4th. edition (DSM-IV), Washington, DC: American Psychiatric Association.

BLOCH, I. (n. d., presumably 1933) *Anthropological Studies on the Strange Sexual Practices of All Races in All Ages*, New York: Anthropological Press.

BOZON, M. and LERIDON, H. (1996) 'The social construction of sexuality', in BOZON, M. and LERIDON, H. (Eds) *Sexuality and the Social Sciences*, Aldershot: Dartmouth.

BRANDT, A.M. (1987) *No Magic Bullet. A Social History of Venereal Disease in the United States since 1880,* New York: Oxford University Press.

BRUNDAGE, J.A. (1994) 'Canon law and sex', in BULLOUGH, V.L. and BULLOUGH, B. (Eds) *Human Sexuality: An Encyclopedia*, New York: Garland.

BULLOUGH, V.L. (1994) 'Art: painting, sculpture, and other visual art', in BULLOUGH, V.L. and BULLOUGH, B. (Eds) *Human Sexuality: An Encyclopedia*, New York: Garland.

BUSS, D.M. (1994) *The Evolution of Desire. Strategies of Human Mating,* New York: BasicBooks.

COLEMAN, E. (1991) 'Compulsive sexual behaviour: new concepts and treatments', in COLEMAN, E. (Ed.) *John Money: A Tribute*, New York: Haworth Press.

COMFORT, A. (1972) *The Joy of Sex*, New York: Crown.

DAVIS, K.B. (1929) *Factors in the Sex Life of Twenty-two Hundred Women*, New York: Harper and Brothers.

DIRTY COMICS (n.d.) *A History of the Eight Pagers* (n.p.).

FRAZER, S. (1994) 'Anthropology: influence of culture on sex', in BULLOUGH, V.L. and BULLOUGH, B. (Eds) *Human Sexuality: An Encyclopedia*, New York: Garland.

GAGNON, J. (1988) 'Sex research and sexual conduct in the era of AIDS', *Journal of AIDS*, **1**, pp. 593–601.

GAGNON, J.H. and SIMON, W. (1973) *Sexual Conduct*, Chicago: Aldine Publishing Company.

GAGNON, J.H. and SIMON, W. (1987) 'The sexual sampling of orogenital contacts', *Archives of Sexual Behavior*, **16**, pp. 1–25.

GRONEMAN, C. (1995) 'Nymphomania. The historical construction of female sexuality', in TERRY, J. and URLA, J. (Eds) *Deviant Bodies. Critical Perspectives on Difference in Science and Popular Culture*, Bloomington: Indiana University Press.

HART, J., COHEN, E., GINGOLD, A. and HOMBURG, R. (1991) 'Sexual behaviour in pregnancy: a study of 219 women', *Journal of Sex Education and Therapy*, **17**, 1, pp. 86–90.

HOFSTEDE, G. (1991) *Cultures and Organizations. Software of the Mind*, London: Harper Collins.

HOWELLS, K. (1986) 'Sex roles and sexual behaviour', in HARGREAVES, D.J. and COLLEY, A.M. (Eds) *The Psychology of Sex Roles*, London: Harper and Row.

IRVINE, J.M. (1995) 'Regulated passions: the invention of inhibited sexual desire and sexual addiction', in TERRY, J. and URLA, J. (Eds) *Deviant Bodies. Critical Perspectives on Difference in Science and Popular Culture*, Bloomington: Indiana University Press.

JOHNSON, A.M., WADSWORTH, J., WELLINGS, K. and FIELD, J. (1994) *Sexual Attitudes and Lifestyles*, Oxford: Blackwell.

KEARNY, P.J. (1982) *A History of Erotic Literature*, London: Macmillan.

KINSEY, A.C., POMEROY, W.P. and MARTIN, C.E. (1948) *Sexual Behavior in the Human Male*, Philadelphia: W.B. Saunders.

KINSEY, A.C., POMEROY, W.P., MARTIN, C.E. and GEBHARD, P.H. (1953) *Sexual Behavior in the Human Female*, Philadelphia: W.B. Saunders.

KLINE, P. (1987) 'Sexual deviation: psychoanalytic research and theory', in WILSON, G.D. (Ed.) *Variant Sexuality: Research and Theory*, London: Croom Helm.

KRONHAUSEN, P. and KRONHAUSEN, E. (1978) *The Complete Book of Erotic Art*, New York: Bell.

LANE, H.C., HOLMBERG, S.C. and JAFFE, H.W. (1991) 'HIV seroconversion and oral intercourse', *American Joural of Public Health*, **81**, p. 658.

LAUMANN, E.O., GAGNON, J.H., MICHAEL, R.T. and MICHAELS, S. (1994) *The Social Organization of Sexuality. Sexual Practices in the United States*, Chicago: Chicago University Press.

LEVINE, M.P. and TROIDEN, R.R. (1988) 'The myth of sexual compulsivity', *Journal of Sex Research*, **25**, pp. 347–63.

MESSIAH, A. and PELLETIER, A. (1996) 'Partner-specific sexual practices among hetero-sexual men and women with multiple partners: results from the French national survey, ACSF', *Archives of Sexual Behavior*, **25**, 3, pp. 233–47.

OLIVER, M.B. and HYDE, J.S. (1993) 'Gender differences in sexuality: a meta-analysis', *Psychological Bulletin*, **114**, 1, pp. 29–51.

PERSON, E.S. (1987) 'A psychoanalytic approach', in GEER, J.H. and O'DONOHUE, W.T. (Eds) *Theories of Human Sexuality*, New York: Plenum.

POMEROY, W.B., FLAX, C.C. and WHEELER, C.C. (1982) *Taking a Sex History: Interviewing and Recording*, New York: Free Press.

REINHOLTZ, R.K. and MUEHLENHARD, C.L. (1995) 'Genital perceptions and sexual activity in a college population', *Journal of Sex Research*, **32**, 2, pp. 155–65.

REINISCH, J.M., ZIEMBA-DAVIS, M. and SANDERS, S.A. (1990) 'Sexual behavior and AIDS: lessons from art and sex research', in VOELLER, B., REINISCH, J.M. and GOTTLIEB, M. (Eds) *AIDS and Sex. An Integrated Biomedical and Biobehavioral Approach*, New York: Oxford University Press.

RUSBRIDGER, A. (1986) *A Concise History of the Sex Manual*, London: Faber and Faber.

SAFILIOS-ROTHSCHILD, C. (1977) *Love, Sex, and Sex Roles*, Englewood Cliffs: Prentice-Hall.

TOFT, M. and FOWLIE, J. (1969) *Stillinger*, Copenhagen: Stig Vendelkaers Forlag.

VAN DE VELDE, T.H. (1930) *Ideal Marriage, its Physiology and Technique*, New York: Random House.

Chapter 5

The Europeans and Their Sexual Partners

Henri Leridon, Gertjan van Zessen and Michel Hubert*

Introduction

The aim of this chapter is to provide basic comparative information about the numbers of sexual partners reported in the various population surveys recently carried out in Europe. Studying who has sex with whom, and with how many partners, can be done for different purposes and from different perspectives that will not all be explored in this paper.

For prevention, understanding how sexual practices and ways of adapting to HIV risk vary according to the characteristics of the partners (their age, gender, level of education, race, religion, and so on) and the dynamics and social context of their relationships, has become a key issue (Peto *et al.*, 1992; Parker and Gagnon, 1995; Van Campenhoudt *et al.*, 1996). We need to know how the risk of HIV has influenced the relational strategies of individuals and, on the contrary, how relations between partners have been reorganized in the era of AIDS (Giami, 1995). This is particularly important for identifying the riskiest situations and focusing preventive messages on what is really problematic from the point of view of HIV transmission. Few surveys, however (van Zessen and Sandfort, 1991; Marquet, Peto and Hubert *et al.*, 1995; Laumann *et al.*, 1994), have adopted such a 'relational' approach. Therefore cross-national analyses of data cannot be made on a large scale.[1]

Estimating the proportion of the population with a potential risk for HIV infection is another aim for which knowing the number of sexual partners in

*The authors would like to thank Anne Johnson (UC London Medical School), who assisted in the preparation of this chapter and processed specific data analyses from the British National Survey of Sexual Attitudes and Lifestyles (NATSAL). Meni Malliori (Athens University Medical School) also participated in the preparation of this chapter and kindly provided us with the data file from her survey on Partner Relations and Risk of HIV Infection carried out in Athens in 1990.

a population is useful (see also Chapter 6 on risk behaviour and risk contexts). But, for this estimate to be precise, one has to know the prevalence of HIV, the kinds of sexual practices (including protections) people have with each of their partners, and these partners' behaviours. Not much was asked on this last issue in the European surveys because there is a general suspicion that the reliability of answers to questions such as whether a respondent's particular partner has other partners (see Chapter 11), how he/she behaves with these partners (taking more or fewer risks, for instance), what his/her current serological status is, and so on, will be low since these answers may reflect the image the respondent has of his/her partner rather than the partner's actual behaviour. Data on types of partners and partner selection can, however, be used to study sexual network formation, but the methodology is not yet fully developed and including more than three attributes in mathematical models proved to be very complex (van Zessen and Jager, 1994).

Data about sexual partners are also necessary for modelling HIV transmission, although relevant indicators for such an approach have not been sufficiently developed in many population surveys (Catania *et al.*, 1996a). The number of partners seems to be more important than the frequency of sexual contacts between partners (Peterman *et al.*, 1988), possibly because on the one hand infected individuals are not infectious immediately and permanently after infection, and on the other hand some individuals may be more vulnerable to acquiring HIV than others. Actually, what is wanted is not the total number of partners over some period of time, but the number of new partners per unit of time (May and Anderson, 1987). This question was asked in only three of the 13 surveys under study in this chapter (France–ACSF, Great Britain, Switzerland), but it has been shown (Leridon, 1998) that estimates of the number of new partners can be derived from data available on the numbers of partners over two different periods of time (for example five years and twelve months) under conditions of unchanged behaviour over these periods of time. Let us stress here only that the number of new partners in one year must not be confused with either the total number of partners over the same period or the number of current partners (at time of survey). To take an example, in France (ACSF) the three parameters for men aged about 30 were 0.3, 1.3 and 0.9, respectively.

Studies and mathematical modelling of HIV spread have also shown that the variance in the number of partners is an important parameter. In the formulation by May and Anderson (1987; Anderson and May, 1988), the 'reproduction rate' of an epidemic (the number of new infections produced by each infected individual) is proportionate to: $m + (\sigma^2/m)$ where m and σ^2 are the mean and variance, respectively, of new sexual partners per unit of time. Given the same average number of (new) partners per unit of time, the epidemic will develop much faster in a population where a few individuals have a very large number of partners than in a population with a small variance (for instance, when people have no more than two or three partners).

One aspect of this variance problem is the difference between the ages of the two partners: the greater the difference, the more the generations of the two partners overlap and the faster the epidemic will spread through the population (Anderson and May, 1988; Knolle, 1990). This factor will be significant in populations where the age difference between partners is wide, as in many African countries (Brouard, 1994), but in every population some specific subgroups, such as sex workers and their clients, may also contribute to this spreading across generations.

The contribution of the 'outliers' who report a large number of partners and account for a large part of the variance may be significant. It is likely, however, that people who have a large number of partners choose partners who share this characteristic. In the French ACSF survey (1992), for example, 10.2 per cent of the male respondents with at least 10 partners in the last five years thought that their last partner had other partners as against 3.4 per cent of men with fewer than five partners; for the penultimate partner the proportions were respectively 21.1 per cent and 4.3 per cent. One way of addressing this issue in epidemiological studies is to split the population into several groups, each defined by a specific behaviour (the 'compartmental approach') (see, for example, Anderson, 1993; Bongaarts, 1988). One difficulty is that to take the diversity of behaviours fully into account one would need a whole picture of sexual partner selection within a population and the network of all sexual relations between individuals (Anderson *et al.*, 1991; Blanchard, 1993). Such data are not available, and the surveys analyzed here had no such ambition.

In this chapter, the variations in numbers of sexual partners will first be analyzed over different periods of time according to the respondent's and his/her partner(s)' genders. More specifically, the gap between males' and females' declarations will be examined in detail. We shall then concentrate on multiple partnership, because this is a key issue in the context of AIDS. Couples where both man and woman are seronegative and have no sexual relationships with anyone else are not exposed to sexual transmission of HIV. The virus spreads in a population only if some proportion of individuals changes partners over time (or has several partners at the same time) *and* has unprotected sexual intercourse. Unfortunately, it is not possible to isolate in surveys respondents living under such conditions because we do not know much about the partner's sexual activity. We shall tackle this issue by studying the respondents who had two or more partners over different periods of time. By doing this, we do not pretend to grasp all the risky situations (for example some monopartners – people who have had only one sexual partner over a certain period of time – may run more risk because of their partner's multiple relations), nor do we think that all the individuals who have more than one partner are at risk. Characteristics such as age, level of education, place of residence, cohabitation status (currently living with a sexual partner) and relational status (involvement in a steady relationship for more than one year) will be examined in detail. Males' experiences of commercial sex will also be studied.

The Data Used

The number and type of wording of the questions about sexual partners in surveys gives a good idea of how relations between partners are represented in a society. As Giami (1995) showed, what is new in the sex surveys that have been carried out in France in the era of AIDS – but this can be extended to most surveys in Europe – is that conjugality is no longer the main dimension used to define partners and relationships, nor is heterosexuality self-evident.

Most of the surveys included questions on the numbers of partners. Ten surveys asked about the total number of partners over life, but only half of them asked for the partner's gender as well. The situation regarding the number of partners over the last 12 months is comparable (the numbers of homo- and heterosexual partners are available separately in Belgium, France–ACSF, Great Britain, Netherlands and Norway). Some surveys referred to other periods of time, for example last five years, three years, or two years; last two months, or four weeks. The number of current partners was also sometimes asked for. Since all these data cannot be compared on a large scale, we shall concentrate in this chapter on the number of partners over life and in the last 12 months (with a brief glance at the last five years).

Referring to the same periods of time is not enough to ensure full comparability of the data between countries. The wording of questions is also a crucial issue. The way interviewees were asked how many partners they had during a certain period of time was similar in all surveys. The question wording was: 'How many different people [or 'men/women' in surveys where this information was collected separately] have you had sex [or 'intercourse' or 'sexual intercourse'] with in your life [or 'five years' or any other period of time]?' The only exception was the Swiss survey, where the question was: 'How many people have you slept with?' A count of the total number of partners over a certain period of time was asked of the respondent him/herself,[2] with several surveys (Belgium, France–ACSF, Great Britain, Netherlands, Norway) stressing the importance of including all partners, that is the spouse or co-habitant as well as casual partners. Three surveys (Belgium, France–ACSF, Netherlands) stressed, before asking for an overall count, that sex workers and prostitutes were also partners.

The main inter-survey differences in question wordings are differences in what is meant by 'having sex' (see Table 5.1). Exact descriptions of the kind of sexual practices requested for counting a partner as a 'sexual partner' were offered in three of the 11 surveys, namely, Belgium, Finland and Great Britain. Having sex was defined in these surveys as practising either oral, vaginal or anal penetration. In the Finnish survey stimulating the genitals by hand was also presented as a kind of sexual intercourse. In the eight other surveys no explicit definition was given, although specific questions on sexual practices such as oral sex or mutual masturbation were asked in the questionnaire. In the French ACSF survey these specific questions were asked before the questions

Table 5.1 *Wording of the main survey questions on partners and sexual activity*

Country	Partner	Sexual activity
Athens–PR (90)	1. 'I am now going to ask you questions about your husband [wife] and/or "regular partner". By a "regular partner", I mean a person (a man or a woman) with whom you had sex for more than one year. He or she could be someone with whom you had sex for less than one year but with whom you intend to continue having sex. He [she] may be your husband [wife]; he or she may be someone you live with; or be someone who does not live in the same house' 4. 'How many different people have you had sex with in your life?'	[No explicit definition of sexual intercourse] 2. 'Have you ever had sexual intercourse? If NO, I mean have you ever had oral sex, anal sex, or vaginal sex? (Yes/No).' 3. [Sexual orientation]
Belgium (93)	3. 'We are now going to speak about the people with whom you have (or have had) sex. Please understand that in speaking about 'sex partners' we mean both the person with whom you may be living as well as other regular or chance partners. For example, prostitutes are also sex partners. 4. 'With how many people of the opposite sex [then of the same sex] have you had sex in the past 12 months?'	1. 'By "sex" we mean intimate contact with (vaginal, anal, or oral) penetration.' 2. 'Have you already had intimate contact without penetration?'
Finland (92)	[Definitions given to read] 1. 'Steady relationship: a regular relationship (marriage, cohabitation or a relationship with partners living apart)' 2. 'Partner: a steady or temporary sexual partner' 5. 'Sexual relationship: a relationship involving intercourse' [Questions]. 6. 'Altogether, in your life so far, with how many partners have you had intercourse?' 7. 'Which of the following experiences have you had with a sexual partner of the same sex? (Arousing fondling without touching genitals, stimulation of genitals by hand or by mouth, anal intercourse).'	[Other definitions] 3. 'Sexual intercourse: a man's penis entering a woman's vagina.' 4. 'Intercourse: sexual interaction in vaginal, oral or anal intercourse or stimulation by hand.'

Table 5.1 *(cont.)*

Country	Partner	Sexual activity
France–ACSF (92)	5. 'We are now going to talk about the people with whom you have had sexual intercourse. This involves the person with whom you live as well as other regular partners. Prostitutes are also sexual partners.' 6. 'All in all, in your lifetime, how many women [men] have you had sex with?' 7. 'Now I am going to ask questions about the last person you had sexual intercourse with.' 8. 'Would you call him/her your "main partner"?'	*[No explicit definition of sexual intercourse]* 1. 'Have you ever had sexual intercourse?' 2. (*Probe: if NO*) 'Have you ever made love or had sex?' 3. *[Sexual orientation]* 4. 'Have you ever [...] engaged in the following sexual activities?' (*masturbation, licking of genitals or anus, penis entering anus . . .*) 9. *[Same questions for last sexual intercourse]*
West Germany (90)	1. 'I am now going to ask you questions about your spouse and/or "regular partner". By a "regular partner", I mean a person (a woman or a man) with whom you have had sex for more than one year. She or he could be someone with whom you had sex for less than one year but with whom you intend to continue having sex. She or he may be your spouse; she or he may be someone you live with; or someone who does not live in the same house.' 2. 'How many different people have you had sex with in the last 12 months?'	3. 'The following is a list of things that people do when they are having sex (*Use colloquial terms*). Tell me if you have ever done it' (*Kissing, licking of genitals, penis in mouth, vagina or anus*)
Great-Britain (91)	*[Definitions given to read:]* 1. 'Partners: people who have sex together – whether just once, or a few times, or as regular partners, or as married partners.' *[Cont.:2]*	*[Other definitions]* 2. 'Genital area: a man's penis or woman's vagina – that is, the sex organs. 3. Vaginal sexual intercourse: a man's penis entering a woman's vagina.

9. 'These questions are about the number of people you have had sex with at different times in your life. Please include everyone you have ever had sex with, whether it was just once, a few times, a regular partner or your wife/husband.'

10. [*Men*] 'Altogether, in your life so far, with how many women have you had sexual intercourse (vaginal, oral or anal)?'

10. [*For women*] 'Altogether, in your life so far, with how many men have you had sexual intercourse (vaginal, oral or anal)?'

11. [*Men*] 'Altogether, in your life so far, with how many men have you had sex (that is oral, anal or other forms of genital contact?)'

11. [*For women*] 'Altogether, in your life so far, with how many women have you had sex (that is oral sex or other forms of genital contact)?'

Netherlands (89)

3. 'A steady relationship is one where you see someone at least once a week and sexual contacts takes (took) place regularly. One needn't be married or living together. (*If the respondent hesitates because the relationship has just begun, it's considered a steady relationship when there is a mutual intention to continue to see each other for a longer period of time.*)'

4. 'Have you had sexual contact during the past year? (*If necessary, probe in case of denial*)' [*See 5*] '*Take your time and probe if necessary. E.g.: suggest vacation contacts, one-time/one-off contacts, prostitution, contacts with men and women.*'

6. 'How many were that in total [*number of men, number of women*]?'

4. Oral sex (oral sexual intercourse): a man's or a woman's mouth on partner's genital area.

5. Anal sex (anal sexual intercourse): a man's penis entering a partner's anus (rectum or back passage).

6. Genital contact NOT involving intercourse: forms of contact with the genital area NOT leading to intercourse (vaginal, oral or anal), but intended to achieve orgasm; for example, stimulating by hand.

7. Any sexual contact or experience: this is a wider term and can include just kissing or cuddling, not necessarily leading to genital contact or intercourse.' [*End of definitions*]

8. [*For men*] 'When, if ever, was the last occasion you had sex with a woman? This means vaginal intercourse, oral sex, anal sex'.

8. [*For women*] 'When, if ever, was the last occasion you had sex with a man? This means vaginal intercourse, oral sex, anal sex'.

12. [*Sexual orientation*]

1. [*Questions on first time 'fell in love', 'petted', 'had sexual intercourse'*]

2. [*Sexual orientation*]

5. [*For sexual partners over past year*] 'Sexual contact here is at least touching the genitals of the other person (the other/yourself being jacked off or fingered).'

Table 5.1 (*cont.*)

Country	Partner	Sexual activity
Norway (92)	3. 'How many sexual partners have you had altogether until now? (Including spouse/cohabitant if applicable)'	[*No explicit definition of sexual intercourse*] 1. 'Have you ever had sexual intercourse?' 2. 'Have you ever had any form of sexual contact with a person of your own sex?' 4. [*Questions on 'oral sex (i.e. penis in mouth)' and anal sex*]
Portugal (91)	1. 'I am going to ask you questions about your wife [husband] and/or "regular partner". By a "regular partner", I mean a person (a woman or a man) with whom you have had sex for more than one year. She or he could be someone with whom you had sex for less than one year but with whom you intend to continue having sex. She [he] may be your wife [husband]; she or he may be someone you live with; or be someone who does not live in the same house.' 3. 'How many different people have you had sex with in your life?'	[*No explicit definition of sexual intercourse*] 2. 'Have you ever had sexual intercourse?' 4. [*Sexual practices*]
Spain (92)	2. 'During your lifetime, how many people do you remember having had sexual relations with?'	[*No explicit definition of sexual intercourse*] 1. [*Sexual orientation*] 3. [*Sexual practices*]
Switzerland (92)	1. 'What is the situation in which you are living? (*Lives with husband/wife; lives alone – no steady relationship; lives alone with steady heterosexual relationship; lives alone with steady homosexual relationship; lives with heterosexual partner; lives with homosexual partner*)' 2. 'Have you ever slept with anyone (other than your steady partner) on the spur of the moment?' 3. 'With how many partners in the past six months?' 4. 'With how many partners in your whole life?'	[*No explicit definition of sexual intercourse*]

Note: The numbers refer to the order in which the questions appear in the questionnaire

on numbers of partners. In the Dutch survey no explicit definition was given of sexual intercourse when age at first intercourse with someone of the opposite sex was asked, but this question came just after the age at which the respondent fell in love and petted for the first time; when it came to 'sexual contact' with someone of the same sex or anyone other than the steady partner (for example number of partners during the last 12 months), it was defined extensively as 'at least touching the genitals of the other person (the other person/yourself being jacked off or fingered)'. In Athens–PR 1990, a definition (oral, vaginal or anal penetration) was given only to the respondents who answered 'no' to the question 'Have you ever had sexual intercourse?'

We believe that these differences in definitions may lead to differences across countries in reported numbers of partners. Logically, these numbers should be slightly smaller in surveys where no definition was given because some respondents might have felt they were not allowed to declare as sexual partners people with whom they had oral sex only, without vaginal or anal penetration, while they should be slightly higher in surveys where stimulation by hand was explicitly defined as sexual intercourse. But things are probably not so clear-cut and may work differently for men and women. It depends also on the different meanings 'having sex' has in the different European cultures. From this point of view, 'having sex' is probably too rough a translation of terms such as 'having sexual intercourse', 'having sexual relations' or 'making love' that are used more often in other languages.

In most surveys, a distinction is made between 'regular', 'steady' or 'main' partners and other partners ('occasional', 'casual') and specific questions are asked accordingly. In a few surveys (Belgium, Great Britain, France–ACSF) this distinction was not put to the respondents explicitly, but can be reconstructed on the basis of the qualification the respondent is asked to give about each of his/her relationships (status, duration, and so on).

In all countries, a few respondents reported a very large number of partners, especially over life. The means are sometimes strongly influenced by these few cases, and the comparability of the data between countries can be affected. This is why, in addition to the means, we provide the medians and maxim. Finally, the last table in the chapter (Table 5.12) shows the means for people reporting fewer than 20 partners over life. We preferred to keep the original distributions (even for the computation of the means), instead of defining an arbitrary ceiling (such as 200 partners), because some of the large answers will be realistic (individuals who actually had a very large number of partners) and some may be overstated, and we have no way to distinguish between these two categories. The problem of the tails is, at least in part, real and cannot be eliminated simply by truncating the distributions.

Data on paying for sex is also available in a majority of surveys. We included here only the surveys with data on lifetime and previous year's experience of paying for sex. These data were culled from questions such as 'Have you ever paid money for sex with a man (or with a woman)?' (Great Britain), 'Have you ever paid anyone in exchange for sexual contacts?'

(Netherlands, Norway), 'Have you ever used male or female prostitution?' (Spain), or 'Have you ever had contacts with a prostitute or visited a massage parlour?' (Switzerland). Sometimes the question was not limited to the exchange of money but also included 'gifts, favours or economic advantages' (Finland, West Germany, Netherlands, Portugal). The French survey (ACSF) included paying or being paid for sex in the same question, but the first category is very likely to be larger than the second one, since sex workers were almost absent from the sample.

The 'no answers' have been left out as missing values in all tables. Their numbers were small but usually higher among men than women and in surveys where the questions on partners were self-administered. In questions on sexual orientation over life the 'no answer' rates (for both genders) were less than or equal to 1 per cent in eight out of 10 surveys and close to 4 per cent in two surveys (Finland and Great Britain). These rates were higher for sexual orientation over the last 12 months, ranging from 0 to 7.8 per cent for men and from 0.1 to 9.5 per cent for women. The ranges were also rather large for the various questions on numbers of partners (from about 0 to 8 per cent for men and 0 to 6 per cent for women), with rather similar 'no answer' rates for lifetime and last 12 months despite the difficulties of recall that one could expect for the lifetime data. No answers to the sex for money questions were consistently below 5 per cent.

Confidence intervals will not be given in the cells, which are too numerous in most tables. The 95 per cent confidence interval can be estimated by the usual formula:

$$p \pm 1.96 \left[p(1-p)/N \right]^{1/2},$$

or, for the French – ACSF survey, due to sample design specificities:

$$p \pm 1.96 \left[2p(1-p)/N \right]^{1/2}.$$

Partners and Gender

Sexual Experience and Orientation over Life

Sexual experience is almost universal in all populations investigated, for by the age of 30 or 35, nearly 100 per cent of the male and female respondents reported some previous sexual experience. When we look at the breakdown by age and gender (table not shown), the proportion reporting previous sexual experience approaches 100 per cent for at least some generations (often a majority of those aged 30 or more) in all countries except West Germany.

Table 5.2 shows the overall proportions of persons (aged 18 to 49) who reported never having sex at all in the various surveys. A high rate might mean either that a significant proportion of the population remains sexually inactive over life (this seems to be the case in the West German survey), or, more frequently, that the first experience happens later than in other countries. This is especially true for women in Athens, Portugal and Switzerland, since all women aged 35 in these countries had been sexually active. In addition, in the Swiss survey, where the upper age limit was 45 years, the youngest age group – who never had sex – made up a larger proportion of the sample than in the other surveys, which may have skewed the data somewhat. Data from Chapter 2 on sexual initiation confirm late entry into sexual life for women in Portugal and Athens: 51 per cent of the female respondents aged 25–29 at time of survey in Portugal, 58 per cent in Athens, and 70 per cent in Switzerland reported having had their first intercourse, compared with from 75 to 95 per cent in the other countries.

Table 5.2 also shows experience of homosexual sex (this topic is explored in more detail in Chapter 3). Men reported partners of the same sex much more frequently than women did, the only exception being West Germany (1990 survey). In all countries, respondents who reported exclusively homosexual relationships were only a minority of all those reporting some homosexual experience. This finding is consistent across countries. One explanation of the discrepancy between the two rates is that homosexual experiences are often concentrated in adolescence or the early part of adult life, and that these relations either cease or continue in parallel to heterosexual life thereafter. An alternative or complementary explanation is that some individuals may start with heterosexual experiences, are perhaps ambivalent as to their sexual preferences for part of their life, and later decide to switch to strict homosexuality. These two assumptions might be tested by comparing the prevalence of homosexual activity in the recent past (last 12 months, for instance) and over life: if the former rate is much lower than the latter, we could conclude that homosexual experiences happened mainly in the rather remote past; if the difference is rather small, then the second assumption would be more valid. Table 5.8 shows that the first hypothesis is supported more in Belgium, the Netherlands and Norway, and the second one in France and, above all, Great Britain.

Fewer than 1 per cent of males reported homosexual partners exclusively (over life) in all surveys except West Germany, the Netherlands and Finland (with a high of 2.7 per cent in this country). From 1 to 5 per cent of the respondents reported bisexual experience in all the surveys except those in the Netherlands and Finland, where the rates were in the 6 to 10 per cent range. The higher reported rates of bisexuality in these two countries are probably partly due to a broader definition of sexual relations, and hence of sexual partners, for in most surveys a sexual relation explicitly or implicitly

Table 5.2 *Sexual experience (hetero-, homo- and bisexuality) over life*

	Athens PR 1990	Belgium[1] 1993	Finland 1992	France ACSF[2] 1992	Germany West 1990	Great Britain[2] 1991	Netherlands 1989	Norway 1992	Portugal 1991	Switzerland[3] 1992
MEN										
No sex at all	5.3	6.5	3.4	4.9	8.2	4.2	6.2	7.7	5.1	7.0
Hetero partners only	93.2	87.8	87.8	92.2	87.8	91.6	82.1	87.5	94.0	88.4
Homo partners only	0.1	0.8	2.7	0.4	1.2	0.4	2.2	0.5	0.1	n.a.
Partners of both sexes	1.3	4.8	6.1	2.5	2.8	3.8	9.6	4.3	0.8	4.4[3]
N	816	1328	787	6533	1126	6408	418	1787	1223	1337
WOMEN										
No sex at all	8.0	5.7	3.5	6.5	10.0	3.3	3.7	4.2	14.4	7.0
Hetero partners only	91.5	92.0	89.0	91.8	85.8	94.8	91.9	92.1	84.8	93.0[4]
Homo partners only	0.0	0.3	1.4	0.1	0.7	0.1	0.0	0.2	0.5	n.a.
Partners of both sexes	0.5	1.9	6.2	1.6	3.5	1.9	4.4	3.5	0.4	n.a.
N	960	1479	742	7462	1279	8048	571	2242	1245	1312

Base: all respondents (18–49 years), except Switzerland (18–45 years)
Notes:
[1] Belgium: the category 'partners of both sexes' might be slightly overestimated because of possible misunderstanding by respondents of the answer categories
[2] France and Great Britain: the proportions of people reporting homosexual experience are based only on the numbers of partners reported, and differ from the published data (which used other information from the questionnaire that resulted in higher estimates)
[3] The category 'partners of both sexes' includes also 'homosexual partners only'
[4] Percentage of women who ever had sex (no information on the gender of the partner)

implied vaginal, anal or oral penetration, whereas the definition of sexual relations in the Dutch and Finnish surveys was extended to include stimulation by hand. The country-to-country rate differentials might also result, in part, from the differences in 'no answer' rates, if the probability of no answer was related to actual behaviour. Actually, the 'no answer' rates ranged from 0 (the Netherlands and West Germany) to 4.3 per cent (Finland). The two extremes were indicated by the countries where the estimates of homosexual experience are the highest. Consequently, the effect of no answers does not seem to be significant.

The rates of bisexuality reported by women were roughly half of those of men, except in West Germany and Finland. Exclusive homosexuality is rare (under 1 per cent), except in Finland (1.4 per cent) but the difference is not statistically significant. Finland also recorded the highest value for female bisexuality (6.2 per cent), which is significantly different from the rates reported in the other countries, which ranged from 0 to 4.4 per cent (the Netherlands). Thus, the same two countries emerge again from the pack, for the reason already given above.

On the whole, the prevalence of homosexual experience recorded in these surveys (as well as in the United States) is below the widely held expectations of one in ten adults that were based on the Kinsey report findings (which did not derive from a representative sample of the population). Actually, it would be better to speak of guesses rather than expectations, since the proportions derived from the surveys used here are often the first estimates from a representative sample for each country. These estimates are probably minima, since reporting of homosexual behaviour depends on the respondent's ability to accept and assert his/her sexual identity in a social context where this behaviour is not always legitimate. This is why the self-reported rate of homosexuality rises when a survey question is enhanced by an introduction that presents homosexuality in a more favourable light or as common behaviour (Catania *et al.*, 1996b).

Number of Lifetime Partners

As Table 5.3 shows, the arithmetic means and even the distributions of the total numbers of partners in lifetime are remarkably consistent between countries for each gender (the figures in this table refer to all relations, both homo- and heterosexual). For males, the average number of reported partners is close to 12 in four countries. The higher value for the Netherlands (19.7) is due to a small number of individuals reporting several thousand same-sex partners. When the class '200+' (which accounts for one per cent of the male population, or twice as much as in most of the other surveys) is removed, the mean comes much closer to those of other countries. No detailed distribution

Table 5.3   *Lifetime numbers of partners (both genders)*

No. of partners	Finland 1992	France ACSF 1992	Great Britain 1991	Netherlands 1989	Norway 1992	Spain[1] 1992	Switzerland 1992
of MEN
0	4.3	5.4	4.2	6.3	8.2	6.2	7.5
1	12.4	17.6	17.9	16.8	17.6	20.2	15.7
2	8.0	8.3	10.4	9.2	7.6		6.6
3–4	14.4	14.2	19.0	18.5	14.3	33.9	14.8
5–9	16.2	14.7	21.4	18.5	19.4		19.2
10–19	20.8	22.2	14.9	12.7	15.5	27.1	19.8
20–49	18.8	13.1	9.6	13.1	12.6	12.6	11.5
50–199	4.3	3.9	2.4	3.9	4.4		4.6
200+	0.8	0.5	0.3	1.0	0.5		0.2
N	741	6495	6409	411	1684	436	1273
Median	n.a.	5	5	4	5	n.a.	5
Mean	*ab.15*	12.0	11.7	19.7	11.9	*ab.10*	11.7
S.D.	n.a.	31.5	106.8	150.9	27.1	n.a.	28.9
Maximum	n.a.	1001	5000	3000	600	n.a.	999
of WOMEN
0	6.3	6.9	3.3	3.7	4.5	12.5	6.5
1	20.8	38.0	36.3	35.2	26.3	44.4	25.5
2	11.9	14.8	17.5	19.1	12.0		13.4
3–4	20.4	16.1	20.1	21.9	18.2	27.2	23.0
5–9	22.8	12.9	14.8	12.4	22.2		16.7
10–19	11.7	8.3	5.9	4.4	12.3	10.9	10.4
20–49	5.1	2.7	1.9	2.3	4.0	5.0	4.5
50–199	0.8	0.4	0.2	0.9	0.4		0.1
200+	0.1			0.2	0.1		
N	725	7433	8049	571	2117	423	1253
Median	n.a.	2	2	2	3	n.a.	3
Mean	*ab.6*	3.8	3.8	6.0	5.6	*ab.5*	4.7
S.D.	n.a.	6.9	12.0	50.7	11.7	n.a.	6.5
Maximum	n.a.	500	1000	1200	300	n.a.	96

Base: all respondents (18–49 years) except Switzerland (18–45 years)
Notes:
General: the proportions of the first line ('0 partner') may differ from the percentages 'never sex at all' given in Table 5.2, because of non-responses to the question on number of partners
[1] Spain: categories are 0, 1, 2–5, 6–20 and 21+ partners

is available for the Spanish survey data, but the mean number of partners is likely to be slightly below the European average (around 10). In contrast, the mean for Finland is likely to be higher (around 15). The medians are five in all countries except the Netherlands, where it is four.

A minority of men – between one-fifth and one-eighth of male survey respondents – reported exactly one sexual partner over life. The percentages of men reporting five or more partners are close to 50 per cent in most surveys, with again the two exceptions of Spain (40 per cent) and Finland (60 per cent).

For females, the means (and the medians) are roughly half of those for men, sometimes even less. The means range from 3.8 to 6.0, and the missing values for Spain and Finland are likely to fall within these limits. The medians are all equal to two or three. Only a minority of women reported exactly one partner over life. Paradoxically, the number of women reporting five or more partners was more variable than among men, ranging from 16 per cent in Spain to 40 per cent in Finland and Norway.

A way of measuring the distance between the means for men and for women is to express the value for women as a percentage of the value for men. In France, Great Britain and the Netherlands, this ratio is close to 30 per cent; in the other countries, it is between 40 and 47 per cent. This large gender difference in the numbers of partners (lifetime) calls for an explanation. In principle, if sexual contacts abroad are discounted, the means should be equal if the samples are representative of both populations and if all partners are of the opposite sex. We shall see in the next section that restricting the reference group to heterosexual partners does not narrow the gap greatly. The minimum age for inclusion in the surveys – 18 years for both genders – might explain some of the difference as follows: since usually men have younger female partners, those aged 18–20 years (or above) may report relationships with younger women (under 18) who are not included in the samples. However, a check on the Dutch data (where the age of the partners are known) has shown that the gap is not reduced when the partners whose age is not within the sample's range are excluded (data not shown).

Paying for sex may offer another source of bias. Men use sex workers much more frequently than women do. On the other hand, professional sex workers are not likely to be represented in the surveys, as a result of which these relations are likely to be underestimated on the female side of the surveys. However, using survey data and estimates of the frequency of paying for sex in the population of Paris, Lagrange (1991) concluded that the bias due to the under-reporting of these relationships by men was likely to be more important than the bias due to the under-representation of sex workers in the sample. A similar conclusion had also been reached by Smith (1988) using US data. What, then, can explain this pattern? We shall come back to this issue later.

Heterosexual and Homosexual Partners

A few surveys asked respondents for the number of partners of each gender. When we take heterosexual partnerships only into account, the means are lowered only slightly for men, and almost unaffected for women (Table 5.4). This holds true for the standard deviations as well. Similar computations for homosexual relationships lead to very low values because the proportions of

Table 5.4 *Lifetime numbers of heterosexual partners*

No. of heterosexual partners	France ACSF 1992	Great Britain 1991	Norway 1992
of MEN			
N	6551	6414	1684
Median	5	4	5
Mean	11.5	10.4	11.7
S.D.	29.3	84.0	25.0
Maximum	1000	4574	600
of WOMEN			
N	7777	8049	2116
Median	2	2	3
Mean	3.8	3.7	5.5
S.D.	6.7	12.0	10.8
Maximum	500	1000	299

Base: all respondents (18–49 years)

people reporting homosexual partners are always small. It is thus more efficient to base the statistics on all individuals having had at least one homosexual partner. These calculations are shown in Table 5.5.

For male respondents, the means numbers of partners are much higher for the 'bisexual' than purely heterosexual respondents in France and Great Britain (strictly speaking, these figures would compare better with the numbers of heterosexual partners for men reporting at least one partner in this category, but the figures in Table 5.4 would be changed very little by such a condition). The low mean for Norway is due to the fact that exclusive homosexuality was proportionately less frequent in this country than in the other two (see Table 5.2) for as a rule in this series of countries the largest numbers of partners were usually reported by a fraction of the population with homosexual experience only.

The situation is different for women, for the mean number of homosexual partners reported by women declaring same-sex experience is lower than the average number of heterosexual partners in the whole female population, regardless of the country.

Number of Partners in Last Five Years and Last 12 Months

The lifetime number of partners does not yield information on recent behaviour, except for the youngest segment of the population. Most surveys also

Table 5.5 *Lifetime numbers of homosexual partners*

No. of homosexual partners	Finland 1992	France ACSF 1992	Great Britain[1] 1991	Norway[2] 1992
of MEN				
% reporting at least one homo partner	8.8	2.9	4.2	4.8
N	34	199	249	71
Median	n.a.	3	2	2
Mean	n.a.	17.2	35.3	4.9
S.D.	n.a.	63.5	321.8	12.3
Maximum	178	1001	5000	100
of WOMEN				
% reporting at least one homo partner	7.6	1.7	2.0	3.7
N	35	156	153	78
Median	n.a.	2	1	1
Mean	n.a.	2.8	2.0	4.6
S.D.	n.a.	2.8	2.3	12.6
Maximum	8	25	20	90

Base: those (of each gender) who ever reported a homosexual partner (except first row where the base is all respondents)
Notes:
General: values of the first line come from Table 5.2
[1] Great Britain: mean influenced (approximately doubled) by a few individuals with many partners
[2] Norway: for homosexuals, total number of partners (both sexes)

focused on various time periods before the survey. The choice of the 'best' reference period is not easy. On one hand, we may think that the shorter the period, the more reliable the recall; on the other hand, too short a period will not yield much information, because the average number of partners will be close to one! Consequently, two periods are often used: five years and twelve months.

For three out of the four surveys including questions on the number of partners over the last five years (Belgium, France, and Great Britain), the means (computed on those who ever had sex) are remarkably consistent, ranging from 3.1 to 3.7 for men and from 1.5 to 1.8 for women (data not shown). In the fourth country, the Netherlands, the means are a little higher, that is, 4.4 and 3.1 respectively, with the latter figure resulting from a couple of 'outliers' (sex workers) in the sample. The relative difference between the answers of men and women is still high (the mean for women is roughly half of the mean for men), but the absolute difference is rather small. The gap is found mainly among the younger individuals; above the age of about 30, the reported means are much more consistent. As an example, let us consider the case of France. Men aged 25 reported a mean of 5.0 partners in the past five years versus 2.1 reported by women of the same age; the means were 2.6 and 1.5, respectively, at the age of 35, and 1.8 and 1.4, respectively, at the age of 45. Both absolute and relative distances decreased markedly. We will show that the distance is even smaller when a shorter time frame is used (12 months).

Most respondents who had already started their sexual lives reported a partner over the last five years: fewer than 2 per cent (of men or women) reported no sexual activity during that period. About 40 per cent of the male and fewer than 30 per cent of the female respondents reported more than one partner over this period. The data usually did not allow for separating concurrent partners from successive ones, but when that was feasible, the majority of partnerships appeared to be successive, especially among young people. For instance, in the French survey, only 2.2 per cent among the men aged 20–24 reported more than one current partner, whereas 25.2 per cent mentioned more than one partner over the last 12 months and 19.1 per cent reported more than one new partner during the same period.

Table 5.6 shows the distributions and means of partners over the last 12 months. The means range from 1.3 to 1.9 for men and from 1.0 to 1.4 for women. Both the country-to-country and male/female variations are much smaller for this time frame than for longer reference periods. Some differences in the distributions are, however, statistically significant. The relative number of men reporting no sexual partner in the previous year, for instance, varied from about 1 per cent (Athens and Finland) to 7.4 per cent (the Netherlands). These differences might be due in part to variations in the effectiveness with which each survey included respondents with no sexual activity in the past or distinguished between a sexual partner and a cohabiting partner (especially for older respondents).

The number of people reporting more than one partner in the past year is a very important figure in the context of AIDS. This is often the definition taken for 'multipartnership' and, as mentioned in the introduction, this number can be used to derive estimates of the number of new partners over the same period. In Finland, Spain and Portugal, the 'multipartnership' rate was quite high for men, about one-third of whom reported two or more partners. Finland and Spain also reported high multipartnership rates for women (17 per cent). Among the other countries, the rate varied from 11 to 19 per cent for men and from 2 to 8 per cent for women, with Norway holding the middle ground. The role of homosexual partnerships in these results is shown in Table 5.8.

As shown above for longer durations, restricting the analysis to hetero-sexual partners only does not change the means much (Table 5.7). For homosexual partnerships, the results shown in Table 5.8 once again take into account only those reporting at least one such relation over life. Two contrast-

Table 5.6 Numbers of partners over last 12 months

No. of partners	Athens PR 1990	Belgium 1993	Finland 1992	France ACSF 1992	Germany West 1990	Great Britain 1991	Netherlands 1989	Norway 1992	Portugal 1991	Spain[1] 1992	Switzerland[2] 1992
of MEN											
0	1.2	1.9	0.7	4.1	3.0	5.6	7.4	5.5	3.7	3.7	3.7
1	87.8	81.9	70.0	80.4	85.1	77.4	74.0	73.6	63.1	62.8	80.6
2	5.7	6.9	12.5	8.9	4.8	9.6	8.7	10.1	15.0	26.9	6.6
3–4	3.4	6.1	9.9	4.2	3.4	5.1	5.4	7.0	12.9		6.3
5–9	1.2	2.1	4.4	1.6	2.8	1.7	2.8	3.0	3.8	6.6	2.0
10–19	0.1	0.9	2.0	0.5	0.6	0.4	0.8	0.6	1.2		0.4
20–49	0.5	0.2	0.6	0.1	0.2	0.1	1.0	0.1	0.2		0.3
50–199	0.0	0.0	0.0	0.0	0.1	0.0	0.0	0.1	0.1		0.1
200+	0.0	0.0	0.0	0.0	0.0	0.0	0.0	0.0	0.0		0.0
% 2+	11.0	16.2	29.3	15.5	11.9	17.0	18.6	20.9	33.2	33.5	15.7
N	755	1247	706	6229	971	6162	392	1540	1106	409	1132
Median	1	1	1	1	1	1	1	1	1	n.a.	1
Mean	1.3	1.4	1.9	1.4	1.4	1.4	1.5	1.5	1.8	n.a.	1.5
S.D.	2.2	1.8	2.6	4.1	2.4	7.1	3.1	3.4	2.6	n.a.	2.8
Maximum	40	30	30	211	52	500	41	120	50	n.a.	64
of WOMEN											
0	1.3	4.1	1.3	4.7	1.2	5.8	7.4	4.0	7.1	7.0	2.2
1	97.2	90.0	81.1	88.3	93.6	86.5	85.1	83.3	88.0	75.9	91.5
2	1.2	4.3	8.2	5.1	3.1	5.5	4.9	7.3	3.3	13.8	4.5
3–4	0.2	1.2	6.1	1.4	1.5	1.9	1.8	3.9	1.1		1.5
5–9	0.1	0.3	2.8	0.4	0.5	0.3	0.5	1.2	0.2	3.2	0.4
10–19	0.0	0.1	0.5	0.1	0.1	0.0	0.0	0.2	0.2		0.0
20–49	0.0	0.0	0.0	0.0	0.0	0.0	0.2	0.0	0.0		0.0
50–199	0.0	0.0	0.0	0.0	0.0	0.0	0.0	0.0	0.0		0.0
200+	0.0	0.0	0.0	0.0	0.0	0.0	0.0	0.0	0.0		0.0
% 2+	1.5	5.9	17.5	7.0	5.2	7.7	7.5	12.7	4.9	17.0	6.4
N	843	1387	673	7067	1110	7801	551	2045	1039	370	1102
Median	1	1	1	1	1	1	1	1	1	n.a.	1
Mean	1.0	1.0	1.4	1.1	1.1	1.1	1.1	1.3	1.0	n.a.	1.1
S.D.	0.3	0.6	1.3	0.6	0.6	0.7	2.1	2.4	0.6	n.a.	0.5
Maximum	6	10	15	16	10	25	49	101	12	n.a.	6

Base: all respondents (18–49 years) who ever had sex, except Switzerland (18–45 years)

Notes:
[1] Spain: categories are 0, 1, 2–5, 6+ partners
[2] Switzerland: estimated from the number of stable partners over one year and unstable partners over six months

Table 5.7 *Numbers of heterosexual partners over last 12 months*

No. of heterosexual partners	Athens PR[1] 1990	Belgium 1993	France ACSF 1992	Germany West[2] 1990	Great Britain 1991	Netherlands 1989	Norway 1992	Portugal 1991
of MEN								
N	743	1233	6252	927	6134	392	1454	1102
Median	1	1	1	1	1	1	1	1
Mean	1.2	1.4	1.4	1.4	1.3	1.2	1.5	1.8
S.D.	1.0	1.6	4.1	2.3	2.2	1.2	3.5	1.9
Maximum	20	30	211	52	200	10	120	25
of WOMEN								
N	839	1380	7403	1056	7790	551	1944	1031
Median	1	1	1	1	1	1	1	1
Mean	1.0	1.0	1.1	1.1	1.1	1.1	1.2	1.0
S.D.	0.2	0.6	0.6	0.5	0.7	2.1	1.0	0.6
Maximum	3	10	15	7	25	49	20	12

Base: all respondents (18–49 years) who ever had a heterosexual partner
Notes:
[1] Athens: base is 'every man/woman who presents herself as heterosexual'; all partners are included
[2] West Germany: same as Athens

Table 5.8   *Numbers of homosexual partners over last 12 months*

No. of homosexual partners	Belgium	France ACSF	Great Britain	Netherlands	Norway
	1993	1992	1991	1989	1992
of MEN					
% reporting at least one homo partner lifetime	5.6	2.9	4.2	11.8	4.8
N	89	199	255	49	71
Median	0	0	0	0	0
Mean	0.9	1.2	3.4	3.1	0.4
S.D.	3.1	3.2	32.1	8.1	0.8
Maximum	30	30	500	41	4
of WOMEN					
% reporting at least one homo partner lifetime	2.2	1.7	2.0	4.4	3.7
N	39	155	154	25	78
Median	0	0	0	0	0
Mean	0.3	0.3	0.3	0.1	0.4
S.D.	0.5	0.5	0.6	0.3	0.8
Maximum	3	6	3	1	5

Base: all respondents (18–49 years) who ever reported a homosexual partner (except first row where the base is all respondents)

ing situations emerge: in Great Britain and the Netherlands, on the one hand, the mean number of partners exceeded three (for men), which is twice the mean number of heterosexual partners in the same countries; in Belgium, France and Norway, on the other hand, the means were lower (even under one in Belgium and Norway). The mean for Great Britain may, however, have been heavily influenced by a few individuals reporting a very large number of partners.

Characteristics of Respondents with Multiple Opposite-sex Partners

In presenting the data on multipartner respondents (defined as people who had two or more partners over a certain period of time) we shall focus on heterosexual partners only, because of sample size limitations. Fewer than 100 men (or women) reported some homosexual experience over their lifetime in all but two of the surveys. It was thus not possible to carry out any significant differential analysis within these subpopulations.

The Mean Number of Partners by Age

One can expect to see the mean number of partners over lifetime increase with age. The relation may, however, be obscured by generational effects, for the older persons belong to older generations whose behaviour may have been different from younger ones. In addition, the oldest individuals might have more substantial difficulties recalling behaviour that occurred long ago and/or declaring activities about which they may feel more social disapproval than the youngest respondents.

Detailed data on the numbers of partners over lifetime are available in four countries; they are shown in Figure 5.1. To eliminate random fluctuations, the crude data for each group were first smoothed with a three-year average (with weights 0.25, 0.5 and 0.25), then adjusted on a third order polynomial function. Both curves are shown. For males, the mean starts in each country from a value of three to four at the age of 18 – the minimum age of respondents in most surveys. It increases rapidly from this age up to an age which differs widely among the countries: the peak seems to be reached by the age of 27–28 in the Netherlands, somewhere between 30 and 35 in France and Norway, and not before 40 in Switzerland, with the maximum value being close to 15 partners in all countries. Afterwards, the trends are not similar: in Norway the mean levels off; in France and Switzerland it drops slightly; and in the Netherlands the decline is steeper, but the random fluctuations are quite

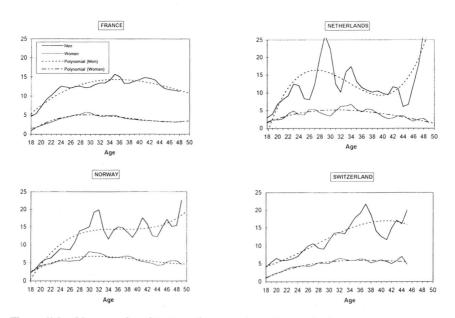

Figure 5.1 *Mean number of partners (by age and sex of respondent)*

important. Note that a decline in the mean number of partners with increasing age reveals a generational effect. A memory bias could also be suspected for the oldest generations, but it is less likely when the decline starts as early as age 30.

In France and Switzerland, the mean number of partners for men exceeds four by the age of 18; about as many more are accumulated between 18 and 25 years, after which the picture is very different: in France the mean levels off rapidly and only two additional partners are reported, while in Switzerland the average at age 25 is only half of the maximum value. In the two other countries, the greatest number of partners seems to be accumulated between ages 18 and 25 (the random variations somewhat obscure the analysis). Overall, we may conclude that there is a period of at least 10 years of great instability after sexual initiation, during which the risks of contracting or transmitting HIV may be elevated if these contacts (especially with new partners) are not protected. It is thus important to pay attention to the sexual behaviour of this specific population.

For women, the results differ less between countries: by the age of 18, the mean number of partners is close to one or two, and the maximum (or plateau) reached around the age of 30 is about five – a value much smaller than the one for men, as already mentioned. It is worth noting here that in France and Switzerland a three- to four-partner difference between men and women is already observed at the age of 18, and the gap does not widen much thereafter. In the other two countries the difference is found mainly between the ages 18 and 25. We may assume that men, particularly the youngest ones who are in the phase of asserting their masculine identity, are keen to count all relationships that tend to have some sexual connotation (from kissing to one-off intercourse), whereas women tend to count only the relationships that are of importance to them.

Who are the Multipartner Respondents?

The proportion of individuals reporting more than one partner during the previous 12 months is – as stressed above – a good indicator of the potential exposure to the risk of HIV, especially because the number of new partners is strongly related to the number of partners above one (there is most often a regular partner among those enumerated). This is the index used in Table 5.9 to analyze some differentials.

Overall, between 10 and 18 per cent of male respondents and between 1 and 11 per cent of female respondents reported more than one heterosexual partner over the past year (the only exception in this table is Portugal, with a rate close to 33 per cent for men, but a similar proportion was observed in Finland and Spain (see Table 5.6)). The gender gap is quite consistent with the

Table 5.9 *Proportions of respondents with two or more heterosexual partners over last 12 months by age, cohabitation, place of residence and education / %*

	Athens	Belgium	France ACSF	Germany West[1]	Great Britain	Netherlands	Norway	Portugal
	1990	1993	1992	1990	1991	1989	1992	1991
MEN								
All	10.9	15.2	14.9	11.5	16.3	13.7	17.5	33.4
Age								
18–19	22.0*	39.9	34.0	5.1*	40.3	13.3	18.8	41.4
20–24	24.1	26.0	27.6	22.7	30.5	17.2	25.4	45.7
25–29	16.7	13.2	17.4	15.4	17.8	16.9	21.3	43.7
30–39	6.6	10.4	10.1	9.2	10.8	13.2	14.1	33.3
40–49	3.5	11.9	8.9	4.7	8.4	9.8	13.2	18.3
Cohabitation								
Cohabiting	n.a.	7.3	6.8	n.a.	6.4	3.7	9.1	20.3
Not cohabiting	28.2	33.0	34.6	n.a.	36.3	30.7	30.8	50.6
Place of residence								
Rural	n.a.	7.6*	11.0	9.3	13.0	0.0	12.5	n.a.
Small towns	n.a.	13.1	13.6	8.3	15.4	12.1	18.9	n.a.
Towns	n.a.	17.5	17.6	14.1	15.9	20.3	21.9	n.a.
Large cities	10.2	25.7	19.8	14.7	23.4	n.c.	n.c.	n.a.
Education								
Low	6.0	13.2	10.3	8.9*	13.0	16.7	15.2	31.7
Medium	9.8	15.7	17.0	12.8	16.9	11.4	21.8	35.4
High	15.7	16.1	18.1	13.2	16.4	18.6	17.5	33.0
WOMEN								
All	1.5	5.7	6.6	5.3	7.6	6.8	11.3	5.0
Age								
18–19	3.6	27.0	14.1*	9.1*	23.1	26.7	24.5	24.4*
20–24	4.4	10.8	11.7	7.3	15.6	16.7	18.5	8.3
25–29	1.3	6.0	7.6	8.5	7.5	5.2	9.5	7.9
30–39	1.3	4.5	5.3	3.8	5.4	3.0	8.5	4.1
40–49	0.4	2.7	3.7	3.0	3.1	2.7	7.8	0.3
Cohabitation								
Cohabiting	n.a.	2.7	3.3	n.a.	2.9	2.4	4.7	0.9
Not cohabiting	7.5	16.2	17.1	n.a.	19.9	18.6	28.2	13.4
Place of residence								
Rural	n.a.	9.5*	4.3	3.0	5.3	3.3	8.7	n.a.
Small towns	n.a.	4.5	6.4	4.0	7.6	5.2	11.7	n.a.
Towns	n.a.	6.3	7.4	3.9	6.0	12.1	13.9	n.a.
Large cities	n.a.	10.1	9.2	9.4	10.8	n.c.	n.c.	n.a.
Education								
Low	0.0	2.3	3.9	3.9	5.9	4.0	8.9	3.3
Medium	1.4	7.3	6.3	5.0	7.9	5.2	13.1	5.8
High	3.8	6.2	10.9	10.1	9.6	12.0	12.7	7.1

Base: all respondents (18–49 years) with at least one heterosexual partner over life
n.c.: = not computable
n.a.: = not available
Notes:
[1] West Germany: all partners (including homosexual). Base: every respondent presenting himself as hetero- or bisexual
* Between 15 and 50 cases in the cell; for sample sizes, see Table 5.7

results described already. The age effect is the same for both genders: the proportion of multipartner respondents declines – sometimes at a very rapid pace – with increasing age. For men, however, the proportion was sometimes lower at age 18–19 than at age 20–24, because of their later entry into sexual life. Not surprisingly, people living with a steady partners are less likely to report at least two partners than those not cohabiting. We must, however, remember that the 'non-cohabiting' group is younger, so that the proportion for the non-cohabiting group is often close to the proportion of the 18–19 (or 20–24) years group. In Norway and the Netherlands, however, and to a lesser degree in Athens, France and Portugal, the proportion of non-cohabiting men with multiple partners exceeds the mean proportion of multiple partners for all age groups. A possible explanation is that a part of the adult population is choosing an independent way of life to remain free to change sexual partners.

In all countries, it is significantly more frequent to have two or more partners in large cities than in rural areas (Table 5.9); indeed, the rate is often multiplied twofold. Clearly, the possible differences in age structures and cohabiting patterns cannot explain the differences. The gradient from rural areas to large cities is not the same in all countries. This is probably due to differences in definitions (the limits, and hence the size, of the cities are not defined the same way everywhere) and in traditions of urbanization between countries. In any case, the opportunities for finding new partners and the social acceptability of frequent changes are obviously much greater in cities than anywhere else.

Education is often a very powerful variable to enable social scientists to identify differentiated behaviours. In the surveys under review it is still powerful for females, but not for males: the proportion of multipartner females increased twofold or threefold over the education range but no more than twice (and often much less) among men. If one admits that the social pressures on women's sexuality are much stronger than on men's and leaves women less freedom to 'choose' their sexual behaviour, one interpretation might be that a higher level of education increases women's sexual and relational autonomy, whereas men do not need such an asset to behave as they wish. Note that the relation is not an artefact of age (young women usually being more educated than older ones), since when the French survey data are cross-tabulated for age and education, the effect of the latter variable persists at all ages (data not shown).

Table 5.10 estimates the amount of 'non-monogamy' in some populations by selecting the people involved in a steady relationship for at least one year as the base (note that this definition does not imply cohabitation). Having more than one partner for someone involved in a steady relationship with one person may refer to various situations, for example having a permanent relationship with another person, having one (or more) occasional partners, visiting sex workers, and so on. It may also mean having homosexual experiences for people engaged in a heterosexual couple. Men and women reporting a homosexual or bisexual orientation are much more likely to be non-monoga-

Table 5.10 *Proportions of people in a steady relationship with two or more partners in previous year, by gender and sexual orientation in the last 12 months / %*

	Belgium	France ACSF[1]	Great Britain[1]	Netherlands	Norway	Portugal
	1993	1992	1991	1989	1992	1991
MEN						
Hetero only	9.2	7.5	5.2	6.5	10.2	21.6
Homo/bi	52.3*	20.2*	47.4*	55.6*	20.0	n.a.
All	9.8	7.6	5.6	8.2	10.3	n.a.
N	1013	1020	3576	269	1074	747
WOMEN						
Hetero only	3.4	3.8	2.2	2.6	5.6	1.1
Homo/bi	60.7*	17.2*	38.5**	0*	15.4	n.a.
All	3.8	3.8	2.3	2.6	5.6	n.a.
N	1214	882	4935	429	1574	833

Base: all respondents (18–49 years) with a current steady relationship that has lasted at least one year
n.a.: = not applicable
Notes:
[1] France and Great Britain: cohabiting partnerships only
*Between 15 and 50 cases in the cell; **fewer than 15 cases

mous over one year in all countries: reported multipartnership exceeded 50 per cent in Belgium (for both genders) and the Netherlands (for men) and was around 20 per cent elsewhere. For the heterosexual population, the figures are much lower, except for men in Portugal.

Men and Sex Workers

Sex work is often considered to be a potential source of HIV infection. In Europe, however, it is not regarded as playing a major role in the epidemic (as might be the case in other regions, such as sub-Saharan Africa), because sex work is usually relatively marginal and a majority of sex workers request that their customers use condoms (Padian, 1988). In many European countries, visiting a sex worker used to be (but is no longer – see Chapter 2 on sexual initiation) a common way of initiating males sexually. It may now be a more frequent means of obtaining sex during time spent out of union. When this is the case, the number of men reporting having paid for sex over their 'lifetimes' can be much higher than for a shorter period, such as the last 12 months. Table 5.10 shows that Norway, Switzerland and, to a lesser extent, the Netherlands probably come into this category, as almost 20 per cent of heterosexual men (13 per cent in the Netherlands) reported paying for sex sometime in their life, but only around 2 per cent over the previous last year. Spain

Table 5.11 *Proportions of males who paid for sex during lifetime or during previous year, by sexual orientation in the same period of time / %*

	Finland	France ACSF	Germany West	Great Britain	Netherlands	Norway	Portugal	Spain	Switzerland[1]
	1992	1992	1990	1991	1989	1992	1991	1990	1992
During lifetime									
Hetero only	9.7	n.a.	n.a.	6.1	13.4	19.7	n.a.	38.1	17.8
Homo/bi	16.7	n.a.	n.a.	18.2	20.4	21.2	n.a.	48.1	35.2
All	9.9	n.a.	n.a.	6.6	14.3	11.3	n.a.	38.6	18.7
N	664	n.a.	n.a.	6053	392	1617	n.a.	409	1260
During previous year									
Hetero only	n.a.	1.1	4.3	0.5	2.8	1.6	4.7	9.9	2.3
Homo/bi	n.a.	1.9	21.9	6.4	2.1	6.3	–	29.6	5.3
All	n.a.	1.1	4.6	0.6	2.8	1.8	4.9	11.0	2.4
N	n.a.	6361	1034	5728	363	1523	1094	409	1267

Base: males (18–49 years) who ever had sex, except Switzerland (18–45 years)

n.a.: = not applicable

Note:
[1] Switzerland: last six months (18–45 years) instead of last 12 months

is an exception, with 38 per cent of men reporting some experience with sex workers in their lives and 10 per cent in the previous 12 months.

Sex work is more common among those reporting homosexual partners, and the contrast between the two reference periods is even greater for this subgroup than for heterosexual men. However, the proportions of homo-sexual or bisexual men having paid for sex during the previous year are not that high, that is between 2 and 6 per cent, except in West Germany, where the rate exceeds 20 per cent, and in Spain, where it is close to 30 per cent. The reasons for such differences are hard to find. The laws concerning homo-sexual behaviour do vary among the countries: in some countries, discrimina-tion on grounds of homosexuality is explicitly forbidden (the Netherlands, Norway, Spain), and unions between partners of the same sex are more or less accepted (the Netherlands and Norway). However, no obvious association between the more or less liberal policies and the prevalence of sex work can be found in Table 5.11. Furthermore, sexual contacts that men of the 'homo/bisexual' group have paid for may be heterosexual contacts: in Great Britain's survey men were asked only about paid relations with women; in France, the lowest rate of paying for sex over the last five years was recorded by men who engaged in homosexual relations only in the past five years, and none of the exclusive homosexuals over the last 12 months reported paying for sex in that same period.

Because of the specific behaviour of homosexual or bisexual males, who usually have more partners than heterosexual males, and the finding that men reporting paying for sex often have large numbers of such contacts, the comparisons of the distributions and means of the numbers of partners between countries could be heavily influenced by the rates of prevalence of these partnerships in the various populations of Europe. Table 5.12 attempts to control for this effect. First the mean number of partners during lifetime is shown for two different age groups (18–29 and 30–49 years). Then the mean is computed for those who reported fewer than 20 partners in their lifetimes (75 to 85 per cent of the male population: see Table 5.3). The resulting means were about half the value of the overall mean for the younger group, and one-third or one-fourth of the overall mean for the older one. Restricting the group further to heterosexuals only does not make any significant difference. Finally, if we subdivide the last group (fewer than 20 partners) into those reporting having ever paid for sex and the others, we see that the mean is significantly higher in the first group, sometimes twice as high. It follows that, even after the 'high partner turnover' group is removed, men paying for sex do report more partners than the others.

Table 5.12 also sheds some light on the gender dimension. When men reporting 20 or more partners are left aside, the means come much closer to those for women (see Tables 5.3, 5.4 and 5.5). Two hypotheses, both of which may hold true, can be put forward here in addition to the specific role of sex work: 1) the men giving a very large number of partners are greatly over-estimating their actual behaviour, and the 'gender gap' is due to a reporting

Table 5.12 *Mean numbers of partners over lifetime (for males only), by age group, <20 partners, sexual orientation and payment for sex*

	France ACSF 1992	Great Britain 1991	Netherlands 1989	Norway 1992	Switzerland[1] 1992
18–29 years					
All	11.1	9.0	12.6	9.2	7.1
<20 partners over life	5.7	5.2	5.3	5.4	4.8
Heterosexual, <20 partners	5.7	5.2	4.9	5.7	n.a.
Heterosexual, <20 p., ever paid for sex	7.2	7.8	8.6	9.9	7.5
Heterosexual, <20 p., never paid for sex	5.7	5.1	4.7	5.5	4.4
30–49 years					
All	13.5	14.4	26.5	18.6	15.6
<20 partners over life	5.5	5.1	4.6	6.8	5.6
Heterosexual, <20 partners	5.4	5.0	4.4	6.8	n.a.
Heterosexual, <20 p., ever paid for sex	9.3	8.1	7.9	11.9	7.0
Heterosexual, <20 p., never paid for sex	5.4	4.8	4.1	6.2	5.3

Base: all males (18–49 years) with at least one partner over life
Note:
[1] Switzerland: means are not restricted to heterosexuals. Age groups are 18–29 and 30–45 years

bias (perhaps also fueled by women under-reporting multiple partnerships); 2) these numbers are in most cases 'real' and the gap must be explained by gender-specific differences in perception of what a sexual partner is, especially in the first years of sexual activity.

Conclusions

Although many differences have been highlighted in this chapter, many general patterns were remarkably similar across European countries. This is true, for example, for differences between men and women, sexual preferences, or distributions of the numbers of partners over various time periods. Generally speaking, existing, and sometimes large, differences in sexual cultures (norms and values, legislation, sexual health services, access to contraception, and so on), as noted by Jones *et al.* (1986), appear not to be reflected in striking differences in adult sexual conduct. In areas where national differences were found, as in the reported prevalence of male same-sex behaviour or the use of sex workers, it is still unclear whether these findings reflect actual behavioural (culturally related) differences or differences in a willingness to report these behaviours. Questions like these cannot be solved via behavioural reports only and need more comprehensive analyses that include indicators for sexual cultures, such as permissiveness.

An important conclusion to which our cross-national analyses have led is that the gap between men and women in the declaration of numbers of partners is a general phenomenon across Europe, as it is on other continents (Laumann *et al.*, 1994; Caraël, 1995). We have shown that the greater use of sex workers by men, the gender-related age differences between partners leading to non-sampling of the partners at both age limits of the samples, and the larger number of 'outliers' among men who declare having had a large number of partners cannot explain the whole gap. Obviously, we are dealing here with something that has also to do with masculine and feminine cultural identities: men and women count differently. That is to say, they do not define their partners the same way: women may tend to take into account only those partners who were really important to them and thus tend to underestimate the number of their partners, whereas men may feel having had a large number of partners is proof of their virility and thus tend to overestimate the number of their partners and/or to include partners they just kissed or petted with. This seems particularly true for young men asserting their masculinity.

More important for the spread of HIV is the variance in the numbers of partners. The sexual behaviour of the small groups of respondents who declared very large numbers of partners is probably more important for the spread of HIV and other STDs than the sexual behaviour of the population at large. It is important to draw attention to the high frequency of partner change in a segment of the homosexual male population consisting of gay men who are concentrated in a few areas, with a very dense sexual network, and with a steady in- and outflow of visitors (van Griensven, 1989; Van Zessen and Jager, 1994). The effectiveness of their sexual practices in spreading HIV, together with the need to consistently practise safer sex, is a key issue for prevention.

Since there has been no substantial heterosexual epidemic in Europe so far, the question is whether and how HIV can spread widely in the heterosexual population. The main lesson of our cross-national analyses is that, in all the surveys under review, homosexual relations often run parallel to, or alternate with, heterosexual relations, at least in some phase of the lifecourse. We have also shown that the point of sexual initiation is followed by a period of at least ten years of great instability in terms of number of partners, during which the risk of acquiring HIV may be high if these contacts (especially with new partners) are not protected.

Notes

1 See some comparisons between Belgium, France and the Netherlands about the normative context of the relationships in Chapter 11.
2 The number of partners over the last 12 months in Switzerland had to be estimated by adding the number of stable partners over one year to the number of casual partners over 6 months, since this information was gathered using two different questions.

References

ANDERSON, R.M. (1993) 'AIDS in developing countries: heterogeneity in potential demographic impact', in MANN, J. and DUPUY, C. (Eds) *Sida, santé et droits de l'Homme*, Lyon: Fondation M. Merieux.

ANDERSON, R.M and MAY, R.M. (1988) 'Epidemiological parameters of HIV transmission', *Nature*, **333**, pp. 514–29.

ANDERSON, R.M, MAY, R.M., BOILY, M.C., GARNETT, G.P. and ROWLEY, J.T. (1991) 'The spread of HIV-1 in Africa: sexual contact patterns and the predicted demographic impact of AIDS', *Nature*, **352**, pp. 581–9.

BLANCHARD, P. (1993) 'Modelling HIV/AIDS dynamics', Bielefeld: BiBos W.P., no. 580.

BONGAARTS, J. (1988) 'Modeling the spread of HIV and the demographic impact of AIDS in Africa', New York: Center for Policy Studies (Population Council), Working Paper no. 140.

BROUARD, N. (1994) 'Aspects démographiques et conséquences de l'épidémie de Sida en Afrique', in VALLIN J. (Ed.) *Populations africaines et Sida*, Paris: La Découverte and CEPED.

CARAËL, M. (1995) 'Sexual behaviour', in CLELAND, J. and FERRY, B. (Eds) *Sexual Behaviour and AIDS in the Developing World*, London: Taylor & Francis.

CATANIA, J.A., MOSKOWITZ, J.T., RUIZ, M. and CLELAND, J. (1996a) 'A review of national AIDS-related behavioural surveys', *AIDS*, **10** (suppl. A), S183–S190.

CATANIA, J.A., BINSON, D., PETERSON, J. and CANCHOLA, J. (1996b) 'The effects of question wordings, interviewer gender, and control on item response by African-American respondents', Paper presented at the conference Researching Sexual Behaviour: Methodological Issues, Bloomington, Indiana: The Kinsey Institute, Indiana University, 26–28 April.

GIAMI, A. (1995) 'Représentations de la sexualité et représentations des partenaires à l'époque du sida', in BAJOS, N., BOZON, M., GIAMI, A., DORÉ, V. and SOUTEYRAND, Y. (Eds) *Sexualité et sida*, Paris: Agence Nationale de Recherches sur le Sida (ANRS), 'Sciences Sociales et Sida Collection'.

JOHNSON, A.M., WADWORTH, J., WELLINGS, K. and FIELD, J. (1994) *Sexual Attitudes and Lifestyles*, Oxford: Blackwell Scientific Publications.

JONES, E.F., DARROCH FORREST, J., GOLDMAN, N., HENSHAW, S., LINCOLN, R., ROSOFF, J.I., WESTOFF, C.F. and WULF, D. (1986) *Teenage pregnancy in industrialized countries*, New Haven/London: Yale University Press.

KNOLLE, H. (1990) 'Age preference in sexual choice and the basic reproduction number of HIV/AIDS', *Biometrical Journal*, **32**, pp. 243–56.

LAGRANGE, H. (1991) 'Le nombre de partenaires sexuels: les hommes en ont-ils plus que les femmes?', *Population*, **46**, 2, pp. 249–77.

LAUMANN, E.O., GAGNON, J.H., MICHAEL, R.T. and MICHAELS, S. (1994) *The Social Organization of Sexuality: Sexual Practices in the United States*, Chicago: University of Chicago Press.

LERIDON, H. (1998) 'Les nouveaux partenaires: estimation de leur nombre et de l'évolution au cours des années récentes dans une enquête "transversale"', in BAJOS, N., BOZON, M., FERRAND, A., GIAMI, A. and SPIRA, A. (Eds) *La sexualité aux temps du sida*, Paris.

MARQUET, J., PETO, D. and HUBERT, M. (1995) 'Sexual behaviour and HIV risk: towards a relation-based approach', in FRIEDRICH, D. and HECKMANN, W. (Eds) *AIDS in Europe – The Behavioural Aspect, Vol. 2: Risk Behaviour and its Determinants*, Berlin: Editions Sigma.

MAY, R.M. and ANDERSON, R.M. (1987) 'Transmission dynamics of HIV infection', *Nature*, **326** (12 March), pp. 137–42.

PADIAN, N.S. (1988) 'Prostitute women and AIDS: epidemiology', *AIDS*, **2**, pp. 413–19.

PARKER, R.G. and GAGNON, J.H. (Eds) (1995) *Conceiving Sexuality. Approaches to Sex Research in a Postmodern World*, New York and London: Routledge.

PETERMAN, T.A., STONEBURNER, R.L., ALLEN, J.R., JAFFE, H.W. and CURRAN, J.W. (1988) 'Risk of HIV transmission from heterosexual adults with transfusion associated infections', *JAMA*, **259**, pp. 55–63.

PETO, D., REMY, J., VAN CAMPENHOUDT, L. and HUBERT, M. (1992) *SIDA: l'amour face à la peur. Modes d'adaptation au risque du SIDA dans les relations hétérosexuelles*, Paris: L'Harmattan, 'Logiques sociales' collection.

SMITH, T.W. (1988) *A Methodological Review of Sexual Behavior Questions on the 1988 GSS*, Report 58, University of Chicago.

VAN CAMPENHOUDT, L., COHEN, M., GUIZZARDI, G. and HAUSSER, D. (1996) *Sexual Interactions and HIV Risk. New Conceptual Perspectives in European Research*, London: Taylor & Francis.

VAN GRIENSVEN, G.J.P. (1989) *Epidemiology and prevention of HIV infection among homosexual men*, Thesis, Amsterdam: University of Amsterdam.

VAN ZESSEN, G. and SANDFORT, T. (1991) *Seksualiteit in Nederland; seksueel gedrag, risico en preventie van aids*, Amsterdam/Lisse: Swets & Zeitlinger.

VAN ZESSEN, G. and JAGER, J.C. (1994) *Analyse van seksuele netwerken (analysis of sexual networks)*, Bilthoven: RIVM.

Part 2

Sexual Transmission of HIV

Chapter 6

Risk Behaviour and Risk Contexts

Per Magnus

Introduction

This chapter will discuss the concept of risk and present data on selected high-risk practices from the European sexual surveys conducted between 1987 and 1993. The prevalence of these practices are analyzed with respect to age group and gender and compared between countries. In addition, one of the practices (having had more than five partners during the past year) is analyzed within countries with respect to cohabitational status, place of residence and gender of the sexual partner; the degree of association with these background variables is then compared between countries. The prevalence of risk-related practices can be seen as estimates of the proportions of the population with a potential risk of becoming infected with HIV. The extent to which such estimates actually correlate with the occurrence of HIV infection is discussed.

In epidemiological terms, the risk of acquiring a disease is the probability that a subject belonging to a particular population may develop a certain disease over a certain time period. In longitudinal studies it is expressed as the number of people who fall ill (or contract an infection) over the total number of subjects under observation. This proportion is called the cumulative incidence. In the case of HIV, the relative risk of infection following a specific type of exposure, for instance a certain behaviour, can be calculated by dividing the cumulative incidence of infection in the exposed group by the cumulative incidence in the unexposed group.

An HIV risk indicator is a variable that has been found to be statistically associated with HIV infection in cohort or case-control studies. The present cross-sectional surveys do not directly relate sexual practices to actual HIV infection. Rather, these look at whether people engage in practices which might put them at risk of contracting HIV. Thus, only potential risk, not actual risk, can be estimated from the surveys. It would have been informative to combine the risk indicators per country into risk indices for sexually transmitted diseases (Stigum and Magnus, 1997). Unfortunately, this was not done for the surveys discussed here because of the difficulties generated by the non-standardized approaches taken across Europe.

What, then, are the risk indicators for HIV infection? After the first descriptions of AIDS, case-control studies of subjects first with and without AIDS, later with and without HIV seropositivity, demonstrated HIV's main transmission routes, namely, unprotected sex, infected blood and blood products, and perinatal transmission. Cohort studies of initially seronegative people gave more precise relative risks of infection for various sexual practices. Also, partner studies of HIV-discordant couples added to the knowledge of risk indicators for HIV infection. Many studies of homosexual men, from the first case-control studies of AIDS patients (Marmor *et al.*, 1984) on, have shown that the number of sexual partners and receptive anal intercourse are related to risk of infection. For injecting drug users (IDUs), sharing needles increases the risk of infection. IDUs may also be at increased risk of being infected through sexual intercourse (Des Jarlais *et al.*, 1992). For heterosexual transmission, injecting drug use among sexual partners increases the risk for both men and women, whereas sex work and sexual intercourse with a bisexual male have been found to increase risk among women (Haverkos and Edelman, 1989). In studies of HIV-discordant heterosexual partners, the practice of anal sex has been found to increase risk of infection (European Study Group, 1989).

Before we turn to the data available in the surveys, some comments on risk context are needed. The probability of becoming infected with HIV in connection with a specific sexual practice will differ across populations, a main determinant being the prevalence of infection among sexual partners. This means that the same practices from surveys across Europe are associated with diverse probabilities of infection. It is less often appreciated that the magnitude of the relative risk of infection associated with a certain practice will also differ across populations and may even change during the follow-up of a cohort (Brookmeyer and Gail, 1994). This will happen if the prevalence of HIV infection changes over time (as the epidemic runs its course) and the change in prevalence differs between sexual partners of subjects with and without a specific practice.

The individual risk context may be very complex and varied, meaning that average statistics may be misleading with respect to a specific sexual practice for a certain individual. The individual selection of partners, the co-occurrence of risk-prone sexual practices (for instance, both unprotected sex and sharing of drug injection equipment), presence of co-factors for transmission, as well as the use of safe sex practices will all modulate the actual risk for an individual. The risk of HIV infection can be subdivided into risk of exposure and risk of virus transmission given exposure. The risk of exposure is dependent on the number and types of sexual partners, the probability of HIV infection in the selected partners and the use of safe sexual practices,

including use of condoms. The conditional risk of transmission given exposure may depend on the presence of certain co-factors such as other STDs, the
partners' genetic and immunological factors and characteristics of the virus.
Recently, it has been reported that some subtypes of HIV may be associated
with higher transmission rates than others (Kunanusont *et al.*, 1995). Except
for the presence of other STDs, which is discussed in the following chapter,
co-factors are not available for analysis in the present context. Therefore,
this chapter will focus on the first risk component, that is, the risk of exposure
as it can be deduced from the surveys of sexual behaviour examined in
this book.

The Data

The presentation of risk indicators starts with some specific practices (sex with
an injecting drug user, anal sex), continues with an analysis of the proportion
of subjects reporting many partners and then examines the question of
paying for sexual intercourse. Finally, in spite of this book's focus on sexual
behaviour, a non-sexual practice, to wit, injecting drug use with the sharing of
needles, is presented. Condom use influences the risk situation and this
practice will be referred to in the text to the extent that it can be analyzed for
subjects with at-risk practices. We have not included blood transfusion among
the risk indicators since this has not been a major problem in Europe since the
late 1980s. Other risk situations, for instance sexual intercourse with people
living in areas of the world with a high prevalence of HIV infection, have been
included in too few studies to be compared in this chapter.

However, some of the variables that are presented here are also based on
a small number of surveys and are of uncertain quality. For instance, only four
of the surveys we examined included questions on sexual intercourse with an
IDU. Although this may be an important pathway for the spread of HIV in
Europe, it is difficult to obtain valid data about this practice. A substantial
proportion of subjects who did have sex with an IDU probably did not know
of their partner's history of drug use, while the ones who did know may not
have been willing to reveal this information or did not know their partner's
serological status. Besides this, the four countries all used different time
periods for their questions (last intercourse, last six months, last 12 months
and ever), making cross-national comparisons complicated. Also, the questions on anal sex in the various countries' surveys were not comparable. In
Norway, anal sex during the last year and at last intercourse was reported, but
only for non-cohabiting persons and cohabiting persons who reported additional partners. In the Netherlands, the questions concerned the last 12
months, whereas in France, they covered the respondent's lifetime as well as
for the last intercourse. Finally, in Belgium, the question was whether the

respondent had ever (that is in his/her lifetime) had anal sex with any of the partners with whom he/she had had intercourse in the preceding 12 months.

The study of the prevalence of injecting drug use is not ideal in these surveys. The surveys were designed to study sexual behaviour, not drug use, and it seems obvious that the surveys will not reach the heavy drug addicts. Many of the respondents who reported injecting drugs may have merely experimented on just one or a few occasions. To make the data comparable across countries (in Norway, only sexually active subjects were asked about drug use), only subjects who had experienced sex were included in the denominators for this variable.

For the variable frequent partner change (five or more partners during the past 12 months), the denominators consist of all persons who have ever had sex. The operational definition of the cut-off for high partner change is somewhat arbitrary and will depend on the diseases studied. For a disease such as gonorrhoea, which has a period of infectivity of a few months, several partners each year would be needed to pass the disease on with sufficient frequency. We chose to use a relatively high cut-off since it has been argued that the proportion of the sexually active population with high partner change (the core group) determines whether a sexually transmitted disease will be endemic (have a stable prevalence) in a population or not (Yorke, Hethcote and Nold, 1978).

The basic reproductive ratio is a measure of the number of persons infected by the average infected subject during that subject's period of infectiousness. If the ratio is one, then the disease will be endemic in the population. Assuming proportional mixing between the core group and the remaining sexually active part of the population, it has been shown that the basic reproductive ratio is close to one for gonorrhoea when 3 per cent of the sexually active population has unprotected sex with more than five partners per year (Stigum, Falck and Magnus, 1994). Since the number of partners was reported in all surveys, cross-national comparison of the proportions reporting five or more partners per year was possible. The proportions were sufficiently high to permit analysis of the correlation with background variables within each country. The reader is referred to Chapter 5 on number of several partners for a discussion of the methodological importance of the underlying variable.

It is possible that the response pattern to the surveys may reflect more pronounced liberal attitudes towards sexuality in the Nordic countries than in the rest of Western society (Schmidt, 1989). In addition, response bias may be of nonsimilar types and strengths from one country to the next. Also, the surveys relied on different data collection methods and phrasings of questions. These methodological differences may limit the validity of comparisons between countries (see Chapter 1).

The 95 per cent confidence intervals are presented in each table for the total percentages and have to be taken into account when comparing differences between countries. A difference will not be considered as statistically significant if the confidence intervals in one group overlaps with the estimate of the proportion in another group.

Risk Indicators

Sex with Injecting Drug Users

Data about sex with injecting drug users are available in Athens, France, Norway and West Germany. The Athens 1990 study asked if the respondent had had sex with an IDU during the past six months. Six of 1661 subjects (0.4 per cent) responded 'yes'. Of these six, four responded to a subsequent question on condom use on these occasions as follows: one answered 'always', two 'sometimes' and one 'never'. In France, the question concerned the past 12 months. The weighted percentage of subjects responding 'yes' to having sex with an IDU was 0.6 (base 3949). Among the subjects who reported having sex with an IDU in the past 12 months, 68.4 per cent (base 27) reported condom use during the same period of time in contrast to 44.4 per cent (base 3849) among those who did not report sex with an IDU. In Norway, the questions focused on the last intercourse. Single subjects or subjects reporting extramarital sex outside their current steady relationship answered a question on sex with an IDU and use of condoms. Four of 3604 subjects (0.1 per cent) reported that their last partner was an IDU, and none of these persons had used a condom in the last intercourse. The West German study of 1990 likewise asked whether the respondents had ever had sex with an IDU. The following percentages of male respondents who had ever had sex answered this question affirmatively: 18–19 years: 2.3 per cent (base 44); 20–24 years: 3.2 per cent (190); 25–29 years: 3.4 per cent (233); 30–39 years: 2.3 per cent (305); and 40–49 years: 2.5 per cent (238). Among females, the corresponding percentages were: 3.0 per cent (33), 3.3 per cent (212), 3.5 per cent (202), 3.0 per cent (403) and 1.9 per cent (266). The overall affirmative response rate was 2.8 per cent for men compared with 2.9 per cent for women.

Experience of Anal Sex

In Norway, 9.5 per cent of men and 10.1 per cent of women reported anal sex during the last 12 months (Table 6.1). In the Netherlands, the proportions

Table 6.1 *Experience of anal sex during the last 12 months by age*

		Netherlands 1989		Norway[1] 1992	
		Men	Women	Men	Women
All	%	3.9	4.5	9.5	10.1
	CI	1.9–5.9	2.7–6.3	7.2–11.8	7.6–12.6
	N	363	512	619	566
18–19	%	7.1	0	7.5	11.4
	N	14	26	53	79
20–24	%	4.7	5.1	13.1	14.9
	N	64	79	160	148
25–29	%	6.6	1.1	11.1	12.9
	N	61	95	117	85
30–39	%	2.8	5.1	10.7	4.9
	N	142	176	140	143
40–49	%	2.4	6.6	4.0	7.2
	N	82	136	149	111

Base: all respondents (18–49 years) who ever had sex
CI: 95% confidence interval
Note:
[1] Norway: only non-cohabiting and cohabiting subjects with extramarital partners answered

were 3.9 per cent for men and 4.5 per cent for women, which is lower than in Norway. Note that the sample studied in the Netherlands was less selective than the Norwegian in that the Dutch study included cohabiting persons without additional partners. However, it is not clear what the difference between the Dutch and Norwegian findings signifies. Table 6.2 shows that 5.1 per cent of the male respondents and 4.2 per cent of the female respondents to the French survey reported anal sex in the last intercourse. These numbers are significantly higher than the figures in Norway, although it must be noted that the denominators are not exactly the same in the two surveys. In Belgium, the lifetime prevalence of anal sex (with one of the partners of the last 12 months) was 16.6 per cent (CI: 14.5–18.7, base 1218) for men. This is lower than the percentage reported by women, which was 19.4 per cent (CI: 17.3–21.5, base 1309). The Netherlands survey analyzed the data on anal sex during the last 12 months by gender of sexual partners. Anal sex was reported by 1.5 per cent (base 340) of the heterosexual males compared with 39.1 per cent (base 23) of the homo/bisexual males. In Norway, the percentages were 6.8 per cent (base 630) and 57.1 per cent (base 21), respectively. If last intercourse only was considered, 1.9 per cent (base 637) of the heterosexual male respondents in Norway reported anal sex, compared with 35.0 per cent (base 20) of the homo/bisexual men. Again, for the Norwegian data one must bear

Table 6.2 *Experience of anal sex during last intercourse by age*

		France 1992		Norway[1] 1992	
		Men	Women	Men	Women
All	%	5.1	4.2	3.1	2.8
	CI	4.2–6.0	3.2–5.2	1.8–4.4	1.5–4.1
	N	2146	1701	699	637
18–19	%	6.7	6.6	5.1	3.6
	N	129	109	59	83
20–24	%	6.4	4.2	4.5	4.9
	N	481	410	176	162
25–29	%	4.4	6.2	3.7	0
	N	473	353	134	98
30–39	%	5.3	4.9	3.7	3.1
	N	652	527	164	160
40–49	%	4.2	2.1	0	1.5
	N	411	302	166	134

Base: all respondents (18–49 years) who ever had sex
CI: 95% confidence interval
Note:
[1] Norway: only non-cohabiting and cohabiting subjects
with extramarital partners answered

in mind that only single men and cohabiting men who had extrarelational partners were included in the denominator. In Norway, 20.8 per cent (base 24) of the men reporting anal sex in last intercourse reported condom use in that intercourse, compared with 18.4 per cent (base 745) of the men not reporting anal sex in the last intercourse. In France, 33.3 per cent (base 131) of the males reporting anal sex the last time they had intercourse did report condom use as opposed to 21.8 per cent (base 2015) of the men who did not report anal sex the last time they had sex.

Five or More Partners During the Past 12 Months

Table 6.3 shows that the proportion of men who reported more than five partners ranged from 2.0 per cent in France and West Germany to 7.0 per cent in Finland. Former East Germany, Spain and Portugal also reported a relatively high proportion of sexually experienced respondents with five or more partners during the last 12 months. The proportion was generally highest for men between 20 and 24 years of age. Exceptions to this trend are found in

Table 6.3 *Proportions of male and female respondents reporting five or more partners during the last 12 months by age*

		Belgium	Finland	France ACSF	Germany East	Germany West	Netherlands	Norway	Portugal	Spain[1]
		1993	1992	1992	1990	1990	1989	1992	1991	1990
MEN										
All	%	3.2	7.0	2.0	6.2	2.0	4.6	3.6	5.1	6.6
	CI	2.3–4.1	5.1–8.9	1.4–2.6	3.9–8.5	1.1–2.9	2.5–6.7	2.7–4.5	3.8–6.4	4.2–9.0
	N	1246	704	2256	434	918	392	1540	1163	409
18–19	%	12.6	3.0	3.4	8.7	0	0	6.5	3.8	11.3
	N	62	33	137	23	31	19	62	121	53
20–24	%	5.7	9.3	5.3	9.7	5.3	8.8	8.8	5.6	5.9
	N	202	97	512	62	113	68	251	236	152
25–29	%	4.1	10.3	2.3	3.6	3.1	6.0	4.3	6.1	
	N	182	116	500	56	193	67	281	126	
30–39	%	2.3	5.8	1.1	8.6	1.0	3.4	2.3	5.7	6.4
	N	398	240	676	162	382	148	521	386	125
40–49	%	1.0	6.0	0.9	2.3	1.0	3.3	1.2	4.1	5.1
	N	402	218	431	130	199	90	425	294	79

WOMEN

		0.5	3.3	0.4	0.9	0.2	0.7	1.5	0.4	3.2
All	% / CI	0.1–0.9	2.0–4.6	0.1–0.7	0.8–1.0	0.0–0.5	0.0–1.4	1.0–2.0	0.1–0.7	1.4–5.0
	N	1387	672	1831	343	1102	551	2047	1219	370
18–19	%	2.2	7.1	0.1	6.3	0	6.5	4.0	2.9	4.8
	N	51	28	115	16	35	31	99	122	62
20–24	%	1.4	4.5	0.6	1.8	0.7	1.2	3.4	0	3.9
	N	191	111	439	55	146	84	350	212	128
25–29	%	0	7.7	0.6	0	0.5	1.0	0.5	0.7	2.7
	N	224	104	379	65	217	103	377	153	111
30–39	%	0.1	1.7	0.4	0.8	0	0	1.2	0	
	N	489	230	558	119	466	186	692	405	
40–49	%	0.6	1.5	0.2	0	0	0	0.8	0	1.4
	N	432	199	340	88	238	147	529	327	69

Base: all respondents (18–49 years) who ever had sex

CI: 95% confidence interval

Note:

[1] Spain: the age categories are 19–21, 22–28, 29–38, 39–50

Spain and Belgium, where the proportions were highest for 18–19-year-old men. However, due to the small numbers involved, the values in the age strata have wide confidence intervals. The percentages of women reporting five or more partners during the past 12 months were much lower (Table 6.3) than for men. The sex ratio is above five for most countries, the exceptions being Norway (ratio: 2.4), Finland (2.1) and Spain (2.1). In most countries, the largest group of subjects with many partners was to be found among the women aged 18–19 years.

The percentage of subjects with more than five partners per year was highest in towns and large cities (Table 6.4). This tendency is found both for males and females. Men living without a sexual partner (non-cohabiting males) reported having more than five partners more frequently than cohabiting men (Table 6.5). For cohabiting men, most countries reported percentages below one. However, Finland, East Germany and Portugal reported percentages above two. For cohabiting women, only Finns had percentages above one (Table 6.5). Thus, it appears that non-cohabiting subjects under 25 living in towns or large cities are the group that has the largest fraction of subjects potentially at high risk of contracting sexually transmitted diseases. Among subjects who have had exclusively heterosexual relations in the past 12 months, the proportion of subjects reporting five or more partners is lower than for the group reporting homosexual or bisexual relations (Table 6.6). The denominators are small in many surveys, and for this table (as opposed to the preceding tables) only subjects who reported having sexual partners during the last year are included.

Regarding condom use, West Germany (1993) included a question asking 'how often condoms were used recently'. Only 4.2 per cent of the male respondents who reported having had five or more partners during the past 12 months versus 48.9 per cent of the males reporting having had one partner replied 'never' to this question. In the West German study of 1990, 91.7 per cent (base 36) of the men who reported five or more partners in the past 12 months had ever used a condom in their lives as compared with 75.8 per cent of men reporting one partner. In the France–ACSF study, 79.0 per cent (base 140) of the men who reported five or more partners in the last 12 months stated they had used condoms in the past year compared with 48.9 per cent (base 2029) of the men with fewer partners and 37 per cent (base 139) of the men with more than five partners reported use of a condom during the last intercourse, whereas 21 per cent (base 2019) of the males with one to four partners in the past 12 months used a condom. Still in France, 64.6 per cent (base 40) of the female respondents who had five or more partners reported using condoms in the past year and 20 per cent (base 39) at last intercourse compared with 55.5 per cent (base 1704) and 14 per cent (base 1654), respectively, of the women with fewer partners. All these data show a clear trend for subjects with more than five partners per year to report more frequent condom use.

Table 6.4 *Proportions of men and women reporting five or more partners during the last 12 months by place of residence*

		Athens 1990	Belgium 1993	Finland 1992	France ACSF 1992	Germany East 1990	Germany West 1990	Netherlands 1989	Norway 1992
MEN									
Rural	%		0	5.2	1.1	1.1	0	11.1	2.3
	N		39	268	503	91	131	9	475
Small towns	%		1.7	6.3	1.9	6.8	1.6	2.8	3.9
	N		630	252	487	265	505	283	711
Towns	%		8.4	10.6	2.4		3.9	9.0	4.6
	N		186	180	755		212	100	350
Large cities	%	1.9	4.5	–	3.4	4.9	2.7	–	–
	N	755	391	–	511	163	70	–	–
WOMEN									
Rural	%		0	1.7	0.2	0	0	0	0.8
	N		41	235	391	76	185	30	598
Small towns	%		0.4	3.6	0.4	0.5	0.3	0.8	1.5
	N		684	248	405	200	574	377	949
Towns	%		0	4.7	0.2		0	0.7	2.4
	N		199	191	656		256	144	468
Large cities	%	0.1	1.7		0.9	1.4	0		
	N	843	463		379	148	87		

Base: all respondents (18–49 years) who ever had sex

Table 6.5 *Proportions of men and women reporting five or more partners during the last 12 months by cohabitational status*

		Belgium	Finland	France ACSF	Germany East	Germany West	Netherlands	Norway	Portugal
		1993	1992	1992	1990	1990	1989	1992	1991
MEN									
Cohabiting	%	0.6	3.8	0.8	3.3	0.2	0.4	0.5	2.4
	N	832	498	1063	395	557	236	1064	649
Not cohabiting	%	9.2	14.6	4.7	13.0	4.7	10.9	10.5	8.1
	N	308	206	1191	108	358	156	476	513
WOMEN									
Cohabiting	%	0	1.8	0.1	0	0	0.3	0.2	0
	N	1028	494	914	373	774	396	1576	739
Not cohabiting	%	2.2	7.2	1.2	6.8	0.6	1.9	5.8	0.6
	N	260	180	917	44	327	155	469	477

Base: all respondents (18–49 years) who ever had sex

Table 6.6 *Proportions of men and women reporting five or more partners during the last 12 months by sexual orientation*

		Belgium	Finland	France ACSF	Germany East	Germany West	Netherlands	Norway	Portugal
		1993	1992	1992	1990	1990	1989	1992	1991
MEN									
Hetero	%	2.9	6.4	1.9	5.9	3.5	2.6	3.7	5.2
	N	1198	654	2095	376	931	340	1361	1058
Homo/bi	%	27.4	66.7	16.0	27.3	9.7	39.1	9.5	44.4
	N	20	3	94	22	31	23	21	9
WOMEN									
Hetero	%	0.5	2.7	0.4	0.9	0.5	0.8	1.2	0.5
	N	1310	625	1708	318	1042	505	1869	957
Homo/bi	%	3.7	9.1	5.0	0	4.5	0	19.0	0
	N	11	11	39	9	44	5	21	5

Base: all respondents (18–49 years) who ever had sex in the last 12 months

Table 6.7 *Proportions of male respondents having paid for sex during the last 12 months*

		France ACSF 1992	Germany West 1990	Netherlands 1989	Norway 1992	Spain[1] 1990	Portugal 1991
All	%	1.1	4.8	2.8	1.8	11.0	5.4
	CI	0.7–1.5	3.5–6.1	1.1–4.5	1.2–2.4	8.0–14.0	4.0–6.8
	N	2176	990	363	1523	409	993
18–19	%	0.1	2.3	0	1.4	11.3	0
	N	130	43	14	73	53	68
20–24	%	2.2	7.5	1.6	1.6	10.5	5.7
	N	487	186	64	251	152	163
25–29	%	1.4	4.0	1.6	2.5	–	6.1
	N	479	226	61	277	–	110
30–39	%	1.1	5.6	4.9	1.6	10.4	7.7
	N	661	302	142	506	125	363
40–49	%	0.6	3.0	1.2	1.9	12.7	3.4
	N	419	233	82	416	79	289

Base: male respondents (18–49 years) who ever had sex in the last 12 months
Note:
[1] Spain: the age categories are 19–21, 22–28, 29–38, 39–50

Paying for Sex During the Last 12 Months

Table 6.7 shows the proportions of male respondents who were sexually active in the 12 months preceding the respective surveys who had paid for sex at any point in that period. The prevalence varied across Europe, being highest in Spain (11.0 per cent) and lowest in France (1.1 per cent). In addition to the surveys presented in Table 6.7, the Belgian survey asked male respondents if they had paid for sex in the last five years. The affirmative answer rate was 6.4 per cent (base 1223, CI: 5.0–7.8). The Finnish and Norwegian surveys also gave the percentages of males who reported having paid for their last sexual intercourse, namely, 0.5 and 1.3 per cent of all male respondents to the Finnish and Norwegian surveys, respectively. In the Athens 1990 study, 65 per cent (17/26) who reported having paid for sex during the past 12 months, reported using condoms on such occasions (15 subjects said 'always' and two 'often'). For Norway, 43 per cent (9/21) of subjects reporting sex with a sex worker in the last intercourse reported using condoms on that occasion. Ninety-two per cent (base 74) of the French men who had paid for sex during the past 12 months reported condom use in the past 12 months. So, these data indicate that condoms are used frequently in contacts with sex workers. They do not, however, reveal the gender of the person selling the sexual favours.

Prevalence of Injecting Drug Use

Table 6.8 shows that the fractions of the population who reported ever having injected drugs were remarkably similar across Europe. The highest lifetime prevalence (2.1 per cent) was recorded in Spain and the lowest (0.4 per cent) in the Netherlands. The prevalence was about twice as high for males as for females (except for Finland and the Netherlands), while no systematic age trend emerged. Five countries included a question on injecting drug use in the last 12 months, the answers to which yielded prevalences of about one-tenth of the lifetime rates (Belgium, France and the Netherlands reported one per 1000 and Norway and Switzerland two per thousand). The Athens 1990 survey included a question on injecting drug use during the last six months, where the estimate was less than one in 1000 (1/1661). None of the subjects reporting injecting drug use in Athens or in the Netherlands had ever shared needles, while 8 per cent in France reported sharing needles.

Discussion

These data reflect not only the proportion of the European population that has a potential risk of becoming HIV infected, but also the segments of the population that should be given priority in HIV prevention. If we look at each country, young, non-cohabiting city dwellers probably constitute one of the groups that keep sexually transmitted diseases flourishing, based on the proportion of subjects who reported having more than five partners in the past 12 months. It therefore seems worthwhile to direct particular efforts towards this group. In Britain, STDs and HIV have the highest prevalences in inner London, an area in which the proportion of people reporting more than 10 sexual partners during the last five years was significantly higher than in other parts of Britain (Wadsworth *et al.*, 1996). Thus, examining the geographical pattern of behaviour within a country can reveal a correlation between risk behaviour and disease prevalence.

Regarding the risk indicators presented in this chapter, only four surveys contained questions on sex with an injecting drug user. Very few respondents (less than 1 per cent of the total corpus) reported such behaviour in the past year, past six months or the last time they had intercourse. As pointed out earlier, this is probably an underestimate, but the degree of bias is not easy to determine. However, it seems fair to conclude that this pathway from a group with a relatively high percentage of people who are HIV positive (IDUs) to a larger heterosexual population, although it represents a potential for the spread of infections, is probably narrow. In order to have stable data on sexual

Table 6.8 Proportions of respondents who reported having injected drugs at any time in their lives

		Finland 1992	France ACSF 1992	Germany West 1990	Netherlands 1989	Norway 1992	Portugal 1991	Spain 1990	Switzerland[1] 1992
All	%	1.1	1.3	1.0	0.4	0.7	1.5	2.1	0.7
	CI	0.6–1.6	1.0–1.6	0.6–1.4	0.0–0.8	0.4–1.0	1.0–2.0	1.1–3.1	0.4–1.0
	N	1442	4086	2185	943	3652	2220	859	2678
Gender									
Men	%	1.0	1.7	1.4	0.5	1.1	2.3	2.8	1.1
	N	735	2255	1034	392	1578	1158	436	1360
Women	%	1.3	0.7	0.7	0.4	0.4	0.6	1.4	0.4
	N	707	1831	1151	551	2074	1062	423	1318
Age									
18–24	%	2.1	0.6	0.6	0.5	0.9	1.5	–	0.8
	N	283	1202	491	202	806	507	–	722
25–49	%	0.9	1.6	1.1	0.4	0.7	1.5	–	0.7
	N	1159	2884	1694	741	2846	1709	–	1956
Place of residence									
Rural and small towns	%	0.9	1.4	0.7	0.4	0.7	–		
	N	1050	1786	1028	699	2779	–		
Towns and large cities	%	1.8	1.2	1.3	0.4	0.8	–		
	N	390	2300	1141	244	837	–		

Base: all respondents (18–49 years) who ever had sex in the last 12 months
CI: 95% confidence interval
Note:
[1] Switzerland: only ages 18–45 are included

Table 6.9 Number of new cases of AIDS per million inhabitants in 1994

	Belgium	Finland	France	Germany	Great Britain	Greece	Netherlands	Norway	Portugal	Spain	Switzerland
AIDS incidence	25.2	8.7	98.1	22.5	29.3	21.1	30.3	16.9	66.1	185.2	97.9

Source: The European Centre for the Epidemiological Monitoring of AIDS (1995)

practices within these relationships (for example condom use), other research designs are required.

Anal sex in heterosexual intercourse is not common if we look at findings on last intercourse. In contrast, about half of the male respondents who reported having had sex with men engaged in anal sex in the past 12 months. The findings also suggest that injecting drug use is not widespread in the countries under survey. The percentages of respondents reporting ever having had experience of injecting drug use are very similar across Europe. This is interesting in light of the diversity of approaches taken to limit the use of these substances.

The surveys also show that, in most countries, a relatively low proportion of men pay for sex and, if they do, condoms are frequently used. Thus, sex work is probably not linked to HIV transmission in Europe as much as seems to be the case in parts of Asia and Africa. If we focus on the individual countries, Spain, with relatively frequent injecting drug use, purchase of sex and high proportions of both men and women with many partners, may be the country with the highest risk levels.

Can the potential risk estimates in this chapter be used as indirect measurements of the HIV loads in these same populations? Table 6.9 shows the incidence of AIDS (new cases per million inhabitants) in Europe in 1994 (European Centre, 1995). The numbers for each country have been fairly stable in the last few years. The high incidence in Spain is due largely to a high number of AIDS cases among injecting drug users. This observation fits with our results that the reported lifetime prevalence of injecting drug use is highest in Spain (Table 6.8). It would be preferable to have population-based data on the occurrence of HIV in the same countries, but only sketchy data exist. The prevalence of HIV ranges from 2 and 6 per cent among persons seeking medical care at STD clinics in Belgium (2.5 per cent), France (5.4 per cent), Great Britain (2.8 per cent), the Netherlands (4.2 per cent) and Switzerland (5.3 per cent) (European Centre, 1993). Pregnant women may be used as a surrogate for a population-based sample, since more than 90 per cent of women become pregnant during their child-bearing years, thus forming a relatively unselected general population group of sexually active women. The prevalence of HIV infection among pregnant women has been estimated in surveys of pregnant women (European Centre, 1994). The lowest figures are found in Norway and Finland (less than 1 per 10000 women), while the highest figures are from France (3.4 per 1000), parts of Amsterdam (4.9 per 1000) and inner London (2.6 per 1000). Eight countries (Belgium, Finland, France, West Germany, the Netherlands, Norway, Portugal and Spain) reported proportions of male and female subjects with five or more sexual partners in the past 12 months (Table 6.3) that could be correlated with AIDS incidence. (In this analysis, the West German data were used for correlation with the AIDS incidence in the country as a whole.) A quick glance at Tables 6.3 and 6.9 shows no significant degree of covariance between the specific risk indicator of five or more partners during the past 12 months and AIDS incidence for either men or women. These correlations should be interpreted very cautiously, however, since there may be a long delay between the specific behaviour and onset of AIDS (the average incubation time of AIDS is 10 years) and other indicators related more directly to preventive practices may have yielded other results.

It is difficult to understand the inter-country variability in HIV occurrence in light of the data presented in this chapter. The low prevalence of HIV among pregnant women in Finland and Norway is remarkable when contrasted with the finding in Table 6.3 that these countries, together with Spain, exhibit the highest prevalences of reporting five or more partners during the past 12 months for women. However, the lack of a significant correlation between risk behaviour in a country and that country's AIDS incidence should not discourage attempts to modify risk behaviour, since there appear to be good reasons for not expecting a high correlation in ecological data of this nature. A more detailed comparison of behaviour in France and Britain (Bajos *et al.*, 1995) showed slightly higher prevalences of risk behaviour in France, although the authors of that paper do not believe that these differences can wholly explain why France's AIDS prevalence is three times higher than Britain's. They suggest that factors such as the time of the virus's first arrival, the timing of prevention policies and the social organization of the gay/homosexual community have an impact as well. These issues should be studied in more detail in cross-national studies. Both HIV prevalence and AIDS incidence are to a large extent dependent on the spread of HIV in the early 1980s. Better understanding of the relation between behaviour and the incidence of HIV infection would need representative data on the number of new cases of HIV infection occuring today.

As mentioned earlier, infectious disease epidemiology states that a disease cannot spread in a population unless the basic reproductive ratio is above one. Mathematical models have shown that with the sexual behaviour reported in the heterosexual Norwegian population, the transmission rate per intercourse between an HIV-positive and an HIV-negative person would have to be above one per cent for the basic reproductive ratio to be above one (Stigum *et al.*, 1991). This transmission rate is markedly higher than the empirical transmission rate for heterosexual intercourse between an HIV-positive and an HIV-negative person. Thus, given the patterns of sexual behaviour ascertained to date, HIV cannot spread in the heterosexual population of Norway. This result is consistent with the observations that in Europe, HIV is still mainly a disease affecting certain risk groups and most heterosexually infected people do not transmit the infection to others. Returning to the distinction made in the introduction between the risk of exposure versus the risk of transmission given exposure, the presence of co-factors almost certainly plays a decisive role in the transmission of HIV. As long as the risk of exposure is as low as it is, we cannot expect to find strong correlations between average behaviour and disease incidence. We may also speculate that the more rapid heterosexual transmission of HIV that has been documented in some regions of the world has more to do with the presence of particular HIV subtypes (high relative prevalences of subtype C in Africa, subtype E in Asia and subtype B in Europe) than with sexual practices. However, studies of sexual behaviour in temporally and spatially representative samples of the population are a prerequisite for evaluating the influences of other factors. Further studies of behaviour in Europe that have common aims and standardized protocols are thus needed.

References

BAJOS, N., WADSWORTH, J., DUCOT, B. *et al.* (1995) 'Sexual behaviour and HIV epidemiology: comparative analysis in France and Britain', *AIDS*, **9**, pp. 735–43.

BROOKMEYER, R. and GAIL, M.H. (1994) *AIDS Epidemiology. A Quantitative Approach*, New York: Oxford University Press.

DES JARLAIS, D.C., FRIEDMAN, S.R., COOPANYA, K. *et al.* (1992) 'International epidemiology of HIV and AIDS among injecting drug users', *AIDS*, **6**, pp. 1053–68.

EUROPEAN CENTRE FOR THE EPIDEMIOLOGICAL MONITORING OF AIDS (1993) 'HIV/AIDS surveillance in Europe', *Quarterly Report*, **40**, Saint-Maurice, France.

EUROPEAN CENTRE FOR THE EPIDEMIOLOGICAL MONITORING OF AIDS (1994) 'HIV/AIDS surveillance in Europe', *Quarterly Report*, **44**, Saint-Maurice, France.

EUROPEAN CENTRE FOR THE EPIDEMIOLOGICAL MONITORING OF AIDS (1995) 'HIV/AIDS surveillance in Europe', *Quarterly Report*, **47**, Saint-Maurice, France.

EUROPEAN STUDY GROUP (1989) 'Risk factors for male to female transmission of HIV', *British Medical Journal*, **298**, pp. 411–15.

HAVERKOS, H.W. and EDELMAN, R. (1989). 'Heterosexuals', in KASLOW, R.A. and FRANCIS, D.P. (Eds) *The Epidemiology of AIDS*, New York: Oxford University Press.

KUNANUSONT, C., FOY, H.M., KREIS, J.K. *et al.* (1995) 'HIV-1 subtypes and male to female transmission in Thailand', *Lancet*, **345**, pp. 1078–83.

MARMOR, M., FRIEDMAN-KIEN, A.E., ZOLLA-PAZNER, S. *et al.* (1984) 'Kaposi's sarcoma in homosexual men. A seroepidemiologic case-control study', *Annals of Internal Medicine*, **100**, pp. 809–15.

SCHMIDT, G. (1989) 'Sexual permissiveness in western societies. Roots and course of development', *Nordisk Sexologi*, **7**, pp. 225–34.

STIGUM, H. and MAGNUS, P. (1997) 'A risk index for sexually transmitted diseases', *Sexually Transmitted Diseases*, **24**, pp. 102–8.

STIGUM, H., FALCK, W. and MAGNUS, P. (1994) 'The core group revisited: the effect of partner mixing and migration on the spread of Gonorrhea, Chlamydia, and HIV', *Mathematical Biosciences*, **120**, pp. 1–23.

STIGUM, H., GRØNNESBY, J.K., MAGNUS, P. *et al.* (1991) 'The potential for spread of HIV in the heterosexual population in Norway. A model study', *Statistics in Medicine*, **10**, pp. 1003–23.

YORKE, J.A., HETHCOTE, H.W. and NOLD, A. (1978) 'Dynamics and control of the transmission of gonorrhea', *Sexually Transmitted Diseases*, **5**, pp. 51–6.

WADSWORTH, J., HICKMAN, M., JOHNSON, A.M. *et al.* (1996) 'Geographic variation in sexual behaviour in Britain: implications for sexually transmitted disease epidemiology and sexual health promotion', *AIDS*, **10**, pp. 193–9.

Chapter 7

Self-reported Sexually Transmitted Diseases and At-risk Sexual Behaviour

Josiane Warszawski*

Introduction

Sexual relations are the predominant mode of transmission of more than twenty micro-organisms pathogenic to the human species that are widespread in most regions of the world, particularly in developing countries. Certain sexually transmitted diseases (STDs) influence the AIDS epidemic itself by facilitating the acquisition of HIV (Wasserheit, 1992). A randomized controlled trial in Tanzania recently showed that improvement in the treatment of symptomatic STDs caused the rate of HIV incidence to fall by approximately 40 per cent (Grosskurth *et al.*, 1995). Moreover, although HIV is the pathogen behind the STD epidemic giving most cause for concern at the present time, the high morbidity associated with other infections (female infertility, ectopic pregnancies, genital cancers, systemic complications and neonatal infections) also makes them major public health problems (Holmes *et al.*, 1990).

The prevalence of various risk behaviours has been compared by Per Magnus (Chapter 6). The objective of this chapter is to study similarities and differences in the frequency of STD reporting according to socio-demographic characteristics, since STDs are potential consequences of high-risk behaviours. Analysis of the information collected about STD history in the European surveys reviewed here is limited by the small number of subjects in each sample who reported such infections. The joint study of these data provides an opportunity for interpreting associations that are not statistically significant but tend to be similar in several surveys. We shall thus examine to what extent the results can help us compare the epidemiology of

*The author would like to thank Béatrice Ducot and Laurence Meyer for their judicious advice.

STDs in different European countries and target particularly vulnerable populations.

Background

STDs are a heterogeneous group of bacterial, viral, fungal and parasitic infections. They differ in clinical features, prognosis, and transmission dynamics, which are determined by the biological characteristics of the organism, the host's response to infection, and patterns of sexual contact (Renton and Whitaker, 1991). In Europe, STDs are represented mainly by two well-known bacterial diseases, *Chlamydia trachomatis* (CT) infection and gonorrhoea, and two viral infections, genital herpes and genital warts. Syphilis has become rare (Aral and Holmes, 1990). *Candida albicans* (yeast), one of the commonest genital infections, is not always included in the group of STDs used to define an HIV risk indicator since endogenous factors may also be implicated in recurrent vulvovaginal yeast infections (Sobel, 1993). Viral hepatitis is also sexually transmitted but not exclusively, and does not have genital symptoms. Antibiotics can cure bacterial infections whereas no permanent cure as yet exists for viral infections.

Geographic and temporal variations in the incidence rate of certain STDs may reflect variations in sexual behaviour and perhaps indirectly in the incidence of HIV infection (Renton and Whitaker, 1994). For various reasons, the prevalence and incidence of STDs are difficult to estimate nationally. In Western Europe, STD patients can be seen in many sites: hospitals, specialized clinics (sexually transmitted disease clinics), and private gynaecologists' and general practioners' offices (Renton and Whitaker, 1991). Clinical examination generally is not sufficient to identify the causal pathogen. The diagnosis cannot be certain without an examination of genital or blood samples, although laboratory methods for each STD are not standardized. STDs may be asymptomatic or have too few symptoms to warrant consulting a doctor. Many of them develop unobtrusively and are not detected until complications appear (Holmes *et al.*, 1990). The date of infection generally remains unknown.

New laboratory tests introduced in the early 1980s, especially for *Chlamydia trachomatis* and viral infections, have become more and more specific, sensitive, easy to use and affordable. They allow more intensive screening for STDs, especially in asymptomatic women in whom they might never have been suspected in the past. An increase observed through case-reporting systems can correspond to the spread and improvement of these diagnostic techniques rather than to a real increase in incidence (Renton and Whitaker, 1994). Systematic screening in a given population allows estimation of prevalence, but not incidence. A way for estimating trends without such a misinterpretation is to repeat cross-sectional surveys of systematic screening with similar diagnostic methods in the same population.

The use of laboratory diagnostics explains why most available studies of STDs are based upon targeted groups selected in medical settings (STD clinics, family planning clinics, student medical services, maternity wards or, more rarely, private practices) (Handsfield and Schwebke, 1990; Treurniet and Davidse, 1993; Meyer *et al.*, 1994).

The characteristics of the people using these care facilities and the relative weights of the various segments of the population are generally poorly known and the results cannot be easily extrapolated to the entire population. However, conducting genital or blood tests in a representative sample of the general population is an unlikely prospect for reasons of cost and social acceptability. National surveys can only ask people about their STD history. Omission, memory errors and deliberate under- or over-reporting are potential biases, as is the case for any answer strongly dependent on social norms and expectations. Two more biases are specific to STD questions as opposed to those concerning personal behaviour reporting. First, people can confuse the names of diseases with each other and with other non-venereal genital pathologies. Second, and more importantly, most reported infections were probably diagnosed following clinical signs or suspicion of exposure, that is, shortly after infection, or detected during a physical examination. So, infections that have not been diagnosed cannot be reported (Anderson *et al.*, 1994). The frequency of STD reporting may then increase with the coverage of STD screening. It could even be negatively correlated with the actual incidence of curable STDs. Differences in rates of STD reporting could just as well be ascribed to differences in screening policy and the ability to understand and remember diagnoses, as to differences in level of at-risk sexual behaviour.

Our results will be discussed in the light of these two hypotheses. We shall have also to take into account a *generation effect* due to changes in diagnostic strategies over the last 15 years. With the relatively recent availability of diagnostic methods, the rate of diagnosis may have increased more in people having better access to care systems, for example among women and college graduates. Thus, women tend to use health services and to declare symptoms more easily, even though STDs are less symptomatic in women than in men and require more active screening (Amaro and Gornemann, 1991). Moreover, genital samples can be taken during a routine internal pelvic examination in a similar way to cervical smears (gynaecological check-up or pregnancy monitoring), while urethral samples are rarely taken from men, and the painfulness of the sampling procedure renders it unacceptable in the absence of clinical suspicion. Lastly, women (and their doctors) are perhaps better informed of the usefulness of STD treatment in light of its possible consequences for female fertility. Higher education also favours access to care, risk awareness and dialogue with doctors (Adam and Herzlich, 1994). Links between gender, age, level of education and a self-declared history of STD may then vary with the length of the reporting period.

Methods

The studies undertaken in Norway (1992), the Netherlands (1989), former East Germany (1990), and former West Germany (1990) asked about life STD history ('Have you ever had an STD in your life?'). In Finland (1992), five separate questions concerned life experience of gonococcal infections, *Chlamydia trachomatis* infections, syphilis, genital warts and genital herpes. In France (1992) and in Belgium (1993) the questions concerned the last five years. The last 12 months were also investigated in Finland, France and the Netherlands. Information on the pathogenic agent in question was collected in Finland, Norway, the Netherlands, France and Belgium.

The study population was restricted to sexually active (sexual relations at least once in one's life) persons between 18 and 49 years of age. Overall, STDs were reported by 355 Belgian (290 men and 65 women), 147 Finnish (127 men and 110 women), 704 French (246 men and 458 women), 59 East German (40 men and 19 women), 207 West German (88 men and 119 women), 65 Dutch (34 men and 31 women) and 716 Norwegian (324 men and 392 women) respondents. People who did not respond to STD questions (because they refused to answer or did not know if they had an STD) were excluded (between 2 and 4 per cent in the Nordic countries and under 1 per cent in the other countries).

We compared the percentages of people reporting an STD during their lifetime, in the last five years and in the last 12 months. Confidence intervals were estimated using traditional simple random sampling formulae for all countries except France, where specialized software, SUDAAN, was used (Shah *et al.*, 1993). Two percentages were considered significantly different if their confidence intervals did not overlap. Relative risks (RRs) – the ratio of the STD percentage in one category over the STD percentage in a second (reference) category – were computed to quantify the degree of association between STDs and various exposure factors. The further the relative risk is from unity, the stronger the STD's association with the category considered.

The data were analyzed in three successive stages. The first step checked whether the pattern of STD reporting agreed with the limited data obtained from epidemiological surveillance and whether self-reported STDs were associated with sexual behaviour at risk of HIV. The specific behaviours studied were the number of partners and paying for sex in the same period as that of the STD history, and lifetime homosexual experience broadly defined. For a discussion of cross-cultural differences in definitions and formulations see

Chapters 3 and 5. We also studied STD reporting's association with self-referred HIV testing, which was taken as an indicator of risk perception. Former East and West Germany were excluded since the number of partners and STD history did not refer to the same period. The second step examined whether the history of an STD was associated with gender, level of education, age and place of residence. The relative risks of STDs associated with these factors (for example, with gender) were calculated for the entire group of respondents and for each stratum of number of partners (high, medium and low), the logic being that similar relative risks for each partner level would indicate that the association was independent of the number of partners. The last step studied country-to-country variations in reported STD frequencies with respect to the differences in risk indicator prevalences described in other chapters.

Consistency of Self-reported STDs with Epidemiological Data

Definition of STDs

Epidemiological surveillance has been instituted for a number of specific diseases. Using all STDs as defined by the answer to the broad question 'Have you ever had an STD?' is a makeshift solution. Most of the surveys considered here also asked questions about specific diseases. However, each disease was reported by a very small number of people, making it possible to check only whether the distributions and sex ratios of the four major European STDs (*Chlamydia trachomatis* infections, gonorrhoea, genital herpes and genital warts) at least converged with epidemiological findings, which seems to be a minimum prerequisite if one is to trust in STD declaration.

Tables 7.1 and 7.2 present the proportions of males and females reporting these diseases and their associated relative risks. Males have a higher lifetime report rate for gonorrhoea than *Chlamydia trachomatis*. However, this situation is reversed for more recent reference periods (five years and 12 months). In women, *Chlamydia trachomatis* infections are consistently reported more frequently than gonorrhoea whatever the period studied, but the gap widens as the reference period shortens. These findings reflect the changes in the gonorrhoea/*Chlamydia trachomatis* ratio that have been 'detected' by epidemiological surveillance, namely, that gonococcal infections have been falling steadily for the past 20 years whereas *Chlamydia trachomatis* infections began to be diagnosed in the late 1970s and have since become the most frequent STD in Western Europe. The predominance of males over females in the gonorrhoea (but not *Chlamydia tracomatis*) frequencies (Table 7.2) is also

Table 7.1 *Proportions of men and women reporting a history of one specific STD*

		12 months			5 years			Life		
		Finland 1992	France 1992	Netherlands 1989	Belgium 1993	France 1992	Norway 1992	Finland 1992	Netherlands 1989	Norway 1992
MEN										
Chlamydia trachomatis	%	0.7	0.1	0.8	0.08	0.4	3.7	6.8	0.3	7.6
	CI	0.01–1.4	0.02–0.2	0.3–1.2	0.0–0.2	0.2–0.6	2.8–4.7	5.0–8.6	0.0–7.7	6.3–8.9
Gonorrhoea	%	0	0.07	0.3	0.03	0.3	1.0	7.8	4.4	9.3
	CI	0.0–0.05	0.0–0.2	0.0–0.5	0.0–0.1	0.1–0.5	0.5–1.5	5.9–9.7	2.4–6.4	7.9–10.7
Papilloma virus	%	0.7	n.a.	n.a.	0.03	n.a.	n.a.	5.1	1.6	4.3
	CI	0.08–1.3			0.0–0.1			3.5–8.1	0.3–2.9	3.3–5.3
Herpes virus	%	0.1	n.a.	n.a.	0.08	n.a.	n.a.	1.5	0	1.5
	CI	0.0–0.4			0.0–0.2			0.6–2.4	0.0–0.1	0.9–2.1
WOMEN										
Chlamydia trachomatis	%	0.7	0.1	0.9	0.3	0.6	4.8	6.9	1.1	9.8
	CI	0.01–1.4	0.03–0.2	0.5–1.3	0.0–0.5	0.5–0.7	3.9–5.7	5.1–8.7	0.0–2.0	8.5–11.1
Gonorrhoea	%	0.1	0.01	0	0.01	0.06	0.1	3.4	2.0	4.1
	CI	0.0–0.4	0.0–0.03	0.0–0.07	0.0–0.3	0.0–0.1	0.0–0.2	2.1–4.7	0.6–3.4	3.3–5.0
Papilloma virus	%	1.4	n.a.	n.a.	0.09	n.a.	n.a.	7.7	0.4	4.7
	CI	0.5–2.3			0.0–0.3			5.8–9.6	0.0–0.9	3.8–5.6
Herpes virus	%	0.8	n.a.	n.a.	0.2	n.a.	n.a.	2.2	0.9	2.6
	CI	0.2–1.4			0.0–0.4			1.1–3.3	0.1–1.7	1.9–3.3

Base: all respondents (18–49 years) who ever had sex
CI: 95% confidence interval; upper 95% confidence limit of 0% is calculated with Poisson distribution
n.a.: not available

Table 7.2 *Relative risk of women versus men associated with specific STDs*

	12 months			5 years				Life	
	Finland 1992	France 1992	Netherlands 1989	Belgium 1993	France 1992	Norway 1992	Finland 1992	Netherlands 1989	Norway 1992
RRf/m									
Chlamydia trachomatis	1.0	1.0	1.1	3.3	1.4	1.3	1.0	3.3	1.3
Gonorrhoea	n.c. (0)	0.1	n.c. (0)	0.3	0.2	0.1	0.5	0.5	0.4
Papilloma virus	2	n.a.	n.a.	3.3	n.a.	n.a.	1.4	0.3	1.1
Herpes virus	10	n.a.	n.a.	2.5	n.a.	n.a.	1.4	n.c. (+∞)	1.7

Base: all respondents (18–49 years) who ever had sex
RR: relative risk
n.c.: not computable
n.a.: not available

225

reported in the literature (Aral and Holmes, 1990; Treurniet and Davidse, 1993; Meyer *et al.*, 1994). Genital warts and herpes infections are declared as often as the two bacterial infections (*Chlamydia trachomatis* and *Neisseria gonorrhoeae*) and more often by women than by men, as described in the literature (Aral and Holmes, 1990). Very few cases of syphilis are reported, especially by women. These findings suggest that confusions and classification errors do not constitute a major bias in STD reporting.

Self-reported STDs and Sexual Behaviour

The rate at which new sexual relationships occur in a population is the main determinant of STD spread (Brunham, 1991). The number of partners in a given period is a commonly accepted indicator of the rate of partner change. Table 7.3 shows that the percentage of respondents with histories of STD increases with increasing number of sexual partners reported over the same reference period, that is lifetime, last five years or last 12 months, in all surveys. This association is similarly high for both males and females and observed for each age class and level of education and regardless of locality size. This means that the correlation is independant of various socio-demographic characteristics able to influence response content on the one hand and access to screening on the other. Self-declared STD history thus appears to be a reliable indicator of multipartnership.

Sex work is another classic risk factor of STD and HIV (Aral and Holmes, 1990). Again, in all the countries studied here, STD is clearly more often reported by men who paid for sex at least once in the period under consideration (Table 7.4).

The high prevalence of HIV and other STDs among male homosexuals has been attributed to more prevalent at-risk sexual behaviour (multiple partners, anal sex) and to the fact that most of their sexual partners belong themselves to groups with high STD prevalence (Ostrow, 1990). On the other hand, awareness of the HIV risk and safer sex, which was likely to be accompanied by an increased awareness of STD treatments, took hold earliest in the gay/homosexual community. Table 7.5 shows that, except in Finland, males who have ever had homosexual relations tend to report an STD more often than exclusively heterosexual males. Nevertheless, homosexuals' higher numbers of partners do not appear to be sufficient to explain this association since this association 1. holds in France, Belgium and the Netherlands, whatever the number of partners; 2. is seen for males reporting 10 or more partners in their lives in Norway; 3. applies to males reporting fewer than 10 partners in Finland. Those high rates of self-declared STDs may reflect both at-risk sexual behaviour and effective STD screening.

Table 7.3 Proportions of men and women reporting an STD history by number of sexual partners in the same reference period

	12 months			5 years		Life		
	Finland[1] 1992	France 1992	Netherlands 1989	Belgium 1993	France 1992	Finland[1] 1992	Netherlands 1989	Norway 1992
MEN								
No. of partners								
Low %	0.6	0.8	0	0.8	1.7	4.0	0	6.0
CI	0.0–1.3	0.5–1.1	0.0–0.1	0.2–1.4	1.3–2.1	1.6–6.4	0.0–0.2	4.2–7.8
Medium %	2.7	1.9	1.8	1.6	4.1	9.3	5.3	15.4
CI	0.09–5.3	0.7–3.1	0.0–5.3	0.0–3.7	2.7–5.5	4.1–14.6	0.2–10.4	11.4–19.4
High %	6.3	1.3	5.6	5.5	8.6	30.7	23.8	39.4
CI	0.0–13.1	0.0–3.0	0.0–16.1	2.2–8.8	6.9–10.3	25.7–35.7	16.4–31.2	35.3–43.5
RR high vs low	*10.5*	*1.6*	*n.c. (+∞)*	*6.9#*	*5.1#*	*7.7#*	*n.c. (+∞)*	*6.6#*
WOMEN								
No. of partners								
Low %	1.3	1.6	0.6	2.5	4.2	5.2	1.8	8.1
CI	0.3–2.3	1.3–1.9	0.0–1.3	1.7–3.3	3.7–4.7	3.0–7.5	0.6–3.0	6.5–9.7
Medium %	11.8	5.4	5.6	8.0	8.2	22.1	8.5	22.4
CI	5.3–18.3	3.4–7.4	0.0–13.0	2.0–14.0	6.1–10.3	15.7–28.5	2.0–15.0	18.6–26.2
High %	13.6	8.1	25.0	19.5	18.5	37.2	38.6	50.6
CI	0.0–28.0	0.8–15.4	0.0–67.4	9.1–29.9	14.8–22.2	28.9–45.5	24.2–53.0	45.3–55.9
RR high vs low	*10.5*	*5.1*	*41.7*	*7.8#*	*4.4#*	*7.2#*	*21.4#*	*6.2#*

Base: all respondents (18–49 years) who ever had sex

CI: 95% confidence interval; upper 95% confidence limit of 0% is calculated with Poisson distribution

#: confidence intervals do not overlap

RR: relative risk

n.c.: not computable

Number of partners low/medium/high during life: 1–4 / 5–9 / ≥10; 5 years: 1–2 / 3–4 / ≥5; 12 months: 0–1 / 2–4 / ≥5

Note:

[1]Finland: 'self-reported STD' included exclusively a history of gonorrhoea, chlamydial infection, syphilis, genital warts and genital herpes, while it was not explicitly defined in the other countries

227

Table 7.4 *Proportions of men reporting an STD history vs paying for sex among men in the same reference period*

		5 years		Life		
		Belgium 1993	France 1992	Finland[1] 1992	Netherlands 1989	Norway 1992
Had ever paid for sex						
yes	%	4.9	8.7	45.6	31.5	46.7
	CI	0.1–9.8	5.1–12.3	33.8–57.4	19.0–44.0	39.4–54.0
no	%	1.4	3.0	14.5	5.1	17.1
	CI	0.7–2.1	2.6–3.4	11.8–17.2	2.8–7.4	15.1–19.1
RR yes vs no		*3.6*	*2.9[#]*	*3.1[#]*	*6.2[#]*	*2.7[#]*

Base: all male respondants (18–49 years) who ever had sex
CI: 95% confidence interval
[#]: confidence intervals do not overlap
RR: relative risk
Note:
[1] Finland: 'self-reported STD' included exclusively a history of gonorrhoea, chlamydial infection, syphilis, genital warts and genital herpes, while it was not explicitly defined in the other countries

Although data on the risk of female-to-female sexual transmission of pathogens are scarce, this risk is considered low (Robertson and Schachter, 1981; Ostrow, 1990). Surprisingly, a history of STD tends to be reported much more often by women who have had homosexual relations at least once in their lives than by exclusively heterosexual women (Table 7.5). The association seems stronger among women who have few partners and even disappears (except in Belgium) for women who reported a high number of partners. It is important to observe that most women reporting homosexual relations have had bisexual experience (Chapters 3 and 5). This being the case, the possibility that their male partners belong to high risk groups cannot be ruled out. This warrants further research on the sexual careers of lesbians in relation to HIV prevention, as demanded by some lesbian associations.

STDs are reported more often by those who have voluntarily been tested for HIV at least once in their lives (Table 7.6), whatever the number of partners and country. This could indicate that people who perceive themselves at higher risk are more likely to be tested for both HIV and STDs. However, we cannot exclude the possibility that the HIV test was performed after an STD was diagnosed. Indeed, such a disease may provide an opportunity for an increased self-perception of risk. In any event, present ability to report an STD history is associated with a higher level of sexual risk perception.

Table 7.5 *Proportions of men and women reporting a history of STD by life sexual orientation*

	12 months			5 years			Life	
	Finland[1] 1992	France 1992	Netherlands 1989	Belgium 1993	France 1992	Finland[1] 1992	Netherlands 1989	Norway 1992
MEN								
Sexual orientation								
homo or bi								
%	0	1.3	2.1	5.5	10.4	14.3	25.0	34.6
CI	0.0–10.6	0.0–2.6	0.0–6.1	0.0–11.2	6.2–14.6	2.7–25.9	12.8–37.2	24.2–45.0
hetero only								
%	1.5	0.8	0.3	1.4	3.0	17.3	6.5	19.8
CI	0.6–2.4	0.6–1.0	0.0–0.9	0.7–2.1	2.5–3.5	14.4–20.2	3.9–9.1	17.8–21.8
RR *homo vs hetero*	0	1.6	7	3.9	3.5[#]	0.8	3.8[#]	1.7[#]
WOMEN								
Sexual orientation								
homo or bi								
%	2.5	4.7	8.3	18.4	15.9	22.5	20.8	46.7
CI	0.0–7.3	1.9–7.5	0.0–19.3	3.9–32.9	9.7–22.1	9.6–35.4	4.6–37.0	35.4–58.0
hetero only								
%	3.1	1.7	0.8	3.3	5.2	15.4	4.9	17.8
CI	1.8–4.4	1.4–2.0	0.02–1.6	2.3–4.2	4.7–5.7	12.6–18.2	3.1–6.7	16.1–19.5
RR *homo vs hetero*	0.8	2.8	10.4	5.6	3.1[#]	1.5	4.2	2.6[#]

Base: all respondents (18–49 years) who ever had sex

CI: 95% confidence interval; upper 95% confidence limit of 0% is calculated with Poisson distribution

[#]: confidence intervals do not overlap

RR: relative risk

Homo or bi: ever had sex with a partner of same gender; otherwise: heterosexual

Note:

[1]Finland: 'self-reported STD' included exclusively a history of gonorrhoea, chlamydial infection, syphilis, genital warts and genital herpes, while it was not explicitly defined in the other countries

229

Table 7.6 *Proportions of men and women reporting an STD history by HIV testing (self-referred test)*

		12 months		5 years	Life		
		France 1992	Netherlands 1989	France 1992	Finland[1] 1992	Netherlands 1989	Norway 1992
MEN							
HIV test							
yes	%	3.1	2.0	9.4	36.2	20.0	36.5
	CI	1.2–5.0	0.0–5.9	6.7–12.1	23.8–48.6	8.9–31.1	30.9–42.1
no	%	0.6	0.3	2.7	15.6	7.2	16.8
	CI	0.4–0.8	0.0–8.8	2.3–3.1	12.9–18.3	4.4–10.0	14.8–18.8
RR yes							
vs no		*5.2*	*6.7*	*3.5[#]*	*2.3[#]*	*2.8*	*2.2[#]*
WOMEN							
HIV test							
yes	%	4.9	0	10.5	32.3	8.3	34.3
	CI	3.1–6.7	0.0–10.3	7.8–13.2	20.9–43.7	0.0–17.4	29.0–39.6
no	%	1.6	1.2	5.0	13.9	5.5	16.3
	CI	1.3–1.9	0.2–2.2	4.4–5.6	11.2–16.6	3.5–7.5	14.6–18.0
RR yes							
vs no		*3.1[#]*	*n.c.*	*2.1[#]*	*2.3[#]*	*1.5*	*2.1[#]*

Base: all respondents (18–49 years) who ever had sex
CI: 95% confidence interval; upper 95% confidence limit of 0% is calculated with Poisson distribution
[#]: confidence intervals do not overlap
RR: relative risk
n.c.: not computable
Note:
[1] Finland: 'self-reported STD' included exclusively a history of gonorrhoea, chlamydial infection, syphilis, genital warts and genital herpes, while it was not explicitly defined in the other countries

Socio-demographic Factors and STD Reporting

Gender

A constant of all surveys on sexual behaviour is that men report higher numbers of partners, higher numbers of casual partners, and shorter lengths of acquaintanceship prior to sexual relations than women (Aral *et al.*, 1991; Chapter 5 in this book). If males really had more at-risk behaviour with the same susceptibility to pathogens than females, male predominance in STDs could be expected. Yet we observe the opposite.

Table 7.7 presents the relative risks (RRs) for females versus males in the whole population, and for strata of various factors. Recent STDs (in the last five years and the last 12 months) are reported 1.7 to 2.5 times more often by women than by men. Moreover, these crude relative risks underestimate the true relationship between female gender and self-declared STDs. For a given number of partners reported in a given period, a recent STD is reported 2 to 7 times more often by women than men. For example, among French heterosexuals, the relative risk for women versus men rises from 1.7 (entire population) to around 2.5 in each number-of-partners category. Such a strong correlation is unlikely to be explained by a higher proportion of women engaging in unprotected risky practices with partners belonging to groups poorly represented in the survey sample, for example non-resident foreigners, injecting drug users, and so on. Other explanations have to be found. Gender differences in STD epidemiology still have not been fully elucidated. Some authors have suggested that women may be more easily infected by certain pathogens (*Neisseria gonorrhoeae, Chlamydia trachomatis, Trichomonas vaginalis,* HIV) than men, perhaps due to more lasting contact with the pathogen and/ or to the cervix's hypothesized greater susceptibility to infection (Ehrhardt and Wasserheit, 1991). Unequal access to screening to the advantage of women might be a second explanation, possibly compounding the effects of unequal gender susceptibility. The changes that have occurred in diagnostic methods in the last 15 years could explain why the association is more pronounced for STDs diagnosed recently, while there is no female predominance in lifetime reports of STD (Table 7.7). This generation effect becomes even clearer if age is taken into account. Except in East Germany, the female/male relative risks of lifetime STD tend to be less than unity after age 39, around unity in intermediate age groups and above unity for 18–24-year-olds, that is, for STDs that occurred at most 10 years ago. Nevertheless, for a given number of partners, STDs are always reported slightly more often by females than males, whatever the age class (data not shown).

Age

Table 7.8 shows that peak STD frequencies in men occur between the ages of 25 and 39, even for STDs occurring in a recent period (less than five years ago), and the pattern holds regardless of the number of partners in France, Belgium and the Netherlands. This could be due to the recent spread of preventive strategies among teenagers in Europe. Condom use has been shown to be very high in 18–24-year-olds (Chapter 9), even though youthfulness is traditionally linked to brief relationships with serial partners. We cannot, however, rule out the possibility that the lower frequency among

Table 7.7 Proportions of STD history – relative risks of females vs males RRf/m according to various factors

		12 months			5 years			Life			
		Finland[1] 1992	France 1992	Netherlands 1989	Belgium 1993	France 1992	Finland[1] 1992	Germany East 1990	Germany West 1990	Netherlands 1989	Norway 1992
WHOLE POPULATION											
Gender											
Men	%	1.4	0.8	0.6	1.6	3.3	17.3	7.0	8.6	8.8	20.5
	CI	0.5–2.3	0.6–1.0	0.0–1.3	0.9–2.3	2.8–3.8	14.6–20.0	4.9–9.1	6.9–10.3	6.0–11.6	18.5–22.5
Women	%	3.0	1.8	1.1	3.7	5.3	15.6	5.6	10.4	5.6	19.0
	CI	1.7–4.3	1.5–2.1	0.2–2.0	2.6–4.8	4.8–5.8	12.9–18.3	3.1–8.1	8.6–12.2	3.7–5.7	17.3–20.7
RRf/m		2#	2.5#	2	2.5#	1.7#	0.9	0.8	1.2	0.6#	0.9
HETEROSEXUALS											
RRf/m		2	2#	2.5	2.5#	1.7#	0.9	n.a.	n.a.	0.8	0.9
No. of partners class:											
RRf/m											
Low		2	2	n.c. (+∞)	3.3	2.5	1.3	n.a.	n.a.	n.c. (+∞)	1.4
Medium		5	2.5	3.3	5	2	2.5	n.a.	n.a.	1.7	1.4
High		2	5	5	3.3	2	1.3	n.a.	n.a.	1.7	1.3

Education: RRf/m										
Low	1.1	1.4	–	2	1.5	0.6	1.0	1.4	1.7	0.7#
Medium	2	2#	0.07	3.3	1.5#	0.8	1.4#	0.7	0.5	1.1
High	2	2.5#	2	2	1.9#	1.3	1.1	0.8	1.1	1.0
Age: RRf/m										
18–24	10#	3.3#	n.c. (+∞)	5#	2#	2	2.5#	0.6	2	1.4#
25–34	1.3	1.7#	1.1	1.7	1.4#	0.9	1.1	1.1	0.5	1.0
35–49	0.2	2	n.c. (+∞)	2	2.5#	0.4#	0.9	0.3	0.7	0.5#
Largest cities: RRf/m	2	2	2	2	1.3	0.9	1.1	0.9	0.9	0.9

Base: all respondents (18–49 years) who ever had sex

CI: 95% confidence interval

#: confidence intervals do not overlap

RR: relative risk

n.a.: not available

n.c.: not computable

Note:

[1]Finland: 'self-reported STD' included exclusively a history of gonorrhoea, chlamydial infection, syphilis, genital warts and genital herpes, while it was not explicitly defined in the other countries

233

Table 7.8 *Proportions of men and women reporting an STD history by age*

		12 months			5 years			Life			
		Finland¹	France	Netherlands	Belgium	France	Finland¹	Germany East	Germany West	Netherlands	Norway
		1992	1992	1989	1993	1992	1992	1990	1990	1989	1992
MEN											
All	%	1.4	0.8	0.6	1.6	3.3	17.3	7.0	8.6	8.8	20.5
	CI	0.5–2.3	0.6–1.0	0.0–1.3	0.9–2.3	2.8–3.8	14.6–20.0	4.9–9.1	6.9–10.3	6.0–11.6	18.5–22.5
Age											
18–24	%	0.8	0.9	0	1.5	3.7	11.0	4.8	4.2	3.5	15.0
	CI	0.0–2.2	0.3–1.5	0.0–4.4	0.01–2.9	2.5–4.9	5.8–16.2	1.1–8.5	1.7–6.7	0.0–7.5	11.2–18.8
25–39	%	2.2	1.1	0.9	2.5	4.4	19.7	6.9	11.4	11.4	22.8
	CI	0.7–3.7	0.7–1.5	0.0–2.3	1.2–3.8	3.7–5.1	15.7–23.7	4.3–9.5	8.8–14.0	7.1–15.7	19.9–25.7
40–49	%	0.5	0.4	0	0.6	1.1	17.3	10.0	6.6	7.9	20.5
	CI	0.0–1.4	0.06–0.7	0.0–4.2	0.0–1.3	0.6–1.6	12.3–22.3	4.1–15.9	3.5–9.7	2.3–13.5	16.7–24.3
WOMEN											
All	%	3.0	1.8	1.1	3.7	5.3	15.6	5.6	10.4	5.6	19.0
	CI	1.7–4.3	1.5–2.1	0.2–2.0	2.6–4.8	4.8–5.8	12.9–18.3	3.1–8.1	8.6–12.2	3.7–5.7	17.3–20.7
Age											
18–24	%	6.2	2.6	2.6	6.8	7.2	22.3	3.0	11.6	7.0	22.3
	CI	2.3–10.1	1.8–3.4	0.0–5.5	3.5–10.1	5.7–8.7	15.6–29.0	0.0–7.2	7.6–15.6	2.3–11.4	18.5–26.1
25–39	%	2.9	2.0	1.0	4.0	6.0	18.1	8.0	11.7	5.2	22.2
	CI	1.1–4.7	1.6–2.4	0.0–2.2	2.5–5.5	5.3–6.7	14.0–22.2	4.0–12.1	9.2–14.2	2.6–7.8	19.7–24.7
40–49	%	1.0	0.8	0	1.1	3.0	6.8	3.0	6.5	5.4	9.7
	CI	0.0–2.3	0.4–1.2	0.0–2.5	0.08–2.1	2.2–3.8	3.3–10.3	0.0–6.3	3.6–9.4	1.8–9.0	7.2–12.2

Base: all respondents (18–49 years) who ever had sex
CI: 95% confidence interval; upper 95% confidence limit of 0% is calculated with Poisson distribution
Note:
¹Finland: 'self-reported STD' included exclusively a history of gonorrhoea, chlamydial infection, syphilis, genital warts and genital herpes, while it was not explicitly defined in the other countries

18–24 versus 25–39-year-olds reflects a higher proportion of undiagnosed STDs, since seeking out health care may be limited by poorer perception of the risk of diseases such as gonorrhoea and *Chlamydia* infections, the lack of opportunities for systematic screening and the lack of a family doctor in the case of the younger subjects (Amaro and Gornemann, 1991).

The lifetime, 5-year and 12-month STD reporting rates for women aged 18–24 are greater than, or equal to, those of 25–39-year-old women and much higher than those of the oldest groups of women. This pattern differs from that seen for men. First, cervical ectopy, which is often observed in very young women, may facilitate the acquisition of certain STDs, for example *Chlamydia trachomatis.* Whether the youngest people acquire infections at a faster rate than older people is partly obscured by changes in diagnostic strategies in the past 15 years and new opportunities for screening upon starting contraception. The non-increase in lifetime cumulative STD frequency with increasing age may be partly due to a higher proportion of undiagnosed STDs in the past (Aral *et al.*, 1991). Here again East Germany is an exception, with later peaks of frequency for both men and women.

Level of Education

Table 7.9 shows that a recent STD history is reported more often by college graduates than by poorly educated people (former East Germany is the only country where women with a low level of education reported STDs in their lifetimes more often than women with higher education). This pattern applies to both genders, but the difference is more marked in women. The correlation is also independent of the number of partners. This is unlikely to be explained by a less preventive strategy for a given number of partners, since condom use also increases with level of education (Chapter 9). The explanation may be a better degree of screening and less reluctance to acknowledge STD history among college graduates. The generation effect already discussed with regard to gender may likewise explain why educational status tends to be linked with 1- or five-year STDs but not with lifetime STDs (Table 7.9).

Place of Residence

STD reporting rates are highest among people living in large cities, regardless of the number of partners (data not shown). This could be explained by both

Table 7.9 Proportions of men and women reporting an STD history by education

		12 months			5 years		Life			
		Finland[1]	France	Netherlands	Belgium	France	Finland[1]	Germany East	Germany West	Netherlands	Norway
		1992	1992	1989	1993	1992	1992	1990	1990	1989	1992
MEN											
Education											
Low	%	1.2	0.5	0	1.2	2.0	18.1	6.9	10.2	5.0	21.9
	CI	0.0–2.9	0.1–0.9	0.0–18.5	0.0–2.4	1.3–2.7	12.4–23.9	0.0–16.1	6.6–13.8	0.0–14.6	18.7–25.1
Medium	%	1.1	0.8	1.4	1.1	3.2	18.0	7.3	6.9	7.9	19.8
	CI	0.03–2.1	0.5–1.1	0.2–2.6	0.2–2.0	2.4–4.0	14.2–21.8	4.7–9.9	1.1–4.9	4.5–11.3	15.6–24.0
High	%	2.3	1.3	0.9	2.4	5.2	15.1	5.9	12.0	9.8	19.1
	CI	0.07–4.5	0.8–1.8	0.0–2.6	1.0–3.8	4.2–6.2	9.8–20.4	2.2–9.6	7.1–17.0	4.6–15.0	16.0–22.2
RR high vs low		*1.9*	*2.6*	*n.c. (+∞)*	*2.0*	*2.6#*	*0.8*	*0.9*	*1.2*	*2.0*	*0.9*
WOMEN											
Education											
Low	%	1.4	0.7	0	2.2	3.0	10.2	10.5	10.5	8.0	15.9
	CI	0.0–3.3	0.4–1.0	0.0–14.8	0.6–3.9	2.3–3.7	5.3–15.1	0.8–20.2	7.8–13.2	0.0–18.6	13.4–18.4
Medium	%	2.6	1.7	1.0	3.4	4.8	15.6	4.8	9.7	3.8	22.6
	CI	0.9–4.3	1.2–2.2	0.03–2.0	1.9–4.9	4.0–5.6	11.8–19.4	1.7–7.9	7.2–12.1	1.9–5.7	18.9–26.3
High	%	4.9	3.4	1.6	4.4	9.7	19.3	4.8	14.1	10.7	20.0
	CI	1.9–7.9	2.6–4.2	0.0–3.9	2.7–6.4	8.3–11.1	13.9–24.7	1.1–8.5	7.0–21.2	5.2–16.2	17.2–22.8
RR high vs low		*3.5*	*4.9#*	*n.c. (+∞)*	*2*	*3.2#*	*1.9*	*0.5*	*1.3*	*1.3*	*1.3*

Base: all respondents (18–49 years) who ever had sex
CI: 95% confidence interval; upper 95% confidence limit of 0% is calculated with Poisson distribution
RR: relative risk
n.c.: not computable
Note:
[1]Finland: 'self-reported STD' included exclusively a history of gonorrhoea, chlamydial infection, syphilis, genital warts and genital herpes, while it was not explicitly defined in the other countries

Table 7.10 *Potential influence of different factors upon sexual acquisition of an STD and STD screening*

	Sexual acquisition of an STD	STD screening
Women	↗ because of: greater susceptibility	↗ because of: more opportunities for screening than men better informed easier routine screening
	↘ because of: less at-risk sexual behaviour	↘ because of: less symptomatic infections than men
High level of education	↗ because of: higher number of partners (in fact linked to more younger highly-educated people)	↗ because of: greater recourse to care systems since better informed and having more resources
	↘ because of: more adequate strategy of protection?	
Youthfulness	↗ because of: higher rate of changes in partners greater susceptibility in young women	↗ because of: gynaecological visits at starting contraception in young women
	↘ because of: more frequent use of condom	↘ because of: limited recourse to care systems in young men?
Large cities	↗ because of: more opportunities for at-risk behaviour	↗ because of: more diversified and more anonymous care availability, better dissemination of information

greater at-risk sexual behaviour and higher levels of STD testing (more diversified care availability and better information networks).

We have seen that the frequency of self-declared STDs depends on both the actual incidence rate and coverage by screening. The complex, partly contradictory influences of socio-demographic characteristics upon actual STD incidence and STD screening are summarized in Table 7.10.

Country-to-country Comparisons and Estimations of STD Frequency

Lifetime STDs reporting rates are highest in Norway (20 per cent) and Finland (16 per cent) (Table 7.8). The slightly lower rate observed in Finland could be explained by the restriction of STD history to gonorrhoea, *Chlamydia* infections, syphilis, genital warts and genital herpes, which together account for 88 per cent of STDs reported by men and 91 per cent by women in Norway. The two countries have very similar report rates for each disease considered (Table 7.1). In the case of *Chlamydia trachomatis* infections they are 7 to 10 times greater than those in the Netherlands, France or Belgium with no female predominance (relative risk of women versus men: 1.3). Nearly 1 per cent of both male and female respondents in the Norwegian and Finnish surveys reported a history of *Chlamydia trachomatis* in the last year (corresponding to 1991). In the French survey, the rate is 10 times lower, but the confidence intervals overlap.

In the case of 18–24-year-olds, both lifetime and five-year STD histories are likely to encompass the entire period of sexual activity, thereby permitting Europe-wide comparison of the youngest age group without distinguishing between the two time spans. Accordingly, Table 7.8 shows that the rates of STDs reported by 18–24-year-olds remain three times higher in Norway and Finland than in the other countries. The rates for young men in West Germany, East Germany, the Netherlands and France are around 4 per cent, with little variation; Belgium has the lowest rate (1.5 per cent). In women, the rates vary from 12 per cent in West Germany to 3 per cent in East Germany. The rates of reported histories of STD over the previous 12 months in Finland, France and the Netherlands do not exceed 3 per cent, all ages combined, and do not vary significantly (large confidence intervals), although Finland tends to remain in the lead.

France and Belgium can be more specifically compared, since surveys in these two countries focused on the 'last five years' period using similarly formulated questions about STDs. Overall, France's reported STD rate is nearly twice that of Belgium. The differences between the two countries are more pronounced for men (3.3 per cent versus 1.6 per cent) than for women (5.3 per cent versus 3.7 per cent). A smaller proportion of Belgian men, compared with French men, report an STD, whatever the age group, level of education and number of sexual partners, particularly in the case of *Chlamydia* infections. In the 18–24-year-old age group, the female rates are of the same order (around 7 per cent), while males declare half as many STDs in Belgium as in France. This may reflect a higher proportion of undiagnosed STDs in males in Belgium.

East Germany is unusual in more than one respect. Reported STD rates are higher in men, even among the most recent generations, and in persons with a low level of education. East Germany also has the lowest frequency of

STDs in 18–24-year-old women. This profile may reflect insufficient availability and acceptability of testing.

Conclusions

Our study shows that the self-reporting of STD history is a reliable indicator for identifying subgroups in the general population that are highly exposed to HIV risk through sexual activity. Several trends are common to all the countries. The findings concerning sex ratio and the relative frequencies of the various pathogens match the available data from epidemiological surveillance in industrialized countries. The correlations with HIV risk-related sexual behaviour (multiple partners, paying for sex, homosexuality) are strong and independent of a series of key socio-demographic characteristics. Biases in STD reporting are essentially due to the unknown proportion of undiagnosed infections.

Infected people who do not have easy access to testing or are not reached by screening measures constitute a germ reservoir for their sexual partners and run the risk of developing complications. STD reporting is linked to characteristics that are health care access markers, that is, female gender and high level of education. These findings suggest that the proportion of undiagnosed STDs is higher among men and people with little education, which could justify the implementation of screening programs for these groups. However, the pattern of strong female predominance, independent of the number of partners and the educational status, is worth stressing. There is no doubt that it is partly due to more medical opportunities for diagnosis. However, it also argues for greater female susceptibility to certain pathogens, which is not easy to demonstrate.

As has been shown in other chapters the Nordic countries also break away from the others for the patterns of sexual behaviour, that is, a long-standing, pronounced trend of gender egalitarianism in sex and more liberal attitudes towards sexuality (see Chapter 2 on the age at sexual initiation and Chapter 6 on the highest female prevalence of reporting five or more partners in the last 12 months). Nevertheless, this is not sufficient reason to infer that greater rates of self-reported STDs in Nordic countries actually reflect higher STD incidence rates. First, differences in STD reporting between the Nordic countries and the rest of Europe tend to hold whatever the number of partners. Second, it would be surprising were Norway and Finland to have the highest STD cumulative incidences while boasting the lowest annual AIDS new case indices in Europe in 1992 (European Centre for Epidemiological Monitoring, 1993). In contrast, France, with a much lower rate of self-declared STDs, had one of the highest incidence rates of AIDS. We may rather assume that the higher rates in STD reporting reflect broader coverage by screening programmes and STD surveillance, which are particularly well-developed in the Nordic countries. For example, prenatal examinations and abortions are accompanied by systematic screening for *Chlamydia trachomatis* in Norway (Stray-Pedersen, 1996). However, a direct correlation between STD control and control of the AIDS epidemic across Europe cannot be established, since, on the one hand, the epidemiological conditions of the spread of various sexually transmitted pathogens and HIV are not similar, and, on the other hand, the dates of HIV's introduction are not identical from one country to the next.

References

ADAM, P. and HERZLICH, C. (1994) *Sociologie de la maladie et de la médecine*, Paris: Nathan.

AMARO, H. and GORNEMANN, I. (1991) 'Health care utilization for sexually transmitted diseases: influence of patient and provider characteristics', in *Research Issues in Human Behavior and Sexually Transmitted Diseases in the AIDS Era*, Washington, DC: American Society for Microbiology.

ANDERSON, J., McCORMICK, L. *et al.* (1994) 'Factors associated with self-reported STDs: data from a national survey', *Sexually Transmitted Diseases*, **21**, pp. 303–8.

ARAL, S. and HOLMES, K. (1990) 'Epidemiology of sexual behavior and sexually transmitted diseases', in HOLMES, K., MARDH, P. *et al.* (Eds) *Sexually Transmitted Diseases*, New York: McGraw-Hill.

ARAL, S., FULLILOVE, R. *et al.* (1991) 'Demographic and societal factors influencing risk behaviors', in *Research Issues in Human Behavior and Sexually Transmitted Diseases in the AIDS Era*, Washington, DC: American Society for Microbiology.

BRUNHAM, R.C. (1991). 'The concept of core and its relevance to the epidemiology and control of sexually transmitted diseases', *Sexually Transmitted Diseases*, **18**, pp. 67–8.

EHRHARDT, A. and WASSERHEIT, J. (1991) 'Age, gender, and sexual risk behaviors for sexually transmitted diseases in the United States', in *Research Issues in Human Behavior and Sexually Transmitted Diseases in the AIDS Era*, Washington DC: American Society for Microbiology.

EUROPEAN CENTRE FOR EPIDEMIOLOGICAL MONITORING (1993) 'AIDS surveillance in Europe', *Quarterly Report*, **37**, Saint-Maurice, France.

GROSSKURTH, H., MOSHA, F. *et al.* (1995) 'Impact of improved treatment of sexually transmitted diseases on HIV infection in rural Tanzania: randomized controlled trial', *The Lancet*, **346**, pp. 530–6.

HANDSFIELD, H.H. and SCHWEBKE, J. (1990) 'Trends in sexually transmitted diseases in homosexually active men in King County, Washington, 1980–1990', *Sexually Transmitted Diseases*, **17**, pp. 211–15.

HOLMES, K., MARDH, P. *et al.* (Eds) (1990) *Sexually Transmitted Diseases*, New York: McGraw-Hill.

MEYER, L., GOULET, V. *et al.* (1994) 'Surveillance of sexually transmitted diseases in France: recent trends', *Genitourinary Medicine,* **70**, pp. 15–21.

OSTROW, D. (1990) 'Homosexual behavior and sexually transmitted diseases', in HOLMES, K., MARDH, P. *et al.* (Eds) *Sexually Transmitted Diseases,* New York: McGraw-Hill.

RENTON, A.M. and WHITAKER, L. (1991) *Using STD Occurrence to Monitor AIDS Prevention. Final Report* (Assessing AIDS prevention. EC Concerted Action on assessment of AIDS/HIV preventive strategies), Lausanne: Institut universitaire de médecine sociale et préventive.

RENTON, A.M. and WHITAKER, L. (1994) 'Using STD occurrence to monitor AIDS prevention', *Social Science and Medicine,* **38**, pp. 1153–65.

ROBERTSON, P. and SCHACHTER, P. (1981) 'Failure to identify venereal disease in a lesbian population', *Sexually Transmitted Diseases,* **8**, p. 75.

SHAH, B.V., BARNWELL, B.G. *et al.* (1993) *Sudaan: professional software for survey data analysis for multi-stage sample designs, release 6.34 (September 1993),* Research Triangle Park: Research Triangle Institute.

SOBEL, J.D. (1993) 'Candidal vulvovaginitis', *Clinical Obstetrics and Gynecology,* **36**, 1, pp. 153–65.

STRAY-PEDERSEN, B. (1996) 'Prévention des MST. L'expérience norvégienne', *Contraception Fertilité Sexualité ,* **24**, pp. 213–17.

TREURNIET, H. and DAVIDSE, W. (1993) 'Sexually transmitted diseases reported by STD services in the Netherlands, 1984–1990', *Genitourinary Medicine,* **69**, pp. 434–8.

WASSERHEIT, J.N. (1992) 'Epidemiological synergy. Interrelationships between human immunodeficiency virus infection and other sexually transmitted diseases', *Sexually Transmitted Diseases,* **19**, 2, pp. 61–77.

Part 3

Preventive Practices and the Normative Context

Chapter 8

Sexual Adaptation to HIV Risk

Danièle Peto, Philippe Huynen and Nathalie Bajos

Introduction

The concept of adapting to HIV risk (Peto *et al.*, 1992) emphasizes the diversity of reactions (be they effective or not from the preventive standpoint) that the AIDS epidemic has triggered in the population. These reactions include abstaining temporarily from sex, selecting or avoiding certain partners or meeting places, testing partners before sexual relations, using the condom, talking about the partner's sexual past, and taking an HIV antibody test to reassure oneself and/or permit oneself to continue a certain sexual lifestyle. Taking account of the diversity of reactions to HIV risk is important on more than one score. Not only does such an approach reveal that the condom is far from the only means people use to cope with the risk of the sexual transmission of HIV, it also enables researchers to understand better the roles occupied by other means, such as HIV testing, for the situation is not cut and dry. The various ways of adapting to HIV risk combine different means in varying proportions and derive from various types of logic.[1] Protecting one's health, which means ultimately one's life, is not necessarily the predominant rationale behind an individual's behaviour. Nor is it necessarily the most decisive one. For example, an 'affective logic' may be more predominant for people who are living alone and have been looking for affection and love for months: some of these people may be reluctant to ask that a condom be used, fearing that such a request might cause their prospective partners to leave. A 'separate worlds' logic, for example, establishes a boundary between the circle of familiars to which one belongs – and in which relations are usually based on trust and the condom is rarely used – and the rest of the world, which is perceived as uncertain and thus dangerous, in which relationships are based more on wariness, and where the condom is more of a must. The absence of precautions may also be explained by, among other things, a logic of 'trust' (partners' exclusive love for each other often has problems accommodating the possibility of risk) or the conscious, shared acceptance of a certain degree of risk (Bastard *et al.*, 1992, 1997). Furthermore, adapting to HIV risk does not necessarily result from the sole decision of one of the two partners. It is possible that what happens in sexual interaction will differ from what one and/or the other partner may have decided beforehand, because the characteristics of the relationship and the type of partner may be determinant.

When the first European surveys on sexual behaviour and HIV/AIDS were conducted, such an approach was not yet theoretically very developed. Instead, most of the researchers sought to determine whether or not people had 'changed their behaviour' by asking them directly a question like 'Have you changed your sexual behaviour since people started talking about AIDS?' and, if so, the types of behaviour change that were involved. One of the problems of asking people directly whether or not they have changed their behaviour is that the problem of defining the risk is disregarded. The implicit assumption is that there is general agreement on the existence of a risk and, by extension, on the need to 'change behaviour'. But how pertinent are questions about behaviour changes for, say, a young population that has just begun its sexual socialization and does not know the pre-AIDS era compared with a population whose behaviour does not carry any risk of HIV infection? Moreover, there is no examination here of how the interviewee him/herself has defined the risk and, from there, possible behaviour changes. Indeed, as individuals cannot know or calculate the risk of being infected, they can only imagine the risks they run. Such representations may depend on the epidemiological context as well as on a range of social, cultural, and psychological factors. The gap between representations of risk and objective risk is difficult to gauge, but indubitably subtends risk over- or under-estimation,[2] even risk denial.[3]

In this chapter we shall not pursue this theoretical debate much further, but analyze the ways the issue of 'behaviour change' was approached and operationalized in the various questionnaires. The numbers and characteristics of respondents who said they had changed their behaviour and the types of changes they reported will then be compared cross-nationally. Because some of the variations in the results can be expected in terms of differences in the manner of questioning, we shall focus more on general trends in the associations of certain socio-demographic factors, such as gender, age, marital status, level of education, and number of partners, than on the overall inter-survey differences. On the whole, the analyses presented here, although they are based on behaviour change indicators, will allow us to assess indirectly the diversity of ways of adapting to HIV risk mentioned at the start of this chapter.

Methods

In order to explore the extent to which valid international comparisons can be made, we shall first examine differences in the question wordings used to study behaviour changes in the various surveys. We shall also deal with the problem of measurement time frames and definitions of the reference populations.

Question Wording

The difficulty of formulating 'standard questions' for collecting information on this subject and the multiplicity of behaviours that must be considered, have led researchers to generate a great diversity of questions. In most of the surveys the question about behaviour change was asked in two parts. The first part (consisting of a comprehensive question of the type 'Have you changed?') served as a filter for the second part (picking out specific questions like 'If so, then in what way?'). Two of the questionnaires, namely Finland 1992 and Belgium 1993, omitted the first part of the question and asked questions about specific types of behaviour directly. As a result of this structure, all of the respondents answered these questions. At the opposite end of the scale, the Portuguese survey (1991) used a set of filters before asking even a very broad question about behaviour change,[4] as a result of which even this first question was not put to all of the people included in the survey.

It is also useful to look at the characteristics of three elements in the first question (see 'Behaviour change in general' in Table 8.1), that is, the *qualification* used to raise the issue of change, what was changed or the *object* of change, and the *cause* that was proposed as having triggered the change.

The surveys that tackled the issue of change by means of a general question often spoke simply of 'change'. It should be pointed out, however, that in the Germany 1993 survey the expression 'more careful' qualified change, and that one of the Dutch wordings involved the paraphrase 'to do something to prevent'. One will easily realize that these expressions do not evoke the same references for respondents as 'changing behaviour'. The objects of change were varied and included or did not include a sexual connotation (life, behaviour, sex life or sexual behaviour). Finally, the link between the possible behaviour change and AIDS as a cause of this change was likewise expressed in various ways, from the most tenuous ('since people have been talking about AIDS') to the strongest ('the risk of infection').

The way the second question, regarding the kind of changes that occurred, was tackled also varied greatly in terms of both the characteristics of the questions themselves and different answer modes (see 'Types of changes' in Table 8.1). This is likely to have had an impact on the results. Thus, in some countries the researchers opted for an open question, leav-

Table 8.1 *Behaviour change questions and answer modes*

	Behaviour change in general			Type of change		
	Qualification	Object	Cause	Question type	Number of answers CQ	Number of answers OQ
Athens–PR (1990)	changed	behaviour	what you've heard about AIDS	OQ		3
Belgium (1993)	/	/	/	CQ	2	
Finland (1992)	/	/	/	CQ	7	
France–ACSF (1992)	changed	sexual behaviour	since there's been talk about AIDS	CQ	6	
France–KABP (1992)	changed	sexual behaviour	since there's been talk about AIDS	CQ	7	
East Germany (1990)	changed	sex life	because of AIDS	OQ		1
East Germany (1993)	more careful	sexual matters	risk of infection with HIV	/	/	/
West Germany (1993)	more careful	sexual matters	risk of infection with HIV	/	/	/
Netherlands (1989), a	changed	sex life	–	OQ		
Netherlands (1989), b	has done something to prevent HIV	–	–	CQ	6+	
Portugal (1991)	changed	behaviour	–	OQ		3
Spain (1990), a	changed	life	since you've known about AIDS	OQ		1
Spain (1990), b	changed	sex life	AIDS	CQ	14	
Spain (1990), c	/	/	/	CQ	4	
Eurobarometer	/	/	/	OQ		1

Notes:
OQ = open question
CQ = closed question
/ = the question was not asked in the survey
– = not specified
a = 'First Question' in the referred survey questionnaire.
b = 'Second Question' in the referred survey questionnaire.
c = 'Third Question' in the referred survey questionnaire.

ing it up to each respondent to mention his or her behaviour changes without prompting. The number of allowed answers to such open questions also varied from one (East Germany, Spain) to three (Athens, Portugal). The fact that one person could give three times as many answers in some surveys as in others made comparing the results even more difficult.

Other surveys presented a list (of variable length) of items to which the respondent was supposed to answer 'yes' or 'no'. Obviously, when the respondents are given a little assistance, one gets higher response rates to certain items than if free responses alone are solicited. Finally, an open question is likely to generate a larger set of responses, including some that were not expected by the researcher.

We shall also refer in this chapter to the results of the Eurobarometer surveys conducted in Europe at the request of the Commission of the European Communities. These surveys offer the advantages of being conducted according to a standardized protocol in all European countries over the same time period.[5]

Time Frames

The variable time intervals between the onset of the AIDS epidemic (the reference point of most questions about behaviour change) and the times at which the surveys were conducted are another obstacle to international comparison. The reference periods for observation of changes in behaviour ranged from three to seven years. This automatically influenced the data, since the longer the reference period, the greater the probability of detecting a change in behaviour. Furthermore, beyond the variability in the length of the periods of reference, qualitative changes such as the continuous presence of prevention campaigns and the development of new social norms governing sexuality and AIDS, may have occurred.

As mentioned above, one must also realize that, the present international comparison aside, studying behaviour change from survey data raises problems of temporality in the analysis of certain factors. One must allow for the fact that collecting information about behaviour change is done with regard to a period of time, whereas collecting information about sexual activity refers to specific points in time. Consequently, establishing links between behaviour change and indicators of sexual activity is not always easy. For instance, declaring a smaller number of partners over a one-year period (this is the case for many of the surveys studied here) can just as easily be the result as the cause of behaviour change.

Reference Populations

Finally, from a public health point of view, the number of respondents who report behaviour changes should be assessed against the number of people actually exposed to the risk of sexual transmission of HIV. If the rates of those who are at risk is not the same in the different surveys, any comparison of the proportion of behaviour change across countries referring to the whole populations will be biased. The definition of the population to be studied also raises the issue of the very definition of a risky behaviour. What factors and indicators of risk should be taken into account to define the population who should be concerned by the risk of sexual transmission of HIV? What period should be retained to define the risk exposure? Whereas at a specific time the risk of infection for the overwhelming majority of the population at large is usually very low, a large majority of the population may be considered to have been exposed, if only once, to the risk of sexual transmission of HIV if a period of several years is considered. Per Magnus's earlier chapter on risk exposure offers more light on this discussion. Furthermore, the different ways of adapting to HIV risk do not necessarily concern the same individuals. For example, is resorting to faithfulness relevant only to those respondents who are currently involved in a couple relationship or does it concern everyone who may hope one day to limit him/herself to one partner? Similarly, giving up penetrative practices can concern only those who practised them in the first place.

These considerations led us to take into account only the 'sexually active' respondents, that is, those respondents who stated they had had penetrative sex at least once in their lives, and to concentrate on the 'specific behaviour changes' that are likely to concern this same sexually active population, that is, types of change related to partner selection, partner communication and condom use.

Results

Reported Rates of Sexual Behaviour Changes

Based on the data shown in Table 8.2, we can divide the surveys into three groups: those in which the reported rate of behaviour change was less than or close to 10 per cent (Portugal and Spain); those where this rate was close to 20 per cent (France and East Germany); and those where this rate was well over 30 per cent (West Germany and the Netherlands).

The rates of affirmative answers to the two Spanish questions were

Table 8.2 *Proportions of respondents who reported having changed their behaviour*

	Athens 1990	France ACSF 1992	France KABP 1992	Germany East 1990	Germany East 1993	Germany West 1993	Netherlands[1] a 1989	Portugal 1991	Spain a 1990	Spain b 1990
Yes	20.5	20.3	11.9	20.9	23.5	51.0	39.7	4.5	9.8	10.7
Maybe			4.8							
No	79.5	79.5	83.2	79.1	75.5	48.0	60.3	2.6	90.2	89.3
Won't help								21.9		
I don't need to								71.0		
No answer		0.2			1.0	1.0				
N	1661	3267	1266	917	1145	2040	935	2230	779	779

Base: all respondents (18–49 years) who ever had sex, except for Spain (19–50 years)
Notes:
[1]Netherlands: This question concerns the last 12 months
a,b See Table 8.1

relatively low. What is more, they were fairly close, although only one of the questions clearly mentioned a change in sexual behaviour. Nevertheless, these low rates must be relativized by the fact that the affirmative answer rates to another question in the same questionnaire that mentioned a series of behaviour changes ranged from 7.4 to 35.9 per cent. So the percentage of respondents who reported a change in behaviour must at least approach the maximum rate of 35.9 per cent. For Portugal, on the other hand, the filters that preceded the question about behaviour change most likely depressed the affirmative answer rate. Indeed, the result of asking at a relatively rational level whether a behaviour change 'suffices' to avoid infection and if, what is more, this type of change 'concerns' the respondent, before asking the behaviour change question itself, was that the last question was ultimately put to less than 10 per cent of the sample. If this question had been put to everyone, the affirmative answer rate might have been higher. What is more, these two filter questions relate to two different levels. The first question[6] is exclusively centred on knowledge, whereas the second question,[7] although it gives the illusion of being a continuation of the first one, actually reflects a type of question that deals as much with knowledge as with behaviour. Consequently, the latter refers to all of the issues of subjective representations that orient the responses of the individual who is talking about his/her own behaviour (representations based on his/her own definition of the risk, subjective risk perception, and so on), as well as to the objective aspect of the decision to change behaviour.

In contrast, the 51.0 per cent affirmative response rate for the West German (1993) survey is all the more surprising as the affirmative response rate to the same question asked the same year using the same questionnaire in the neighbouring eastern Länder was only 23.5 per cent. The greater ease of talking about condoms (and by extension, talking about protection during sex) and the more widespread use of and familiarity with the condom in the western as opposed to the eastern Länder seem to indicate how different the histories of sexual relations in the two halves of this formerly divided country are. Risky behaviour may also have been less widespread in East Germany.

Our intention obviously is not to reduce the explanations of the observed differences in results solely to differences in question wordings. It is not possible to measure the exact impact of the differences in question wordings on the survey results. While we mention certain variations as being significant international differences, we also feel it is important to take account of the findings obtained in other frameworks, such as the Eurobarometer surveys, which show, among other things, markedly different results (Huynen, Marquet and Hubert, 1995).[8] For example, the rates of behaviour change reported in Portugal in 1990 were systematically higher than in the other European Union Member States. Moreover, the very high rate (compared with the other surveys examined here) recorded by the Netherlands should be highlighted, for in the 1990 Eurobarometer survey the Netherlands belonged to the group of countries in Europe with 'average' rates of behaviour change (concerning sexual matters).

Still, whatever the reservations concerning the international variations observed and the difficulty of explaining them, it is no less true that behaviour changes linked to the onset of the HIV epidemic are reported by at least one-fifth of the population in the different European countries.

Behaviour Change and Socio-demographic Profiles

Besides the characteristics specific to each national survey that have just been mentioned and which are due in part to the specific natures of the question-naires, there was cause to highlight the trends among the socio-demographic variations that could be generalized to the entire body of results examined in this section.

The results presented in Tables 8.3 and 8.4 clearly show that a (much) higher proportion of men than women reported behaviour changes. Can we conclude from this that men are more likely to have to (or have had to) change their behaviour than women? Without rejecting this interpretation out of hand, if only because using the services of a sex worker is a predomi-nantly male behaviour, we cannot help relating this observation to the fact that proportionately more men also reported having more partners than women did. To the extent that the tendencies would be for women to under-report and/or men to over-report the number of partners (a hypothesis that should be confirmed – see the chapter on sexual partners in this book), it is easier for men – if this is consistent with their discourse – to report having changed their behaviour than for women. Without wanting to put forward here an issue that will be examined more thoroughly in the next chapter, we may also wonder how condom use is perceived by men and women. It is not far-fetched to believe that women may not consider it a behaviour change as much as men, since the behaviour itself can be said to be more that of the man. Consequently, if the man takes the initiative of imposing a condom, it is possible that the woman will not interpret this as being a behaviour change, whereas if condom use is agreed upon at the woman's request, this behaviour is more likely to be perceived as a possible behaviour change by both parties.

In almost all cases, the older the respondent, the lower the rate of reported behaviour change. However, this does not mean that reported be-haviour changes were systematically higher among young people. Thus, in the Athens 1990 and West Germany 1993 surveys the decreases in behaviour change rates did not begin until the 20–24-year-olds, whereas in the East Germany 1993 and Portuguese surveys the rates rose steadily until the 30–39-year-olds and 25–29-year-olds, respectively, after which they began falling. The

Table 8.3 *Proportions of respondents who reported having changed their behaviour by age, class, gender, level of education and cohabitation*

	Athens 1990	France ACSF 1992	France KABP 1992	Germany East 1990	Germany East 1993	Germany West 1993	Netherlands[1] a 1989	Portugal 1991	Spain a 1990	Spain b 1990
All	20.5	20.3	11.9	20.9	23.5	51.0	39.7	4.5	9.8	10.7
Age										
18–19	29.6	37.9	19.9	31.1	9.0	58.0	74.4	2.0	–	–
20–24	32.6	30.6	16.8	25.7	22.0	61.0	58.3	5.1	7.8	12.2
25–29	26.0	21.4	18.2	25.9	25.0	53.0	44.4	7.2	12.5	12.5
30–39	18.0	17.8	10.0	16.2	32.0	52.0	32.3	4.5	11.4	10.2
40–49	12.2	13.6	7.6	18.8	12.0	40.0	27.9	3.6	3.4	6.8
Gender										
Men	27.0	24.5	15.9	23.4	27.5	53.0	42.8	6.3	12.5	11.7
Women	14.9	15.9	7.9	19.4	19.4	48.0	37.5	2.5	6.8	9.5
Education										
Low	9.0	14.6	n.a.	n.a.	n.a.	n.a.	30.2	3.7	10.0	11.0
Medium	19.8	21.4	n.a.	n.a.	n.a.	n.a.	37.9	6.3	8.4	8.9
High	31.1	25.8	n.a.	n.a.	n.a.	n.a.	46.2	2.9	10.4	11.4
Cohabitation										
Cohabiting	11.9	11.9	5.8	18.6	n.a.	n.a.	31.3	3.5	4.6	7.9
Not cohabiting	39.2	39.2	27.8	35.5	n.a.	n.a.	59.5	6.1	14.4	13.1

Base: all respondents (18–49 years) who ever had sex, except for Spain (19–50 years)
Notes:
[1] Netherlands: This question concerns the last 12 months
n.a. = not available
a,b See Table 8.1

'non-cohabiting' respondents reported a proportionately higher rate of behaviour change since (or because of) the risk of AIDS than the 'cohabiting' respondents did.

Living with someone and older age definitely give individuals fewer objective grounds for changing their behaviour. Chapter 5, examining the number of partners, confirms this point. Thus, in referring to these two parameters (cohabitation status and age) one is measuring not so much the question of change, as the pertinence of that question to various situations. The issue of temporality can help us to understand why the youngest age classes do not report markedly higher rates of change, for the period covered by the question is not as obviously one of sexual activity as in the case of the older respondents. Another factor likely to shed light on this phenomenon is the fact that, unlike the older respondents, 18- and 19-year-olds have more of an 'AIDS-prevention culture', as a result of which the concept 'behaviour change' probably does not elicit the same responses in their minds as it does in today's 40-year-olds.

A higher rate of behaviour change was observed for the more highly educated respondents in the Athenian, French and Dutch surveys. This correlation was less obvious in the Spanish and Portuguese data, where the intergroup differences were not statistically significant. These findings reflect a higher potential rate of exposure to the risk[9] and the objective reasons for behaviour changes, as well as the fact that prevention messages are 'perceived' better by these population groups, as is the case in many other areas of health prevention, notably the prevention of cardiovascular diseases (Adam and Herzlich, 1995).

Behaviour Change and Sexual Activity

The relationship between reported behaviour change and reported number of partners, whether the latter covers the lifetime, the last 5 years or the last 12 months, is the same in all countries, namely, the greater the number of current or past partners, the higher the reported behaviour change rate. In the case of respondents who stated they had had no partner (over the last 5 years or 12 months), the percentage who said they had changed their behaviour was very high and in any case systematically much higher than (twice that of) the single-partner respondents covering the same period (these data were available in the French and Dutch surveys only).

Having several partners is known to be a risk factor. People with multiple partners are thus more objectively in a position to change behaviour than people with single partners. The high percentage of respondents without partners who reported having changed their behaviour leads us to wonder whether abstinence is not a way of adapting to risk for a sizable fraction of the

Table 8.4 *Proportions of people who declared having changed their behaviour by number of partners*

	Athens 1990	France ACSF 1992	Germany East 1993	Netherlands[1] a 1989	Portugal 1991	Spain a 1990	Spain b 1990
All	20.5	20.3	23.5	39.7	4.5	9.8	10.7
No. of partners							
Lifetime							
1		6.1		29.9		2.9	3.3
2		8.1		38.1		–	–
2–3–4						9.5	11.4
3–4		22.1		41.1		–	–
5–9		23.4		53.3		17.1	15.9
10+		32.1		42.9		19.7	23.7
5-years							
0		23.0		68.8			
1		7.6		31.1			
2		23.8		55.2			
3–4		41.6		61.8			
5+		45.2		63.1			
12 months							
0	35.0	29.2		73.3		12.2	12.2
1	17.6	16.5	17.4	36.0	3.2	6.1	7.8
2	58.5	43.9	37.3	55.9	6.9	–	–
2–3–4						17.4	16.1
3–4	51.9	56.2	21.2	65.5	10.3	–	–
5+	66.7	51.2	45.8	63.6	16.4	25.6	25.6

Base: all respondents (18–49 years) who ever had sex, except for Spain (19–50 years)
Note:
[1] Netherlands: This question concerns the last 12 months
a,b See Table 8.1

population. To what extent this hypothesis can be validated will be examined later.

It should also be emphasized that, depending on the country, from one-third to one-half of the respondents with multiple partners reported no behaviour change. It would doubtless be worthwhile, with regard to prevention policies, to study their characteristics in greater detail, country by country.

Behaviour Change Besides Condom Use

Of the various preventive behaviours that may be adopted, partner selection is one of the most frequent. Partner-selection behaviour may be based notably on social knowledge of partners ('I have sex only with people I know') or affective knowledge ('I have sex only with people with whom I'm in love'). In the first case homogamy appears to confer a certain immunity, whereas in the second case the so-called protective strength of 'love' appears to come into play. Implementing such behaviours may mean being faithful to one's main partner, reducing the number of one's partners, even embracing sexual abstinence for a while. The mode of prevention based on communication between partners consists in, for example, asking a partner questions about his/her sexual experience or asking him/her to take an HIV antibody test. In such a case, preventive behaviour may be prompted by the responses that are obtained. Finally, the preventive behaviour may rely on protection linked more directly to the sexual practices *per se*, for example, using a condom, giving up anal, vaginal, or oral penetration, or not swallowing semen. The status of a fourth way of adapting to HIV risk, taking an HIV antibody test, may be more ambiguous. In some cases it can be one element of a complex risk-management behaviour. For example, a person embarks on a relationship, after which, based on the two partners' test results, protective behaviours may be dropped. In this case, such a behaviour is related to a communication-based way of adapting to HIV risk. For other people or in other cases it may also help justify the absence of protective measures and/or reassure an individual who tests negative after unprotected sex.

Table 8.5 summarizes the data about the different ways of adapting to HIV risk that are available in a few European surveys. The very high percentages of French survey respondents who reported having adopted one or the other behaviour seems to reflect a methodological specificity, for the French survey was the only one in which different ways of adapting to HIV risk were indicated using a pre-established grid, and then only to the persons who said that they had changed their behaviour.

The various surveys show that individuals devise highly diverse ways of adapting to the risk of sexual transmission of HIV that go well beyond condom use, which is the means of protection promoted by all the national prevention campaigns. These preventive behaviours involve the selection and/or reduction in the number of partners, communication between partners, and changing the scenario of sexual relations (Laumann *et al.*, 1994). This holds true even in the surveys where no way of adapting to HIV was suggested in advance. In all the surveys except the Dutch one, preventive behaviour that relied on partner selection was mentioned as often as, even more often than, condom use. Attention should be given to the fact that taking partner selection to its extreme, that is (temporary) abstinence, was scarcely reported. While in the Athenian and Finnish surveys 'careful selection' or faithfulness achieved levels on a par with condom use, 'having sex with partners whom one knows' was mentioned more often in the French and Spanish surveys.

Preventive behaviours that necessarily involved verbal communication between partners were explored in the French survey only. Here, asking a partner for information about his/her sex life, which doubtless precedes and

Table 8.5 *Preventive behaviours of respondents who reported behaviour change*

	Athens	Belgium	Finland	France	Netherlands b	Spain[1] a	Spain[1] b
	1990	1993	1992	1992	1989	1993	1993
Selection/Reduction							
Abstinence			1.9	7.4	0.7		
Faithfulness	18.2		21.5	63.5	13.7	6.4[4]	
Look for stable relationship					17.8		
Sex if in love				65.7			
Sex if know each other				88.1		24.4	27.2
Get information on the partner	5.6		15.4				
Careful selection	29.7			20.0[3]			
No sex with sex worker	12.4			85.9	12.3		35.9
Fewer partners			12.0	11.8			17.6
Breaking off a relationship		8.4					
Communication							
Speak with partner about his/her sex life				62.6[3]			
Ask partner to take a HIV-antibody test				7.3			

Protection						
Condom	29.4		20.0[2]	72.9	75.3	12.8	
No penetration		4.6		8.2[3]		
Avoid certain sexual practices						
Safer sex			7.4		10.3	
No anal sex						1.3	7.7
Not swallow semen							7.4
N	341	2630	725	210	146	779	779
Type of question	Open	Closed	Closed	Closed	Open	Opened	Closed

Base: all respondents (18–49 years) who reported having changed their behaviour except in Belgium and Finland, where the data refer to the population at large

Notes:

[1] Spain: The Spanish survey has asked two questions about sexual behaviour change, one open ('Has AIDS changed your sex life? If yes explain'), the other closed ('As a result of your knowledge about AIDS, how has your sexual behaviour changed?')

[2] 'Have used a condom more than before', whereas in the other surveys, it was just 'have used a condom'

[3] These figures come from the ACSF survey conducted the same year as the KABP survey. The questions were put to 770 respondents who reported a change in behaviour. All the French data presented in this chapter come from the KABP survey, except for Tables 8.1 and 8.2, where both surveys are presented

[4] Faithfulness to the main partner

a,b See Table 8.1

contributes to the decision to engage in 'safe sex'/to use a condom, was more frequent than asking the partner to be tested. Searching for information may thus make it possible to avoid using a condom. Asking about/for an HIV test also offers a chance to refer explicitly to the fear of contracting a fatal disease, which is known to be particularly difficult to integrate into a predominantly love relationship (Ludwig, 1992).

The data on giving up specific sexual practices are much harder to interpret, given the methodological considerations discussed above. It should be noted, however, that in the Belgian and French surveys, which included clear references to giving up penetration in general, only a minority of the respondents answered affirmatively, whereas the data on sexual practices revealed that all of the sexually active respondents engaged in at least one type of penetration (vaginal penetration in the great majority of cases). Since it is highly unlikely that the interviewees associated penetration with anal sex only, it seems at least that changing the most structuring practice of the sexual scenario of a heterosexual relationship is much more difficult to envisage and implement.

Types of Change and Socio-demographic Profiles

Detailed analysis of the implementation of different ways of adapting to HIV, such as having fewer partners or avoiding penetration, according to various socio-demographic and sexual activity characteristics shows that HIV sexual transmission risk management may also be affected by the individual's social and sexual biographies (Bajos *et al.*, 1997).

Partner-selection behaviours, indicated by affirmative responses to the item 'fewer partners', were not implemented more often by men than by women in the French and Dutch surveys. While a higher proportion of female than male respondents answered 'yes' to this question in the Spanish survey, the opposite trend was observed in the Athenian and Finnish surveys.

Similarly, no particular trends emerged with regard to level of education (no differences in the Spanish and Finnish surveys, opposite trends in the Athenian and Dutch surveys) and cohabitation status (no differences in the Spanish and French surveys, opposite trends in the Athenian and Finnish surveys). In contrast, there was a clear age-related effect. In all of the surveys considered, the youngest respondents (especially the under-25s), that is, those who were in the process of acquiring a sexual repertory in terms of both practices and partners, were the least likely to reduce the number of their partners. In addition, the over-40s who reported having changed their behaviour adopted such preventive behaviour less easily. This may reflect a certain fear of affective solitude given the greater difficulty of starting new relationships for these age groups.

Table 8.6 *Frequency of partner selection (%)*

	Athens PR 1990	Finland 1992	France KABP 1992	Netherlands b 1989	Spain 1990
All	12.4	12.0	85.9	12.3	17.6
Age					
18–19	4.2	9.3	80.8	0.0	–
20–24	9.9	14.9	84.4	12.2	12.9
25–29	9.3	15.6	91.0	13.3	17.0
30–39	16.5	11.9	87.3	16.7	23.3
40–49	15.8	9.0	81.0	5.6	13.9
Gender					
Men	15.3	13.0	85.5	12.5	16.1
Women	7.6	10.8	86.7	12.0	20.2
Education					
Low	19.4	11.6	n.a.	0.0	18.4
Medium	14.1	12.2	n.a.	10.6	18.8
High	8.8	12.9	n.a.	15.5	16.2
No. of partners					
1	n.a.	1.3	n.a.	0.0	6.7
2	n.a.	2.2	n.a	0.0	–
2–3–4					10.3
3–4	n.a.	7.1	n.a.	13.8	–
5–9	n.a.	13.3	n.a.	13.2	25.0
10+	n.a.	23.7	n.a.	15.8	32.1

Base: all respondents (18–49 years) who reported having changed their behaviour, except for Finland, where the data refer to the population at large
Notes:
n.a. = not available
b   See Table 8.1

In the case of the Finnish, Dutch and Spanish surveys, reducing the number of partners is reported more often by individuals who might be described as being highly active sexually in that they have had many partners in their lives. However, this pattern may overlap with the aforementioned age effect, for the older respondents also have had the time to have the most partners. In fact, this correlation does not hold if one takes into account the number of partners over the last five years, with the proviso that such data are available for the Dutch survey only (data not shown).

Giving up penetrative practices is the least frequently reported type of change. The data that can be culled from the French and Belgian surveys show a steady decrease in giving up penetration with increasing age in Belgium, but no trend in France. This type of change is more often reported by Belgian males and does not appear to be linked to the level of education in either

Table 8.7 *Frequency of giving up penetrative sex (%)*

	Belgium 1993	France KABP 1992
All	4.6	8.1
Age		
18–19	13.7	3.7
20–24	8.9	8.8
25–29	5.8	7.2
30–39	2.8	8.3
40–49	2.8	10.0
Gender		
Men	6.8	5.5
Women	2.6	12.4
Education		
Low	4.4	10.4
Medium	5.0	9.6
High	4.3	4.5
No. of partners		
1	–	13.9
2	–	28.5
3–4	–	6.1
5–9	–	7.4
10+	–	6.7

Base: all respondents (18–49 years) who reported having changed their behaviour, except for Belgium, where the data refer to the population at large

country. It is interesting to note that this preventive behaviour was systematically used more frequently by respondents who lived alone, which leads us to wonder whether these data may not reflect the greater rigidity of 'marital' sex. In other words, while it would be possible not to engage in penetration with a more occasional partner, such an option would appear difficult *vis-à-vis* a steady partner with whom penetration is the norm.

Even though the above-mentioned data do not allow us to analyze preventive behaviours' co-occurrence, it is important to stress that the various ways of adapting to HIV may be implemented simultaneously ('I ask my partner questions and, depending on the answers, a condom will or will not be used') or alternatively ('with some partners I use a condom certain days, with others I avoid penetration; at certain moments I put an end to a seductive relationship that might lead to physical contact'). As seen earlier, 'you don't do no matter what, with no matter whom' and, as will be shown in the next chapter, condoms are not used the same way with different types of partners.

Conclusions

The data collected by the European surveys under comparison support Choi and Coates's (1994) thesis that AIDS prevention policies, which are based for the most part on promoting condom use, have fostered important behavioural changes. This would seem to be one of the fastest and farthest-reaching responses to a health problem of all times. However, we must bear in mind that, on the one hand, even respondents who state they take account of the risk of HIV transmission do not necessarily have zero risk behaviour and, on the other hand, people who state having changed their behaviour may not necessarily have been in situations requiring such a change.

Our analyses have revealed some of the general characteristics of the various ways of adapting to HIV risk. However, they often failed to explain the whys and wherefores of such adaptive behaviour. Still, the indicators available in each of the surveys rarely contextualized the behaviour or behaviour change studied. What is more, we might well ask if repetitive observations of behaviour, even if derived from declarations, rather than one-time measurement of stated behaviour changes might not be a more suitable way to capture the behaviour changes triggered by a phenomenon such as AIDS. In a word, the observation dynamics rather than the respondent's memory should reveal the dynamics of the phenomenon. In any event, even if this issue had been tackled from the standpoint of reported changes or the status quo, it is possible to contextualize the behaviour by asking the respondent to explain the reasons for the behaviour change, to situate it systematically in time, or to shed light on (the type of) partner with regard to whom a given behaviour change took place, for example.

It thus seems indispensable to encourage the development of a 'relation-based approach' (Marquet, Peto and Hubert, 1995; Morris and Kretzschmar, 1997) to complement the more individual-orientated approaches, for it is inside relationships that the risks and the ways of coping with them are built. By seeing behaviour in its context (the relationship) and observing this context, a 'relation-based approach' enables the investigator to circumscribe a set of elements (the status of the relationship for the partners and the evolution of the relationship, the norms and balances of power that govern it, the possible concurrency with other relationships, and so on) explaining the behaviour that individual-orientated approaches will not reveal. In this way we give ourselves the means not only to characterize behaviour change within existing relationships, but also to pick up on changes that may occur in the various types of budding relationships.

Notes

1 Logic is the implicit consistency of a series of practices that can be discerned only by the researcher's analysis and helps to give action a certain direction (Remy, Voyé and Servais, 1978, p. 93).

2 The ambiguity surrounding information about obscure risks, such as AIDS at the start of the epidemic, can lead to risk over-estimation, whereas, as cognitive psychology has shown, when objective probabilities are too low, individuals tend to consider them nil (Leplège, 1993). This last phenomenon is doubtless beginning to emerge with regard to heterosexual transmission, the probability of which may be lower than that of other risks such as traffic fatalities, for example (Anonymous, 1993).

3 At the start of the epidemic a certain denial of the risk was seen, notably in some gay circles and parts of the Black African population living in industrial countries. These groups considered their 'risk group' label to be a manifestation of homophobia or racist hostility (see in particular Pollak and Schiltz, 1987).

4 Question 1005: 'Can a person avoid getting AIDS by changing his/her behaviour? That is, by doing certain things and not doing other things?' and question 1008 (if 'yes', to question 1005): 'Do you think that you need to change any of your behaviours to protect yourself from getting AIDS?'

5 Question 68: 'Have the emergence and the spread of AIDS led you personally (yes or no) to . . .
   (a) be more careful about what you touch?'
   (b) seek more stability in your choice of partners?'
   (c) take precautions in sexual intercourse?'
   (d) avoid certain places (areas, establishments)?'
   (e) avoid certain types of people?'

6 Question 1005: 'Can a person avoid getting AIDS by changing his/her behaviour? That is, by doing certain things and not doing other things?'

7 Question 1008: 'Do you think that you need to change any of your behaviours to protect yourself from getting AIDS?'

8 The question about behaviour change used in the Eurobarometer surveys was put to samples of the entire European population older than 15 years, be they 'sexually active' or not.

9 The chapter on partners shows that the highly educated respondents are also more likely to have multiple partners.

References

ADAM, P. and HERZLICH, C. (1995) *Sociologie de la maladie et de la médecine*, Paris: Nathan.

ANONYMOUS (1993) 'How risky is risky sex? Letter to the editors', *Journal of Sex Research*, **30**, 2, pp. 188–91.

BAJOS, N., DUCOT, B., SPENCER, B. and SPIRA, A. (1997) 'Sexual risk taking, socio-sexual biographies and sexual interaction: elements of the French national survey on sexual behaviour', *Social Science and Medicine*, **44**, 1, pp. 25–40.

BASTARD, B. and CARDIA VONECHE, L., with the participation of MAZOYER, A. (1992) *Les choix et les comportements affectifs et sexuels face au sida, Une étude sociologique auprès de personnes séparées ou divorcées*, Paris: Centre de sociologie des organisations.

BASTARD, B., CARDIA VONECHE, L., PETO, D. and VAN CAMPENHOUDT, L. (1997) 'Relationships between sexual partners and ways of adapting to the risk of AIDS: landmarks for a relationship-oriented conceptual framework', in VAN CAMPENHOUDT, L., COHEN, M., GUIZZARDI, G. and HAUSSER, D. (Eds) *Sexual Interactions and HIV Risk. New conceptual perspectives in European research*, London: Taylor & Francis.

CHOI, K.H. and COATES, T.J. (1994) 'Prevention of HIV infection', *AIDS*, **8**, pp. 1371–89.

HUYNEN, P., MARQUET, J. and HUBERT, M. (1995) 'Les Européens et le SIDA: situation actuelle et tendances', INRA, *Les Européens et la santé publique*, Brussels.

LAUMANN, E.O., GAGNON, J.H., MICHAEL, R.T. *et al.* (1994) *The Social Organization of Sexuality. Sexual Practices in the United States*, Chicago: The University of Chicago Press.

LEPLÈGE, A. (1993) 'Relation médecin-malade et Santé Publique: incertitudes et partage de l'information dans la prévention du Sida', in JOB SPIRA, N., SPENCER, B., MOATTI, J.-P. and BOUVET, E. (Eds) *Santé Publique et maladies à transmission sexuelle*, Paris: John Libbey Eurotext.

LUDWIG, D. (1992) *Le sida: étude des représentations du risque. Influence des messages préventifs*, Paris: ANRS.

MARQUET, J., PETO, D. and HUBERT, M. (1995) 'Sexual behaviour and HIV risk: towards a relation-based approach', in FRIEDRICH, D. and HECKMANN, W. (Eds), *AIDS in Europe. The Behavioural Aspect, Vol. 2: Risk Behaviour and its Determinants*, Ergebnisse sozialwissenschafftlicher AIDS-Forschung 16.2, Berlin: Ed. Sigma.

MORRIS, M. and KRETZSCHMAR, M. (1997) 'Concurrent partnerships and the spread of HIV', *AIDS*, **11**, pp. 641–8.

PETO, D., REMY, J., VAN CAMPENHOUDT, L. and HUBERT, M. (1992) *SIDA: l'amour face à la peur modes d'adaptation au risque du SIDA dans les relations hétérosexuelles*, Paris: L'Harmattan, Logiques sociales Collection.

POLLAK, M. and SCHILTZ, M.A. (1987) 'Identité sexuelle et gestion d'un risque de santé. Les homosexuels face au Sida', *Actes de la Recherche en Sciences Sociales*, **68**, pp. 77–102.

REMY, J., VOYÉ L. and SERVAIS, E. (1978) *Produire et reproduire*, Brussels: Editions Vie Ouvrière.

Chapter 9

Condom Use

Françoise Dubois-Arber and Brenda Spencer

Introduction

Early in the course of the AIDS epidemic, condoms were recognized as an effective means of prevention if used properly and consistently. All the European countries from which data are presented in this chapter have included the promotion of condom use in their overall AIDS prevention policies, even if the importance of this element in relation to others, such as promotion of counselling and testing and advocacy of fidelity, has differed according to the different socio-cultural and political contexts. Prevention campaigns addressing the general population have been used more or less extensively, differing in intensity, duration, tone and style (Wellings, 1994), but were present in all countries.

In our comparison of condom use in the various countries, it is important to remember that attitudes to condoms at the beginning of the AIDS epidemic differed from country to country. Condoms have a long history: the first published mention of the device dates back to 1564. Although originally intended for disease prevention, their contraceptive properties were already known in the eighteenth century. The discovery of the vulcanization of rubber in 1839 led to widespread potential availability of the product (Gerofi and Spencer, 1994). However, traditions of use vary considerably from country to country (see Table 9.1), being determined by specific social, political and commercial environments. In some countries, such as the UK, they were for a long period the principal means of contraception, and were obtained both commercially and in birth control clinics. In others, their use was historically much more limited. In France, for example, they suffered from restrictions similar to those imposed on other contraceptive methods until 1967, when birth control finally became officially available. Furthermore, legislation prohibiting their promotion for disease prevention and for contraception was not finally abolished until 1987 and 1991 in the UK and France respectively.

Table 9.1 *Proportions of married women of reproductive age whose partners use condoms in several European countries, 1970–1988*

Year	Country	% use	Country	% use
1970	Denmark	20	Great Britain	31
1971	Belgium	10	Finland	31
1972	France	8		
1975	Denmark	29	Netherlands	10
1976	Italy	16	Great Britain	22
1977	Norway	15	Finland	32
1978	France	7		
1979	Italy	13		
1985	West Germany	6	Netherlands	6
1988	France	4		

Sources: Population Reports, Series H, 6, 1982;
Population Reports, Series H, 8, 1990

Societal acceptance of adolescent sexuality – and with it the degree of access of young people to contraception, including condoms – has also differed (and presumably continues to do so): the very liberal attitudes towards sexuality in the Netherlands are thought to explain the exceptionally low rates of teenage pregnancy in this country (Jones *et al.*, 1985); in Great Britain, campaigns to promote contraception specifically among the under-18s were launched as early as 1976 (Smith, 1978; Cossey, 1980). Finland has also had traditionally high rates of condom use (Population Reports, 1982; Coleman, 1981).

One question at issue concerning condom promotion at the start of the AIDS epidemic was how to deal with the device's dual role (prevention of sexually transmitted diseases and contraception). The usefulness of the condom in preventing disease transmission had ironically earned it a bad reputation and a poor social image. In certain countries commercial companies had spent the years since World War Two attempting to change the image of the product from a prophylactic with 'unsavoury' connections to a contraceptive for married couples, a 'family' product (Spencer, 1987). There was therefore some confusion as to how the situation should now be handled, since AIDS was after all (at least in this context) another sexually transmitted disease. Would this new promotion in some way undo the progress so far made to destigmatize and upgrade the product's image? Another issue was the question of changes in contraceptive methods. The oral contraceptive had not only removed the need for barrier methods (at least in the case of stable relationships), perceived as interfering with the sexual act, but had also given women more control over their fertility. Would the use of condoms be seen as a retrograde step? In this chapter, therefore, we offer a comparison of condom use across several European countries and discuss the differences and similarities encountered.

Methods

Three common indicators of condom use were derived from the studies available for this overview.

Lifetime experience with condoms. This indicator was available in eight countries. In each country's survey (except Athens–PR (1990)), the wording of the question was similar ('Have you ever used a condom?'). In Athens, lifetime use referred to use as a contraceptive method. All the data on lifetime use presented are computed for all respondents who have ever had sexual intercourse. In Switzerland, data related to this indicator come from the 1994 survey on sexual behaviour and not from the 1992 survey, as in the other chapters, since this indicator was first introduced into the routine core questionnaire in 1994.

Condom use in the last 12 months. This indicator was available in three countries. In Belgium and France, the period referred to was the last 12 months, in the Netherlands 'this past year'. In all three cases, the answer was 'yes/no'. The data are computed for persons who had at least one partner during the last 12 months/year.

Condom use during last intercourse. This indicator was available for three countries. In France and Switzerland, the question wordings were similar but not exactly the same (France: 'Did *you or your partner* use a condom the last time you had sexual intercourse?'; Switzerland: 'Did *you* use a condom the last time you had sexual intercourse?'). In Finland, the question was related to the use of a contraceptive method during last intercourse: all the answers other than condom use, including no contraception used, were recorded as 'no'. All the data presented are computed for persons who have ever had sexual intercourse.

It should be noted that indicators of condom use during lifetime and the last 12 months give only an indication of experience of condom use, not the frequency of use. This is because all respondents who used a condom once are in the same group as those who used them regularly, whatever the level of regularity. This point should be kept in mind, especially when we refer to an 'increase' in condom use.

The data presented are weighted data and refer to the general population aged 18–49 (for Switzerland the reference population is 18–45 years old). The 95 per cent confidence intervals are indicated. In some of the tables, particularly those presenting data stratified by age or by number of partners, the number of cases is small and the confidence intervals therefore large. Comparison between categories or countries is then based on the general tendency observed, even if individual differences are not statistically significant.

Results

In the following tables and figures, the data are presented chronologically to take into account a possible time effect in comparing studies, since we note that in certain countries evidence exists of increasing use of condoms between 1989 and 1994. This is the case for Switzerland (Dubois-Arber *et al.*, 1993), France (Moatti *et al.*, 1995), Germany (Bundeszentrale für gesundheitliche Aufklärung, 1993), Scotland (Robertson, 1995) and the Netherlands (de Vroome *et al.*, 1994). For example, in Switzerland (Dubois-Arber *et al.*, 1993), regular condom use with casual partners over the last six months increased from 8 per cent in 1987 to 60 per cent in 1992 among persons 17–30 years old.

Experience with Condoms (Lifetime Use)

This is the broadest indicator of condom use and the one present in most of the studies available (Table 9.2 and Figure 9.1). It gives no information on frequency of use, only on experience of use. The group of 'ever' users is therefore heterogeneous, potentially including, to take an extreme example, both those who have used a condom only once in their lives and regular users over a number of years.

Eight countries gathered data on condom use over life: Athens/Greece (Ath89 and Ath90), Netherlands (NL89), East Germany (EG90 and EG93) and West Germany (WG93), France (FR92), Portugal (P91), Belgium (B93) and Switzerland (CH94). Reported levels of condom use are different between countries. Some countries show high levels of lifetime condom use early in the period covered (NL89), whereas other countries have lower levels later (P91, B93). Nonetheless, we shall see that, taking the countries as a whole, an overall trend of increasing use over time does exist for the younger stratum of the population.

Gender-related Differences in Lifetime Condom Use

As shown in Table 9.2 and Figure 9.2, more men than women report having ever used condoms. This difference between genders, which is also observed

Table 9.2 *Lifetime experience of condom use by gender*

		Ath89	NL89	Ath90	EG90	P91	FR92	B93	EG93	WG93	CH94[1]
All	%	51.0	76.2	68.3	70.0	57.1	62.4	65.0	68.4	88.0	83.4
	CI	46.6–55.4	73.5–78.9	66.1–70.5	67–73	55.1–59.1	60.7–64.1	63–67	65.7–71.1	86.5–89.5	81.9–84.8
	N	503	934	1664	898	2253	3266	2619	1115	1994	2523
Men	%	58.7	79.5	75.7	78.3	65.8	69.1	71.0	75.9	91.0	86.1
	CI	51.9–65.5	75.4–83.5	72.4–78.5	73.9–82.6	63.1–68.5	66.9–71.3	68.5–73.5	72.4–79.4	89.2–92.8	84.2–87.9
Women	%	46.7	74.0	61.9	61.6	48.0	55.5	59.6	60.7	84.0	80.6
	CI	41.1–52.3	70.3–77.6	58.7–65.1	57.6–65.6	45–51	53.1–57.9	57–62.1	56.6–64.7	81.4–86.5	78.3–82.8

Base: all respondents (18–49 years) who ever had sex
Note:
[1] Switzerland: 18–45-year-old respondents

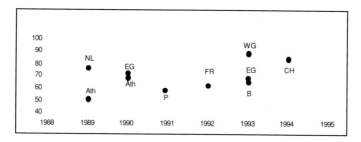

Figure 9.1 *Lifetime experience of condom use*

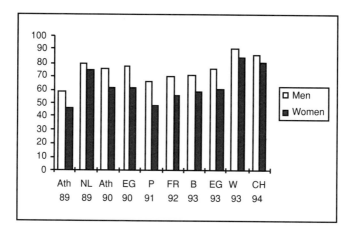

Figure 9.2 *Lifetime experience of condom use by gender*

in the number of partners (see Chapter 5 in this book), is well known. Explanations generally suggested include biases (Wellings *et al.*, 1994) such as:

Sampling bias. Women with high numbers of partners and high levels of condom use, such as sex workers, may be under-represented in the samples. Conversely, men with high numbers of partners and high levels of condom use may be better represented. There may also be systematic gender-related age differences between partners leading to non-sampling of the partners at both age limits of the sample.

Reporting bias. 'Social desirability effects' may lead some subgroups of the population to under-report certain practices. Women may under-report condom use for a number of different reasons: as men are the ones who actually wear the condoms, they may not consider that they themselves used one or may be embarrassed to report use. They may also feel that reporting the use of a condom devalues the relationship, particularly in the case of occasional relationships, which do not fit society's image of female sexuality (Bajos *et al.*, 1997).

Other gender differences in condom use detected in qualitative work, such as the difficulty women encounter in getting men to wear condoms (Gold *et al.*, 1992; Hubert *et al.*, 1993), particularly in casual relationships (Holland *et al.*, 1992; Dubois-Arber *et al.*, 1993), may also have an influence on reported differences between men and women in population surveys. Women may also have greater difficulty than men contemplating condom use in situations where strong emotional commitment is present (Peto *et al.*, 1992) for fear of spoiling the moment or threatening the relationship.

Interestingly, the difference between genders is smaller in the Netherlands, West Germany and Switzerland. These countries are those where lifetime experience of use is highest. In the United Kingdom, lifetime use of condoms is also high and differences between genders small: in 1990–1, for example, 80.9 per cent of men aged 18–59 and 71.9 per cent of women had used a condom at least once in their lives (Bajos *et al.*, 1995). In this respect two types of hypothesis may be made. The first is related to prevalence of use: when the level of use is high, this may mean that the overall acceptability of condoms is high, facilitating both the negotiation and the reporting of their use. The second concerns the use of condoms as a method of contraception: when the condom is used as a contraceptive, less of a difference is seen between men and women because both genders find this reason for use more acceptable and therefore report its use more easily. The latter hypothesis may apply to Great Britain (Wellings *et al.*, 1994) and the Netherlands (see below), where high use of condoms as a contraceptive means is reported. We find further support for this hypothesis in the 1992 Swiss data. Overall, men reported significantly more condom use than women at last intercourse. However, no significant difference in rate of condom use during last intercourse was observed in the subsample of men and women living in a 'stable', 'faithful' relationship[1] and reporting condom use as a contraceptive device (men 58.7 per cent, women 57.9 per cent, p = 0.9).

Age-related Differences in Lifetime Condom Use

Table 9.3 and Figure 9.3 show lifetime condom use by age category. Analysis of these data is complex because in each country studies were conducted at different stages in the epidemic. For each data set it is therefore necessary to consider both the country and the time effect simultaneously.

When we consider the distribution of lifetime experience of condom use according to age, two main patterns would, nonetheless, appear to emerge.

Pattern 1 is characterized by more experience of use in the older age categories. It is observed for two countries in studies conducted in 1989 (the Netherlands) and 1990 (East Germany). This type of distribution suggests a situation where condoms were used as a contraceptive by older generations, particularly at the onset of sexual activity. In subsequent generations, oral

Table 9.3 *Lifetime experience of condom use by age*

		Ath89	NL89	Ath90	EG90	P91	FR92	B93	EG93	WG93	CH94[1]
All	%	51.0	76.2	68.3	70.0	57.1	62.4	65.0	68.4	88.0	83.4
	CI	46.6–55.4	73.5–78.9	66.1–70.5	67–73	55.1–59.1	60.7–64.1	63–67	65.7–71.1	86.5–89.5	81.9–84.8
	N	503	934	1664	900	2248	3266	2619	1115	1977	2523
18–19	%	53.6	56.3	75.3	57.8	73.0	83.7	82.1	75.0	88.0	94.5
	CI	38.3–68.8	42.3–70.3	65.9–84.5	43.4–72.2	66.1–79.8	78–89.4	74.8–89.3	62.2–86.8	80.2–95.1	90.3–98.7
20–24	%	56.5	66.4	64.0	57.4	58.9	66.8	75.2	81.0	90.0	87.4
	CI	46–67	58.9–73.9	58–69.9	49.4–65.4	53.8–64	62.9–70.7	70.9–79.5	75–86.9	86.6–93.4	81.1–93.6
25–29	%	47.9	80.0	69.2	68.4	54.1	54.2	63.7	73.9	92.5	85.9
	CI	37.9–57.9	74–86	63.9–74.5	61.4–75.3	48.1–60.1	49.9–58.5	58.9–68.4	67.8–79.9	88.9–96.1	82.9–88.9
30–39	%	51.1	82.6	68.6	69.2	59.6	62.0	61.7	68.1	86.6	81.7
	CI	43.9–58.2	78.3–86.7	64.8–72.4	64.3–74.1	56.2–63	59.1–64.9	58.5–64.9	63.5–72.7	84.2–89	79.3–84.1
40–49	%	51.1	75.0	68.4	74.7	50.2	61.3	62.5	64.0	84.7	78.6
	CI	40.1–61.3	69.5–80.5	64.2–72.6	68.5–80.1	46.4–54	58.2–64.4	59.2–65.7	58.6–69.4	81.4–87.9	75–82.1

Base: all respondents (18–49 years) who ever had sex
Note:
[1] Switzerland: 18–45-year-old respondents

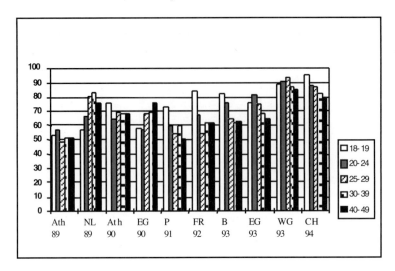

Figure 9.3 *Lifetime experience of condom use by age*
Base: all respondents (18–49 years) who have ever had sex

contraception then progressively displaced the condom as a contraceptive. The pattern evident at this point may now have changed, but data obtained as late as 1989 in the Netherlands show that contraception was still the main reason for current condom use for both younger and older generations. The main reasons given for using condoms during the last year for people aged 18–19 were protection against AIDS (13 per cent), contraception (81 per cent) and protection against STDs (7 per cent); whereas for people aged 40–49 the main reasons were protection against AIDS (17 per cent), contraception (79 per cent) and protection against STDs (0 per cent) (other = 4 per cent) (mutually exclusive answers).

Pattern 2 is characterized by a higher lifetime experience of use in the younger age categories. It has been seen since 1991 in five countries (Belgium, East Germany in 1993, France, Portugal, Switzerland) where we consistently observe higher use by the younger age categories. This suggests use of recent onset by the younger generation, mainly for HIV prevention purposes. Young people have been the first to adapt their behaviour and use more condoms in situations where HIV/STD prevention is especially important. This phenomenon is well illustrated in Figure 9.4, which depicts the rate of regular condom use with casual partners by age group in Switzerland as observed over several years.

Among the Pattern 2 country studies, the higher AIDS-related use by young people is reflected in the reasons given for recent condom use. In France, the reasons given for using condoms over the previous 12 months among people aged 18–19 were protection against AIDS (75 per cent), contraception (53 per cent), and protection against STDs (76 per cent); whereas, for

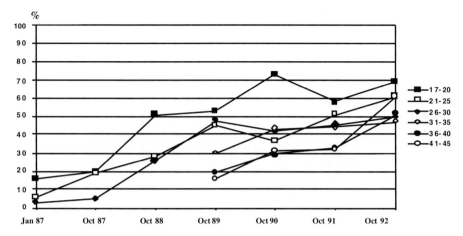

Figure 9.4 *Evolution (1987–92) of condom use (% 'always') with casual partners, by age, in Switzerland*
Base: all respondents (17–45 years) who have ever had sex

people aged 40–49, the reasons were protection against AIDS (3 per cent), contraception (60 per cent), and protection against STDs (43 per cent). In Belgium, the reasons for using a condom over the previous 12 months among 15–24 year olds were contraception (19.5 per cent), AIDS/STD prevention (16.9 per cent), or both (62.9 per cent); whereas, for people aged 35–44, they were contraception (52.2 per cent), AIDS/STD prevention (14.8 per cent), or both (29.1 per cent). In Switzerland, the reasons for condom use in a new relationship begun during the past year among the 17–20-year-olds were protection against AIDS (78.5 per cent), and/or contraception (83 per cent); whereas for people aged 41–45 they were protection against AIDS (86.1 per cent), and/or contraception (32.4 per cent).[2]

In the West Germany study, the picture partially fits Pattern 2 (considerably higher use in the youngest than in the oldest group), but in this case the highest use is seen in the intermediate age category. Condoms also played a significant part in contraception in this country in 1993: 50 per cent of the 18–19-year-olds using a contraception mentioned condoms as (one of) the method(s) used versus 26 per cent of the 40–49-year-olds. In Athens and East Germany, we observe a change of pattern with more use by young people in the second survey.

Finally, if we assume that lifetime use can be considered a surrogate indicator of recent use in the youngest part of the population who recently became sexually active, we see in Europe a general time trend towards higher levels of use (Figure 9.5) than is shown by the data for the population as a whole (Figure 9.1).

This time trend can be accepted as an overall effect of AIDS prevention in a generation with considerable exposure to preventive activities. Use of condoms is a strategy that need not require a limitation of sexual activity, but

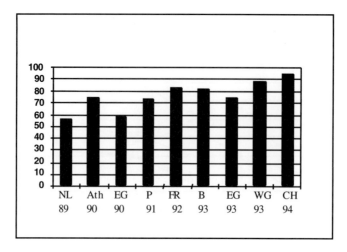

Figure 9.5   *Lifetime experience of condom use among 18–20-year-olds*

does involve some (implicit or explicit) negotiation. For young people who have always experienced their sexuality in the context of AIDS, it is perhaps easier and more 'normal' to speak about sexuality and prevention, because current cultural scenarios of sexuality frequently include condoms (Laumann and Gagnon, 1995).

Education-related Differences in Condom Use

Table 9.4 and Figure 9.6 show the distribution of lifetime condom use by level of education. The trend in almost all the countries is one of higher prevalence of use with increasing level of education. It should be noted, however, that level of education is not a constant for the various age strata, the average level of education of young people being systematically higher. This might confound the relationship between education and condom use. Nevertheless, the link between educational level and condom use in the France–ACSF (1992) data still remains after controlling for age (Ducot and Spira, 1993). In any event, this pattern is similar to that observed for contraceptive use, and indeed reflects what is known about the take-up of prevention in general, that is, higher social classes are more responsive to prevention messages (The Black Report, 1988). It is difficult to comment on the similarities and differences between countries because of the lack of equivalence in the categorization of the three categories. It is, however, notable that the only countries in which no gradient is observed are the Netherlands and Greece (Athens only). The Netherlands is noted for its relative lack of differences in terms of social

Table 9.4 *Lifetime experience of condom use by level of education*

		Ath89	NL89	Ath90	EG90	P91	FR92	B93	CH94[1]
All	%	51.0	76.2	68.3	70.0	57.1	62.4	65.0	83.4
	CI	46.6–55.4	73.5–78.9	66.1–70.5	67–73	55.1–59.1	60.7–64.1	63–67	81.9–84.8
	N	503	923	1664	899	2251	3264	2619	2522
Education									
Low	%	55.9	73.3	57.1	66.1	48.6	50.8	55.7	74.4
	CI	48–63.8	60.4–86.2	51.9–62.3	51.2–80.9	45.4–51.8	47.8–53.8	51.7–59.7	69.2–79.5
Medium	%	45.4	76.8	68.4	65.4	58.7	65.3	66.4	83.9
	CI	38.2–52.6	73.4–80.1	65.3–71.5	60.1–70.2	55.3–62.1	62.8–67.8	63.5–69.3	82.3–85.5
High	%	54.2	75.4	77.1	73.1	71	73.1	69.5	89.2
	CI	46.6–61.7	69.9–80.8	73.2–81	66.9–79.3	67–75	70–76.2	69.5–72.3	85.4–92.8

Base: all respondents (18–49 years) who ever had sex
Note:
[1] Switzerland: 18–45-year-old respondents

Table 9.5 *Experience of condom use in the last 12 months by gender, age and level of education*

		Netherlands 1989	France 1992	Belgium 1993
All	%	26.0	31.6	25.8
	CI	23.1–29	30–33.2	24.1–27.5
	N	868	3162	2535
Gender				
Men	%	32.0	36.2	32.4
	CI	27.2–36.8	33.8–38.5	29.8–35
Women	%	21.8	26.8	19.6
	CI	18.2–25.4	24.6–29	17.5–21.7
Age				
18–19	%	40.0	66.4	61.9
	CI	24.8–55.2	60–73.8	52.6–71.2
20–24	%	32.2	45.1	46.7
	CI	24.5–39.8	40.8–49.4	41.7–51.7
25–29	%	32.7	30.5	26.4
	CI	25.3–40.1	26.4–34.6	22–30.1
30–39	%	26.4	28.3	22.2
	CI	19.5–33.3	25.6–31	19.5–24.9
40–49	%	14.0	22.5	15.0
	CI	9.4–18.6	19.8–25.2	12.5–17.4
Education				
Low	%	11.4	22.3	16.8
	CI	2–20.8	19.7–24.8	13.8–19.8
Medium	%	22.1	33.5	25.7
	CI	9.8–34.4	31–36	23–28.4
High	%	39.1	40.5	31.4
	CI	32.7–45.5	37–44	28.5–34.3

Base: all respondents (18–49 years) who have had at least one sexual partner in the last 12 months

class and level of income. It is tempting to speculate on the part this may play in determining these results, but when one looks at condom use over the past year (Table 9.5) the education gradient observed in other countries also emerges in the Dutch data.

Condom Use in the Last 12 Months

This indicator of recent/current use allows us to identify and compare national condom use trends based on some additional socio-demographic

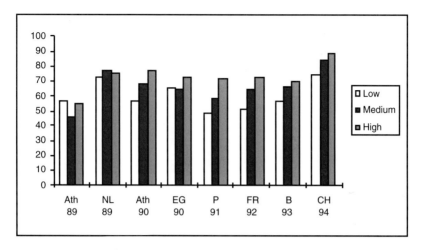

Figure 9.6 *Lifetime experience of condom use by level of education*

characteristics of users, especially as regards the number and nature of their sexual partners. For this variable, data are available for only three countries (NL89, FR92, B93). Unfortunately, we have no comparable data indicating the frequency of use or patterns of use according to type of partner. Table 9.6 shows that recent/current condom use varies according to the same main dimensions (gender, age and education) as lifetime condom use, that is, more use by men, by younger ages, and by the more highly educated.

Table 9.7 shows two other dimensions influencing the use of condoms number of partners and living status (whether or not cohabiting).

In all three countries, condom use steadily increases with the number of partners, but it seems that there is a threshold effect around five partners. At this point, the increase in use is less marked or we can even see a decrease in use (NL89, B93). This 'high partner change' category accounts for less than 3 per cent of the samples and it may be a very heterogeneous population. Nevertheless, a significant part of it is likely to be at high risk of exposure to HIV/ STDs since between a quarter and half of these persons do not use condoms.

Assuming that the relationship between people who live together is in general more stable than one in which they do not live together, the 'cohabiting' indicator may tell us something about the nature (duration and/or fidelity) of the relationship between partners.[3] As expected, condom use is lower for people living with their partners and higher among those living alone and people with multiple partners.

The slightly different pattern exhibited by the Netherlands (smaller age- and living arrangement-related differences) may be due to higher use of condoms as contraception in this country and/or to the fact that the survey was conducted in 1989, before a significant increase in use due to AIDS could occur.

Table 9.6 *Condom use at last intercourse by gender, age and level of education*

		Finland 1992	France[1] 1992	Switzerland[2] 1992
Gender				
Men	%	31.6	16.5	28.1
	CI	28.3–34.9	14.7–18.3	25.5–30.6
Women	%	21.5	11.3	17.9
	CI	18.5–24.5	9.7–12.8	15.7–20.1
Age				
18–19	%	50	41.4	53.8
	CI	38.3–61.7	33.6–49.2	46–61.6
20–24	%	33.5	24.7	34.1
	CI	27.3–39.8	21–28.4	29.5–38.7
25–29	%	25.2	11.5	20.9
	CI	19.6–30.8	8.6–14.4	17.1–24.7
30–39	%	27.9	10.5	18.2
	CI	24–31.8	8.6–12.3	15.7–20.7
40–49	%	19.2	8.5	13.9
	CI	15.6–22.8	6.7–10.3	10.6–17.2
Education				
Low	%	22.1	9.2	12.6
	CI	17.6–26.6	7.4–11	7.7–17.5
Medium	%	27.7	15.7	23.2
	CI	24.5–30.9	13.7–17.6	21.3–25.1
High	%	28.9	17.4	29.8
	CI	24.3–33.4	14.7–20.1	24.1–35.5
N		1476	3120	2359

Base: all respondents (18–49 years) who ever had sex
Notes:
[1] France: respondents who described a last intercourse in the last 12 months
[2] Switzerland: 18–45-year-old respondents

Condom Use at Last Intercourse

Data are again available for only three countries, in this case Finland (FIN92), France (FR92) and Switzerland (CH92). Direct comparisons between these countries are not possible owing to the different wording of the questions: in Finland, the question was related to the type of contraception used during last intercourse; in France and Switzerland the question was related to the use of condoms, whatever the purpose, during last intercourse. In both situations, condom use reflects mainly use with a stable partner, a situation that is much more frequent than casual relationships.

Table 9.7 *Experience of condom use in the last 12 months by number of partners in the same period and by cohabitation status*

		Netherlands 1989	France 1992	Belgium 1993
No. of partners				
1	%	21.7	27.5	21.2
	CI	18.8–24.6	25.8–29.2	19.5–22.8
2	%	49.2	59.8	52.2
	CI	36.7–61.2	53.3–66.3	44.1–60.3
3–4	%	66.7	70.1	72.4
	CI	49.8–83.6	60.5–79.7	63.3–81.5
5+	%	54.5	77.5	71.9
	CI	33.6–75.3	64.5–90.4	58.9–84.9
Cohabitation				
yes	%	20.7	23.4	18.3
	CI	17.5–23.9	21.6–25.2	16.5–20
no	%	33.3	52.1	47.3
	CI	25.3–41.3	48.8–55.4	43–51.6
N		868	3153	2535

Base: all respondents (18–49 years) who have had at least one sexual partner in the last 12 months

Table 9.8 *Condom use at last intercourse by number of partners in the last 12 months*

No. of partners		Finland 1992	France 1992	Switzerland[1] 1992
1	%	25.7	12.8	16.2
	CI	23–28.4	11.6–149	14.5–17.9
2	%	26.6	20.7	37
	CI	19.4–33.8	15.3–26	28.4–45.6
3–4	%	30	25.8	58.4
	CI	21.4–38.6	16.6–35	47.6–69.2
5+	%	26.8	35.4	60.8
	CI	16.5–37.1	20.6–50.2	43.3–78.3
N		1476	3120	2521

Base: all respondents (18–49 years) who ever had sexual intercourse
Note:
[1] Switzerland: 18–45-year-old respondents

Table 9.6 shows condom use at last intercourse by gender, age and level of education. The differences between genders, ages and levels of education display the same characteristics as already seen with lifetime and last year use. In all three countries, condoms were used more by the youngest age group. In

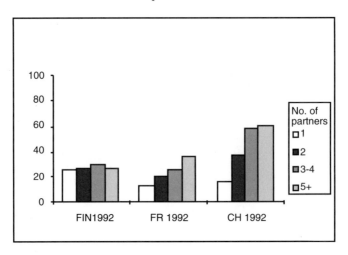

Figure 9.7   *Condom use at last intercourse by number of partners in the last 12 months*

France and Switzerland, the decrease in use related to age is very marked, suggesting an 'AIDS prevention' effect, that is condoms used as protection from HIV transmission, while in Finland this decreasing trend is less marked, suggesting a situation where condoms are being used more for contraception.

The differences between France and Switzerland on the one hand and Finland on the other hand are also apparent when condom use is assessed in relation to the number of partners (Table 9.8 and Figure 9.7): the trend towards an increase in use as the number of partners increases (FR92, CH92) also suggests an 'AIDS prevention' effect that does not seem to be as pronounced in Finland.

Conclusions

Lifetime experience with condoms is relatively high in Europe: between 51 per cent and 88 per cent of the general population, according to the country and the year of the survey, have used condoms at least once in their lives. The highest levels of use are found in the most recent surveys (France, Belgium, Germany, Switzerland; the Netherlands with its high level of lifetime use in 1989 being an exception). In these surveys, use is higher in the younger generations and clearly related to AIDS prevention, while older people use condoms more for contraceptive purposes. High condom use and increasing trends in use among young people have also been observed in the USA (CDC, 1995 a and b). In these cases we can speak of an AIDS prevention effect.

This recent AIDS prevention effect is also reflected in the use of condoms as measured over the past 12 months: in France and Belgium the age pattern of the current level of use during the year is very similar to lifetime use. On the other hand, in the Netherlands this pattern of current use is different. Older users have much lower rates when condom use is measured over the past 12 months (14 per cent) than when it is measured over the respondent's lifetime (75 per cent), suggesting 'historical' contraceptive use. In addition, in several countries with high lifetime use by young people (France, Belgium, Switzerland), the young acknowledge that the main reason for use is related either exclusively to AIDS or to both AIDS and contraception. In these countries condom promotion has essentially been linked to AIDS prevention. In the Netherlands, contraceptive condom use has been promoted and is reported, but AIDS is evidently also a reason for use since, as in France and Belgium, during the last 12 months condoms were used by a higher proportion of people with multiple partners than by those with one partner. These data on young people underline the necessity of making explicit the link between AIDS/STD prevention and contraception in sexual education and AIDS prevention, in order to increase use with all partners.

The level of lifetime use can be used for country comparisons as a surrogate indicator for current use in the 18–20-year-olds who became sexually active in the AIDS era. The range of the difference between lifetime use and last 12 months' use is between 16 and 20 per cent for the three studies where both sets of data are available. Applying this correction to the data on lifetime use, it can be estimated that in Europe between 40 and 70 per cent of this group used condoms at the time of the survey. The highest values are found in the more recent studies in West Germany and Switzerland.

We have no data on lifetime use of condoms for the Nordic countries represented in this data set. The only possible comparisons are based on use at last intercourse. Levels of use are difficult to compare, but patterns of use suggest that some AIDS/STD prevention effect exists in Finland, and that there is a clear effect in France and Switzerland (that is, more use by young people and individuals with multiple partners).

Levels of protection vary considerably between the countries surveyed and additional sources of accurate data are needed to learn more about current condom use and to understand the reasons underlying the differences observed. In particular, further comparative research should investigate in more depth the different patterns of condom use by relationship type and stage and the underlying rationales (such as alternative or complementary protective strategies chosen by individuals) (Marquet *et al.*, 1995). Yet, if we define predominance of use of condoms by the young and people with multiple partners as indicators of positive effects of prevention, we have to acknowledge that this behaviour is apparent in most of the European countries investigated here.

Early doubts about the desirability of choosing to promote condoms in direct association with AIDS, and hence disease prevention, appear to have been unfounded. In fact, the social representation of AIDS seems to be completely disconnected from 'traditional' sexually transmitted diseases. While this disconnection may not always be to the good (Job-Spira, 1990), the combined impact of AIDS education, especially on the young, has associated condoms with a modern phenomenon said to concern all of society. This particular sexually transmitted disease has therefore paradoxically helped to remove the stigma historically associated with condom use. These data illustrate that for the young at least, traditional problems of image do not present a barrier to condom use. For the older generations, image may contribute to the relative delay in necessary behaviour change, although it is certainly not the only factor, there being many reasons why 'you can't teach an old dog new tricks'.

The role of the condom as a contraceptive in the AIDS era remains unclear. Some believe it necessary to recommend taking the pill in addition to using condoms, others feel that this 'belt and braces' approach is not advisable. More research is needed in this area if policy is to be founded on evidence rather than opinion.

Notes

1   The terms used correspond to the wording of the questions in the study.
2   The number of 41–45-year-olds concerned is small.
3   Assuming that the relationship between people who live together is in general more stable than a relationship where they do not live together.

References

BAJOS, N., WADSWORTH, J., DUCOT, B., JOHNSON, A.M., LE PONT, F., WELLINGS, K., SPIRA, A. and FIELD, J. (1995) 'Sexual behaviour and HIV epidemiology: comparative analysis in France and Britain', *AIDS*, **9**, pp. 735–43.

BAJOS, N., DUCOT, B., SPENCER, B. and SPIRA A. (1997) 'Sexual risk-taking, socio-sexual biographies and sexual interaction: elements of the French National Survey on sexual behaviour', *Social Science and Medicine*, **44**, 1, pp. 25–40.

THE BLACK REPORT (1988), in TOWNSEND, P. and DAVIDSON, N. (Eds) *Inequalities in Health*, Harmondsworth: Penguin Books.

BUNDESZENTRALE FÜR GESUNDHEITLICHE AUFKLÄRUNG (1993) 'AIDS im öffentlichen Bewusstsein der Bundesrepublik Wiederholungsbefragung', Köln.

CDC (1995a) 'Trends in sexual behavior among high school students. United States, 1990, 1991, and 1993', *MMWR*, **44**, 7, pp. 124–32.

CDC (1995b) 'Youth risk behaviour surveillance – United States, 1993', *MMWR*, **44**, SS–1, pp. 1–17.

COLEMAN, S. (1981) 'The cultural context of condom use in Japan', *Studies in Family Planning*, **12**, 1, pp. 28–39.

COSSEY, D. (1980) 'Teenage birth control: the case for the condom', London: Brook Advisory Centre.

DE VROOME, E.M.M., PAALMAN, M.E.M., DINGELSTAD, A.A.M., KOLKER, L. and SANDFORT, T.G.M. (1994) 'Increase in safe sex among the young and nonmonogamous: knowledge, attitudes and behavior regarding safe sex and condom use in the Netherlands from 1987 to 1993', *Patient Education and Counselling*, **24**, pp. 279–98.

DUBOIS-ARBER, F., JEANNIN, A., MEYSTRE-AGUSTONI, G., GRUET, F. and PACCAUD, F. (1993) 'Evaluation de la stratégie de prévention du sida en Suisse sur mandat de l'Office fédéral de la santé publique. Quatrième rapport de synthèse 1991–1992', Lausanne: Institut universitaire de médecine sociale et préventive (CahRechDoc IUMSP, 82).

DUCOT, B. and SPIRA, A. (1993) 'Les comportements de prévention du Sida: prévalence et facteurs favorisants', *Population*, **5**, pp. 1479–1503.

GEROFI, J. and SPENCER, B. (1994) 'Condoms', in CORSON, S.L., DERMAN, R.J. and TYRER, L.B. (Eds) *Fertility Control*, Second Edition, London, Ontario: Goldin Publishers.

GOLD, R.S., KARMILOFF-SMITH, A., SKINNER, M.J. and MORTON, J. (1992) 'Situational factors and thought processess associated with unprotected intercourse in heterosexual students', *AIDS Care*, **4**, 3, pp. 305–23.

HOLLAND, J., RAMAZANOGLU, C., SCOTT, S., SHARPE, S. and THOMSON, R. (1992) 'Risk, power and the possibility of pleasure: young women and safer sex', *AIDS Care*, **4**, 3, pp. 273–83.

HUBERT, M., MARQUET, J., DELCHAMBRE, J., PETO, D., SCHAUT, C. and VAN CAMPENHOUDT, L. (1993) 'Comportements sexuels et réactions au risque du SIDA en Belgique. Premiers résultats de l'enquête nationale', Rapport à la Commission des Communautés Européennes (DG V), Facultés universitaires Saint-Louis, Bruxelles.

JOB-SPIRA, N. (1990) 'Une approche commune pour la lutte contre les MST et le Sida', in JOB-SPIRA, N., SPENCER, B., MOATTI, J.P. and BOUVET, E. (Eds) *Public Health and the Sexual Transmission of Diseases*, Paris: John Libbey Eurotext.

JONES, E.F., FORREST, J.D., GOLDMAN, N., HENSHAW, S.K., LINCOLN, R., ROSOFF, J.I., WESTOFF, C.F. and WULF, D. (1985) 'Teenage pregnancy in developed countries: determinants and policy implications', *Family Planning Perspectives*, **17**, 2, pp. 53–63.

LAUMANN, E.O. and GAGNON, J.A. (1995) 'Sociological perspective on sexual action', in PARKER, R.G. and GAGNON, J. (Eds) *Conceiving Sexuality: Approaches to Sex Research in a Postmodern World*, New York: Routledge.

MARQUET, J., PETO, D. and HUBERT, M. (1995) 'Sexual behaviour and HIV risk: towards a relation-based approach', in FRIEDRICH, D. and HECKMANN, W. (Eds) *AIDS in Europe – The Behavioural Aspect*, Vol. 2: Risk Behaviour and its Determinants, Berlin: Editions Sigma.

MOATTI, J.P., GRÉMY, I., OBADIA, Y., BAJOS, N., DORÉ, V. and GROUPE KABP/ACSF (1995) 'Sida: dernière enquête nationale, succès et risques des campagnes de prévention', *La Recherche*, **12**, pp. 30–4.

PETO, D., REMY, J., VAN CAMPENHOUDT, L. and HUBERT, M. (1992) *SIDA, l'amour face à la peur. Modes d'adaptation au risque du SIDA dans les relations hétérosexuelles*, Paris: l'Harmattan, logiques sociales Collection.

POPULATION REPORTS (1982) 'Update on condoms – products, protection, promotion', *Population Reports*, Series H, 6, September–October.

ROBERTSON, B.J. (1995) 'Sexual behaviour and risk of exposure to HIV among 18–25-year-olds in Scotland: assessing change 1988–1993', *AIDS*, **9**, pp. 285–92.

SMITH, W. (1978) 'Campaigning for choice', Family Planning Association Project Report, 1, London.

SPENCER, B. (1987) 'Studies in birth control provision for men', Unpublished PhD thesis, University of Manchester.

WELLINGS, K. (1994), 'General population', *Médecine Sociale et Préventive*, **37**, Suppl. 1, pp. S14–S46.

WELLINGS, K., FIELD, J., JOHNSON, A.M. and WADSWORTH, J. (1994) *Sexual Behaviour in Britain*, London: Penguin Books.

Chapter 10

Voluntary HIV Testing

André Jeannin, Mitchell Cohen and Nathalie Bajos

Introduction

The identification in January 1983 of human immunodeficiency virus's (HIV's) antigen structure opened the door to new means of controlling the spread of the epidemic, notably through the development of specific serotests. The use of these serological tests, which came onto the market in 1985, plays an important role in structuring attitudes and behaviour towards HIV risk for seropositive and seronegative individuals alike. The tests make it possible to identify infected individuals. They also provide, or should provide, a prime opportunity for giving personalized counselling for prevention. As a result, testing is a major public health tool.

With the recent development of new therapies, testing policies must be redefined. The combined administration of several antiretroviral drugs can lead to a marked drop, even the disappearance, of the virus in infected people. Early testing appears to be a public health imperative now more than ever, especially since scientists now commonly believe that people are particularly infective immediately after infection.

Analyzing the socio-demographic characteristics and sexual activity of people who are tested and determining the significance of taking an HIV antibody test thus take on special importance by making it possible to give partial answers to prevention workers and policy-makers' myriad questions. For example, do these whose sexual behaviour places them at the greatest risk of being infected with HIV take the HIV antibody test, and if so, why? Inversely, do people who face an extremely low risk of being exposed to HIV through sexual behaviour get themselves tested repeatedly? What position does the test occupy in risk adaptation strategies? Does announcing one's serological status prompt people to change their sexual behaviour, and if so, in what way? How is the decision to take the test made and in what type of interactional process? The answers to these questions call for data that are not always found in today's surveys, although European surveys on sexuality and AIDS prevention in the general population almost always include one or more items dealing with HIV testing. HIV testing is generally thought of as a meaningful, goal-orientated, behaviour that constitutes part of a person's response to the risk of HIV/AIDS infection.

In its broadest sense HIV testing could be defined as a set of procedures for ascertaining a biological sample's serological status. The individual from whom the biological sample was taken is generally, but not necessarily always, known. In analyzing ways of responding to HIV risk one must restrict the definition of HIV testing to voluntary HIV testing, knowing that the reasons for being tested may be various (to ascertain one's serological status before giving up condom use, before embarking on a new relationship, after being exposed to a risk, and so on). However, this notion of voluntary testing is itself unclear, and attempts to define it have been few and un-satisfactory. For instance, according to Anderson *et al.* (1992), ' "Voluntary tests" include blood tests sought voluntarily from doctors, clinic, or health maintenance organization', which is tautological. The CDC provide a more satisfactory definition, as follows: 'Voluntary tests were HIV-antibody tests that respondents had obtained by their own choice primarily to determine infection status (*i.e.* excludes tests required for blood donation, military induction, employment, insurance, or other purposes)' (Centers for Disease Control and Prevention, 1992). The CDC definition stresses two points, that is, the idea of respondent's own choice and the goal of the test from the respondent's point of view ('primarily to determine infection status'), and specifically excludes giving blood. Some people may, however, use blood donation as an indirect means of determining their own infection status (Berrios *et al.*, 1992; Lefrère *et al.*, 1992; Gill, Meyers and Rajwani, 1994; Lefrère *et al.*, 1996). It would be very important to be able to distinguish between testing of blood donors, where the primary purpose is to determine the blood sample's infection status, and testing as a result of some other motivation, the purpose of which is to determine the respondent's infection status. However, this distinction is not easy to operationalize in quantitative surveys.

In this chapter we shall first review the different procedures used in the European surveys to investigate HIV testing in order to highlight the problems of question wordings and to identify their implications for data comparison. Indeed, analysis of the questionnaire items in the various surveys reveals difficulties in the definition of voluntary testing itself. Then we shall attempt to show that, despite their limited comparability, the data on voluntary HIV testing in the European surveys in our possession nevertheless give a broad picture of the magnitude and main specificities of voluntary HIV testing. Finally, we shall try to propose some guidelines for designing questions on voluntary HIV testing in future surveys.

Methods

The European surveys included in this review dealt with HIV testing in varying depths through a wide range of topics. The subsets of items dealing with HIV testing in each survey indicate how HIV testing is conceptualized, what its dimensions are, and what its place and importance are in the broad range of ways of responding to HIV risk. The items' wordings also delineate the data's potential comparability. Table 10.1 summarizes the themes covered in 10 surveys. Only the items concerning actual HIV testing by the respondents and their partners were taken into account in constructing this table; items dealing with general opinions about testing were ignored.

The data on frequency of testing have many weaknesses. In addition to the well-known difficulties inherent in asking 'threatening' questions about behaviour in surveys (Schuman and Presser, 1981) and problems pertaining to AIDS behavioural research in general (Catania *et al.*, 1990), inconsistent self-reporting of HIV testing has been mentioned specifically (Phillips and Catania, 1995; Lindan *et al.*, 1994). These difficulties compound the differences in survey design, data collection modes, and item wordings and further decrease the data's precision and comparability.

The items selected for comparative analysis show some variation in their wordings and the circumstances of HIV testing that are included. The Norwegian survey provides the most precise and restrictive wording, specifically excluding tests made in connection with blood donation, pregnancy and military service. The Swiss survey excludes blood donation only. The four other surveys do not specify what circumstances of HIV testing should be taken into account in the answer. Thus, the Norwegian survey is likely to provide the most restrictive figures, followed by the Swiss survey, while the other surveys are likely to provide comparatively inflated figures. The most basic information, 'ever tested', was not included in the Athens and Portuguese surveys. In surveys where 'ever tested' is included, it is sometimes not possible to distinguish between tests done in conjunction with giving blood or for other reasons. Few surveys inquire about blood donation *per se*.

The items dealing with the circumstances in which the test – generally the last one – was performed are very heterogeneous. The items on the place where the test was done use different lists of places, few of which are exhaustive. The confidentiality or anonymity provided by the setting is seldom investigated. Nor is counselling, whether pre- or post-test.

Some of the surveys acknowledge that HIV testing does not take place in a motivational vacuum but as a response to the individual's situation or acceptance, for instance, of routine testing offered by a practitioner. The motivation for being tested is dealt with through items on the source of advice and reasons for taking the test, with much overlapping between the two. The

Table 10.1 *Themes regarding HIV testing dealt with in ten European surveys*

Survey	Themes
Belgium 1993	Partner tested as means of protection
	Respondent ever tested,[1] frequency
	Time of last test
	Source of advice to be tested
	Place of last test
	Quality of service at testing place
	Respondent and partner took test before respondent's first sexual intercourse and thereafter
France–ACSF 1992	Respondent ever tested
	Respondent tested within last 12 months
	Number of tests performed in the last year and before the last year
	Intention to take test
	Date and result of the last test
	Asked whether partners had been tested
	Circumstances of tests within last 12 months
Germany (East) 1990	Respondent ever tested[1]
	Intention to take test again
Germany (West) 1989	Respondent ever tested[1] or planning to be
	Respondent and partner tested together
	Respondent planning to be tested before having child
Germany 1993	Respondent ever tested[1]
	Number of tests
	Place[2] of test
	Intention to take test
Netherlands 1989	Respondent ever tested
	Reasons for taking test
	Test result
Norway 1992	Respondent ever tested (excludes blood donation, etc.)
	Number of tests
	Year of first and last test
	Spouse has been tested
Portugal 1991	Intention to take test
	Willingness to know result of test
Scotland 1992	Frequency of blood donation now and 5 years ago
	Respondent ever tested
	Intention to take test
Switzerland 1992	Respondent ever donated blood
	Year of last blood donation
	Respondent ever tested (excludes blood donation)
	Number of tests
	Year of last test
	Place of last test
	Source of advice to be tested
	Reason for taking test
	Pre-test counselling
	Means of communicating test result
	Post-test counselling

Notes:
[1] without specification (no definition given)
[2] includes 'in connection with a blood donation'. 'Intention to take test': subsumes various degrees of intentionallity: from general willingness to definite intention

290

Table 10.2 *Wording of items on HIV testing (lifetime) used for comparison*

Survey	Wording of items
Belgium 1993	'Have you personally had an HIV/AIDS screening test?'
France 1992	'Have you been tested for HIV/AIDS in the last twelve months?'
	if not 'Have you been tested for HIV/AIDS previously to the last twelve months?'
Germany (East) 1990	'Have you ever been tested to check whether you have the virus that causes AIDS?'
Germany (West) 1989	'Have you ever been tested for HIV/AIDS?'
Netherlands 1989	'Have you, yourself, been tested for HIV?'
Norway 1992	'Have you been tested for HIV/AIDS? (Do not include testing in connection with being a blood donor, pregnancy, or military service)'
Switzerland 1992	'Excluding blood donation, have you ever had an HIV/AIDS screening test?'

individual's testing strategy is dealt with through items on the total number of tests in the respondent's lifetime and/or within a given period of time; it is but rarely (French and Belgium survey) linked to specific partners. Intention to test (or to test again) is sometimes included, but motivation for testing again is not; the reasons for not being tested are never investigated. The possibility of outside influences, such as an ongoing advertising campaign at the time of the decision to test, is never investigated.

We then compared the frequencies of HIV testing observed across countries and categories among the sexually active population. The analysis was restricted to the sexually active respondents since we were studying HIV testing as a way of coping with AIDS as a sexually transmitted disease. Having had at least one HIV test in one's lifetime ('ever tested') was the main indicator used. Table 10.2 shows the wording of this indicator in the seven surveys for which comparable data were available. It was used for comparative analysis and a crude assessment of the magnitude of overall HIV testing within the limits of comparability.

A set of common variables to be used in cross-national comparisons has been defined for all of the surveys investigated. Six of the common socio-demographic, behavioural and attitudinal variables were used here, namely, gender, age, education, number of partners during last year, location (with modalities 'large towns' and 'cities' aggregated) and cohabitation status. The prevalence of HIV testing was then cross-tabulated against these common variables. Confidence intervals were computed by normal approximation using simple random sampling formulae for all the countries except France, where specific software was used (SUDAAN: see Shah *et al.*, 1993).

Similarities and Particularities of HIV Testing across Europe

The lifetime HIV testing frequency data in the six surveys included in this comparison show testing to be a widespread, large-scale phenomenon (Table 10.3). The overall proportions of people tested span a wide range, from less than 10 per cent in the Netherlands to about 30 per cent in Western Germany and France. The country rates seem to cluster around three different levels, that is, low overall level of tested people (the Netherlands 9 per cent), medium level (Norway 16 per cent, Belgium 18 per cent, East Germany 20 per cent) and high level (Switzerland 26 per cent, France 29 per cent, West Germany 30 per cent), but are not correlated with the survey date. For example, the oldest surveys (1989) in the data set have both the highest (West Germany) and the lowest (the Netherlands) rates, while the latest survey (Belgium 1993) shows only a medium rate of testing. On the other hand, they are likely to be related to variations in policies and question wordings, which two dimensions are doubtless not independent. Thus, for example, at the time of the Dutch survey people were discouraged from being tested and, as we said before, the Dutch survey also contains the most restrictive question on HIV testing. In any event, these results mean absolute numbers of hundreds of thousands and up, according to country. Voluntary HIV testing is thus truly a mass phenomenon. Although rates vary according to country and subgroup, the data show testing to be widespread, spanning genders, educational levels, rural and urban areas, and age groups.

Differences in the proportions of men and women tested are mostly small and not statistically significant, the largest differences being 7 per cent in the Netherlands (women 6 per cent, men 13 per cent) and France (women 33 per cent, men 26 per cent). In Britain, 4.2 per cent of men and 2.9 per cent of women were tested for 'other reason[s]', that is, presumably voluntary testing (Wellings *et al.*, 1994).

The age-related testing pattern is remarkably similar between countries. Despite differences in levels and gradients, the proportion of people tested increases until ages 25–29, then decreases, to form a rough 'dome pattern' in every country except France. In each country the highest and lowest testing rates (percentage of the population) are in the 25–29 and 18–19 age groups, respectively.

The age-related frequency of testing is not always the same for both genders (data not shown in Table 10.3). The 'dome' seems to have a steeper slope for women. For example, in Switzerland 41 per cent of the women versus 28 per cent of the men aged 25–29 years had been tested, compared with 23 per cent of the men and only 17 per cent of the women in the 40–44 age group. The pattern is similar in West Germany, where 46 per cent of the women aged 25–29 and 17 per cent of the women aged 40–49 had been tested compared with 38 per cent and 21 per cent, respectively, of the men. In East

Table 10.3 *Proportions (%, with 95% confidence intervals) of respondents ever tested in seven European countries*

	Belgium 1993		France ACSF 1992		Germany East 1990		Germany West 1989		Netherlands 1989		Norway 1992		Switzerland[1] 1992	
All	18	±1	29	±1	20	±2	30	±2	9	±2	16	±1	26	±2
Gender														
Men	17	±2	26	±1	22	±4	29	±3	13	±3	17	±2	24	±2
Women	18	±2	33	±1	18	±3	31	±3	6	±2	15	±1	27	±3
Age														
18–19	9	±4	15	±4	19	±14	15	±8	3	±4	5	±3	15	±6
20–24	22	±4	34	±2	24	±8	33	±6	5	±3	19	±3	23	±4
25–29	26	±4	44	±2	26	±6	42	±5	15	±5	20	±3	34	±4
30–39	24	±3	31	±1	21	±4	34	±3	10	±3	18	±2	28	±3
40–49	18	±3	36	±1	13	±3	19	±4	8	±3	10	±2	20	±4
Education														
Low	15	±2	22	±1	17	±6	23	±3	7	±7	14	±2	21	±6
Medium	14	±2	31	±1	18	±3	35	±4	10	±2	18	±3	26	±2
High	24	±2	36	±2	24	±4	32	±4	6	±3	16	±2	27	±5
No. of partners over last year														
0	11	±5	20	±3	19	±6	25	±5	4	±5	16	±6	18	±5
1	19	±1	29	±1	20	±3	29	±2	10	±2	14	±1	25	±2
2	28	±6	37	±4	26	±13	48	±10	10	±8	22	±5	38	±8
3–4	35	±8	42	±6	21	±15	45	±11	6	±8	25	±6	49	±11
5 or more	51	±12	39	±8	64	±33	53	±22	18	±16	41	±10	42	±16
Place of residence														
Rural	24	±8	26	±1	12	±3	28	±5	10	±9	13	±2	22	±3
Small towns	14	±2	30	±2	16	±4	28	±3	9	±2	14	±2	28	±3
Large towns, cities	26	±2	37	±2	30	±4	35	±4	10	±4	23	±3	30	±5
Cohabitation														
Cohabiting	19	±2	30	±1	20	±3	29	±2	10	±2	15	±1	26	±2
Not cohabiting	27	±3	28	±2	19	±5	32	±3	8	±5	18	±2	26	±3

Base: all respondents (18–49 years) who ever had sex

Note:
[1] Switzerland: 18–45-year-old respondents.

Germany the difference is smaller in the 25–29 age group (women 28 per cent, men 25 per cent) than in the 40–49 age group (women 9 per cent, men 17 per cent). The prevalence of testing is higher in women from 20–24 to 30–39 years of age in Switzerland; from 25–29 to 30–39 years of age in West Germany; and from 20–24 to 25–29 years of age in East Germany. These higher female testing prevalences in the most active child-bearing years might be related to partially differing uses of testing. For women in these age brackets the testing rates may reflect both greater access to pregnancy-related screening and greater willingness to be tested before contemplating pregnancy, whereas for men they may be more related to the risk of infection in a general sense.

In the different countries, with the exception of the Netherlands and Norway, lower education is associated with lower proportions of tested people. The trend is not regular, however, perhaps due to differences in educational systems or the way education levels were aggregated for cross-national comparisons. In some countries (Belgium and East Germany) the threshold difference is between the 'medium' and 'high' categories, whereas in other countries (West Germany, Switzerland, and Norway) the threshold is between the 'low' and 'medium' categories.

We may wonder whether these data reflect differences in risk exposure according to social class and/or inequalities in access to health care structures in general and testing centres in particular. The data analyzed by H. Leridon *et al.* in Chapter 5 provide some clues, for they reveal a gradient between level of education and number of partners in the last 12 months in all of the countries except Norway and the Netherlands. We might also wonder if these data do not reflect socially marked preventive attitudes, that is, that people with more privileged backgrounds tend to be more ready consumers of preventive care and clients of care systems, as suggested by the analysis of STDs that is included in this volume (Chapter 7).

There is a strong general association between the reported number of sexual partners in the last 12 months and lifetime HIV testing. The proportions of tested people are highest among those with the highest numbers of partners in all countries except Switzerland, where the highest proportion is found in the second highest category of number of partners. Still, it is important to emphasize that a large proportion of the respondents who reported having many partners had never had access to a screening test.

The percentages of people with five or more partners in the last 12 months who had not been tested (Table 10.3) range from 82 per cent in the Netherlands to 36 per cent in East Germany, although one must allow for the large confidence intervals due to small frequencies. Dubois and Spencer have shown that a sizeable minority (that is 45 per cent in the Netherlands, 22 per cent in France) of persons with five or more partners in the last 12 months had not used any condoms in that time (see Chapter 9). Although there is no information on the co-occurrence of these behaviours (absence of test and condom use in the presence of multipartnership), the possibility of a group of people with high-risk behaviour revealed by the available data is worrisome and deserves further scrutiny.

No clear pattern can be seen regarding the association with location. The proportions of tested people are higher in the large towns and cities in all of the countries except Belgium. Similarly, there is no clear association between cohabiting with a partner and HIV testing.

The data available in these cross-sectional surveys do not allow us to make any assertions about the exact role that testing plays in people's reactions to HIV risk. Testing might follow risk taking, such as unprotected intercourse, but could also result from a desire to stop using condoms in stable, mutually 'faithful' relationships. It is very likely, however, that several explanations are at work concurrently.

Policies regarding HIV testing in Europe have been classified as either 'extensive' or 'selective' (Setbon, 1996). Extensive policies, such as those of Sweden and France, promote widespread testing; in the case of selective policies, such as those of Great Britain, Switzerland, and the Netherlands, the focus and precondition of testing is the availability of proper counselling. General population prevention campaigns have generally not made HIV testing a central message. Wellings (1994) does not even mention this topic in her review of the content of campaign messages in 11 Western European countries.

The aggregate HIV testing pattern revealed by the 'ever tested' indicator is broadly similar in all countries, that is, HIV testing appears to be strongly associated with higher numbers of partners in the last 12 months. This pattern suggests that HIV testing is used in conjunction with risk taking and that this use is similar across Europe. It is very remarkable that this similarity of re-sponding to HIV risk through HIV testing occurred across countries where public health policies have been very different and similar degrees of reliance on testing are seen in countries with different policies, such as in France and Switzerland. This suggests that the same social models of responding to HIV risk through HIV testing have been invented simultaneously yet independ-ently in the various countries.

Designing Questions on HIV Testing for Future Surveys

This analysis leaves a number of questions unanswered, whether from the public health standpoint or in terms of theory and methodology. In particular, the available data are not sufficient to analyze the impact of being tested on preventive behaviour, whether we consider the negative effects of 'false reassurance' or the positive effects of allowing more properly for the risk (Higgens *et al.*, 1991). Nor do they allow us to understand why a large proportion of the subjects who are exposed to the risk because of their multipartner status state that they have never been tested. A major challenge therefore is to design future studies and survey questions that will fill these gaps in our knowledge.

The Test's Status

First of all, the status of the behaviour being studied must be clarified. As we have seen, the notion of 'voluntary' testing is ambiguous. For instance, is testing 'voluntary' when its purpose is to fulfil a job or insurance requirement? What is a free decision, influence, and coercion? Should not testing through giving blood be counted the same as 'voluntary testing' when someone fearing discrimination uses this means to determine his/her serostatus? To avoid the problem, it is suggested that a dichotomy be constructed using the appropriate wording for the item in line with the test's focus (the main 'subject' whose serological status must be known), namely, the blood sample in the case of giving blood and the person him/herself otherwise. Accordingly, 'giving blood' becomes one of the locations where testing is done, and should be followed, in a survey, by items inquiring about the reasons for choosing this particular setting.

Taking the Test: An Interactive Decision-making Process

A central question is how the decision to test was taken. The decision-making process involves several components, including people, networks, and information. Social scientists are very interested in the various people and social networks beyond the individual him/herself that may have been involved, that is, partner(s), doctor, friends, and so on. Under what circumstances involving which players does the decision to be tested crystallize? In the same vein, we should explore the question of not being tested. Rates of voluntary HIV testing reflect an unknown amount of 'failure' to get tested for various reasons (Irwin, Valdiserri and Holmberg, 1996). No analysis of the decision to get tested can be complete without investigating the negative outcome (a decision not to be tested) as well, and surveys focusing on understanding the motivational dimension of voluntary HIV testing should include this. In particular, the fear of potential discrimination, whether real or imagined (Green, 1995; Westbrook, Legge and Pennay, 1993), may lead the individual to use various strategies at the time of the test in order to hide his/her true motive or to avoid some consequences of the test. It is the researcher's responsibility not to be misled and to make as certain as possible that the true constellation of motives is taken into account during the interview.

The information – especially its source and accuracy – upon which the decision was partly based is highly relevant from the public health point of view, as this is where information campaigns or their lack comes into effect. The presence of an ongoing sustained media campaign, especially television advertising, has been shown to have increased testing rates (Ross and Scott, 1993). In surveys where the research question is explaining the decision to get tested, inquiries about the media environment at the time of that decision should be made.

The Significance of Taking the Test

Knowing the number of people in a population who have been tested at some unknown time does not say much about either risk taking or the proportion of people who actually know their serostatus, which may have changed after the last test. It should at least be complemented by the first and last tests' dates. Most important, it would be very interesting to be able to situate the moment of being tested within the subject's life history so as to be able to judge what impact such an act has on behaviour.

This last approach is doubtless easier to conduct using a qualitative methodology. The probable overall link between HIV testing and risk taking may indicate the existence of strategies for dealing with HIV risk set up autonomously by individuals. The identification of such strategies (Peto *et al.*, 1992), their origins, modes of transmission, and impact in terms of risk of transmission should be a concern both for public health and the social sciences.

The various aspects of counselling should also be investigated. This topic is central to the public health aspects of HIV testing as well as to the social science concerns, as it is central to understanding the individual's behaviour after the test (for example, repeated risk taking and repeated testing). It should cover pre- and post-test counselling and some assessment by the individual of the relevance of the received counselling.

The Circumstances of Being Tested

It is very important to identify clearly the circumstances of being tested, since it has been shown that the types of patient using different facilities, their motivations for testing, and thus the demand pattern are very different according to the setting (Van Casteren *et al.*, 1993; Jeannin, Dubois-Arber and Paccaud, 1994; MMWR – Morbidity and Mortality Weekly Report, 1993; Smith *et al.*, 1994). Knowing the circumstances is likely to shed light on the determinants of such behaviour and the decision-making process that culminates in being tested.

When inquiring about the setting where the last test was done, the questionnaire should provide a complete list of places where testing is done, including 'blood donation centre' and 'at a gynaecologist's'. This latter example shows that the place of testing and purpose, such as 'screening before pregnancy', may be closely related. Consequently, there should be some assessment of the reasons for choosing the place.

The motivation or purpose of being tested should distinguish properly between the following cases: routine screening, such as for pregnancy, which may or may not be mandatory; testing done at the request of some institution, for example insurance company or employer; and testing done at the individual's initiative ('voluntary' testing) and linked directly to the risk of infection, whether to avoid a risk (for example to stop using condoms in a regular, faithful partnership) or to ascertain the consequence of a risk (for example unprotected intercourse with a casual partner). The list of motivations should include the benefits perceived by the respondent (Dawson *et al.*, 1993; Meadows, Catalan and Gazzard, 1993a and 1993b; Myers *et al.*, 1993; Wortley *et al.*, 1995).

Other characteristics of the test's setting are relevant in explaining changes in the demand of voluntary testing. In addition to the availability of anonymous HIV testing in the respondent's geographic area (Hirano *et al.*, 1994), privacy concerns have been shown to be important in planning to be tested (Phillips *et al.*, 1995) and the client's awareness of the testing options (confidentiality/anonymity) has been found to have at least a short-term influence on actual testing (Hirano *et al.*, 1994).

Testing and Monitoring

The number of tests done in a specific period, for example, in the last 12 months, provides information that could be used for incidence computations.

Information about the setting where the test (for example the last test) was carried out is important for monitoring, demand assessment and (perhaps) resource allocation by the public health authorities, as well as being an element in the decision-making process. Information about the actual result of the test is not very relevant in broad, population-based surveys because the prevalence of HIV is so low in the general population. On the other hand, clearly stating before the interview that no question will be asked about the test's result may increase the willingness to provide accurate answers.

Conclusions

Despite the limitations due to comparability and data quality issues, a few broad conclusions can still be drawn from this analysis of HIV testing as a way of responding to HIV risk in Europe.

There is a clear need for clarifying the way that the phenomenon is approached in surveys. There is a basic need to identify the relevant items of interest according to the survey objectives. A distinction between voluntary testing and routine testing of blood donors would be the minimum requirement in this respect. The motives for testing and the difficult problem of distinguishing between 'voluntary' and 'non-voluntary' should be given at least conceptual and operational solutions. The individual's 'testing record' and strategies of responding to the HIV risk need to be taken into account if the focus of the survey is gauging the public health stakes of and/or analyzing and understanding HIV testing behaviour from a social science point of view.

HIV testing appears to be a large-scale, widespread phenomenon in all the countries surveyed. Most likely this phenomenon pertains to voluntary HIV testing, not routine testing of blood donors. HIV testing has until now received attention mostly from an atomistic point of view, as an individual's decision or, at best, as a micro-social phenomenon. However, the sheer numbers involved mean that it has become a macro-social phenomenon that should be analyzed as such through, for instance, classical sociological categories such as role, socialization, behavioural models, social differentiation, subcultures, and so on. A further social science challenge, in the absence of mass media campaigns, is the puzzling fact of the simultaneous 'invention' in different countries of a similar response to HIV risk through HIV testing. The magnitude of the phenomenon is striking when contrasted with the relative timidity of the campaigns to promote HIV testing that have been conducted across Europe and calls for further scrutiny.

HIV testing is a major public health challenge. HIV testing is a large-scale phenomenon, most probably generally related to risk-taking, not always occurring with proper guidance from the health authorities, and the consequences of which are still under-researched. Evaluating its impact in terms of risk of infection should be moved to the top of the research agenda.

As Setbon (1996) points out, the test, which is originally a technical tool, acquires another dimension when public controversy leads to public policy decisions defining its use. The HIV antibody test has been the butt of controversy about its use (voluntary, systematic, or mandatory) since it was developed. New treatment strategies are likely to rekindle this debate. Social science research must be on hand to resolve the debate. It must also provide opportunities for thinking about the conditions of access to testing and management of the individual immediately after the diagnosis of seropositivity (Doré, Moatti and Souteyrand, 1996).

References

ANDERSON, J.E., HARDY, A.M., CAHILL, C. and ARAL, S. (1992) 'HIV antibody testing and post-test counselling in the United States: data from the 1989 National Health Interview Survey', *American Journal of Public Health*, **82**, pp. 1533–5.

BERRIOS, D.C., HEARST, N., PERKINS, L.L., BURKE, G.L., SIDNEY, S., McCREATH, H.E. and HULLEY, S.B. (1992) 'HIV antibody testing in young, urban adults', *Archives of Internal Medicine*, **152**, pp. 397–402.

CATANIA, J.A., GIBSON, D.R., CHITWOOD, D.D. and COATES, T.J. (1990) 'Methodological problems in AIDS behavioral research: influences on measurement error and participation bias in studies of sexual behavior', *Psychological Bulletin*, **108**, 3, pp. 339–62.

CENTERS FOR DISEASE CONTROL AND PREVENTION (CDC) (1992) 'HIV counselling and testing services from public and private providers – United States, 1990', *MMWR – Morbidity and Mortality Weekly Report*, **41**, 40, pp. 743–52.

DAWSON, J., FITZPATRICK, R., HART, G., BOULTON, M., McCLEAN, J. and BROOKES, M. (1993) 'Access to HIV testing for homosexually active men', *European Journal of Public Health* (Oxford), **3**, pp. 264–8.

DORÉ, V., MOATTI, J.-P. and SOUTEYRAND, Y. (1996) 'Le dépistage du VIH: une contribution des recherches en santé publique', in *Le dépistage du VIH. Politiques et pratiques*, Paris: ANRS.

GILL, M.J., MEYERS, G. and RAJWANI, A. (1994) 'Use of blood donation history of people with HIV infection to identify recipients at risk', *Canadian Medical Association Journal*, **151**, 8, pp. 1147–51.

GREEN, G. (1995) 'Attitudes towards people with HIV – are they as stigmatizing as people with HIV perceive them to be?', *Social Science and Medicine*, **41**, pp. 557–68.

HIGGINS, D., GALAVOTTI, C., O'REILLY, K. *et al.* (1991) 'Evidence for the effects of HIV antibody counselling and testing on risk behavior', *Journal of American Medical Association*, **266**, pp. 2419–29.

HIRANO, D., GELLERT, G.A., FLEMING, K., BOYD, D., ENGLENDER, S.J. and HAWKS, H. (1994) 'Anonymous HIV testing: the impact of availability on demand in Arizona', *American Journal of Public Health*, **84**, 12, pp. 2008–10.

IRWIN, K.L., VALDISERRI, R.O. and HOLMBERG, S.D. (1996) 'The acceptability of voluntary HIV antibody testing in the United States: a decade of lessons learned', *AIDS*, **10**, pp. 1707–17.

Voluntary HIV Testing

JEANNIN, A., DUBOIS-ARBER, F. and PACCAUD, F. (1994) 'HIV testing in Switzerland', *AIDS*, **8**, pp. 1599–603.

LEFRÈRE, J.J., ELGHOUZZI, M.H., PAQUEZ, F., N'DALLA, J. and NUBEL, L. (1992) 'Interviews with anti-HIV-positive individuals detected through the systematic screening of blood donations: consequences on predonation medical interview', *Vox Sanguinis*, **62**, 1, pp. 25–8.

LEFRÈRE, J.J., ELGHOUZZI, M.H., SALPETRIER, J., DUC, A. and DUPUY-MONTBRUN, M.C. (1996) 'Interviews of individuals diagnosed as anti-human immuno-deficiency virus-positive through the screening of blood donations in the Paris area to 1994: reflections on the selection of blood donors', *Transfusion*, **36**, pp. 124–7.

LINDAN, C.P., AVINS, A.L., WOODS, W.J., HUDES, E.S., CLARK, W. and HULLEY, S.B. (1994) 'Levels of HIV testing and low validity of self-reported test results among alcoholics and drug users', *AIDS*, **8**, pp. 1149–55.

MEADOWS, J., CATALAN, J. and GAZZARD, B. (1993a) ' "I plan to have the HIV test" – predictors of testing intention in women attending a London antenatal clinic', *AIDS Care*, **5**, 2, pp. 141–8.

MEADOWS, J., CATALAN, J. and GAZZARD, B. (1993b) 'HIV antibody testing in the antenatal clinic: the views of the consumers', *Midwifery*, **9**, 2, pp. 63–9.

MMWR – MORBIDITY and MORTALITY WEEKLY REPORT (1993) 'Differences between anonymous and confidential registrants for HIV testing – Seattle, 1986–1992', *MMWR*, **42**, 3, pp. 53–6.

MYERS, T., ORR., K.W., LOCKER, D. and JACKSON, E.A. (1993) 'Factors affecting gay and bisexual men's decisions and intentions to seek HIV testing', *American Journal of Public Health*, **83**, 5, pp. 701–4.

PETO, D., VAN CAMPENHOUDT, L., REMY, J. and HUBERT, M. (1992) *SIDA: l'amour face à la peur. Modes d'adaptation au risque du sida dans les relations hétérosexuelles*, Paris: l'Harmattan, logiques sociales Collection.

PHILLIPS, K.A., COATES, T.J., EVERSLEY, R.B. and CATANIA, J.A. (1995) 'Who plans to be tested for HIV or who would get tested if no one could find out the results?', *American Journal of Preventive Medicine*, **11**, 3, pp. 156–62.

PHILLIPS, K.A. and CATANIA, J.A. (1995) 'Consistency in self-reports of HIV testing: longitudinal findings from the national AIDS behavioral surveys', *Public Health Reports*, **110**, pp. 749–53.

ROSS, J.D. and SCOTT, G.R. (1993) 'The association between HIV media campaigns and number of patients coming forward for HIV antibody testing', *Genitourinary Medicine*, **69**, 3, pp. 193–5.

SCHUMAN, H. and PRESSER, S. (1981) *Questions and answers in attitude surveys. Experiments on question form, wording and context*, New York: Academic Press.

SHAH, B.V., BARNWELL, B.G. *et al.* (1993) *SUDAAN: professional software for survey data analysis for multistage sample designs*, release 6.34, Research Triangle Park: Research Triangle Institute.

SETBON, M. (1996) 'Approche comparative internationale du dépistage de l'infection par le VIH comme politique publique', in ANRS (Agence Nationale de Recherche sur le Sida) (Ed.) *Le dépistage du VIH. Politiques et pratiques*, Paris: ANRS.

301

SMITH, E., WORM, A.-M., VOSS JEPSEN, L., LARSEN, J., BRANDRUP, F., VEIEN, N. *et al.* (1994) 'Patterns and trends of sexual behavior, HIV testing, and HIV prevalence among all sexually transmitted disease clinic attenders in Denmark', *Sexually Transmitted Diseases*, **21**, 2, pp. 97–102.

VAN CASTEREN, V., LEURQUIN, P., BARTELDS, A., GURTNER, F., MASSARI, V., MAURICE-TISON, S. *et al.* (1993) 'Demand patterns for HIV-test in general practice: information collected by sentinel networks in five European countries', *European Journal of Epidemiology*, **9**, 2, pp. 169–75.

WELLINGS, K. (1994) 'General population', *Sozial Präventivmedizin*, **31**, Suppl. 1, pp. 14–46.

WELLINGS, K., FIELD, J., JOHNSON, A.M. and WADSWORTH, J. (1994) *Sexual Behaviour in Britain. The national survey of sexual attitudes and lifestyles*, Harmondsworth: Penguin Books.

WESTBROOK, M.T., LEGGE, V. and PENNAY, M. (1993). 'Attitudes towards disabilities in a multicultural society', *Social Science and Medicine*, **36**, pp. 615–23.

WORTLEY, P.M., CHU, S.Y., DIAZ, T., WARD, J.W., DOYLE, B., DAVIDSON, A.J. *et al.* (1995) 'HIV testing patterns: where, why, and when were persons with AIDS tested for HIV?', *AIDS*, **9**, 5, pp. 487–92.

Chapter 11

Social Networks and Normative Context

Alexis Ferrand, Jacques Marquet and
Luc Van Campenhoudt

Introduction

This chapter illustrates some issues which can be defined as coming under
'the social networks' approach, which is composed of both a general
paradigm (Degenne, 1983; Degenne and Forsé, 1994; Ferrand and Snijders,
1997; Wellman and Berkowitz, 1988) and various kinds of methodologies
(Wasserman and Faust, 1994; Marsden, 1990). In this approach, individuals
are seen as actors who behave intentionally and try to manage the gap between
desires and prohibitions, goals and resources. Their relations, and the networks they form, are effects and conditions of actions – effects when actors
bargain to create or transform relations, conditions when relations provide
resources and alternatives, or impose constraints on actions. Then existing
relations influence some emerging or other existing relations. Another way of
saying this is that some kinds of relations – not all – are interdependent or
form 'systems'.

Sometimes researchers can describe a whole network, that is, all relations
of a given kind amongst a given set of people: pupils in a classroom, subset of
a local elite, and so on. But such a methodology is often limited to the deep
structural description of limited milieus. Sexual research on large populations
uses questionnaires administered to randomly selected, *a priori* unconnected
people. The methodology forbids direct description of the whole network, but
allows the statistical description of 'personal networks' in given populations.
In mass surveys it is possible to ask interviewees to describe some personal
relationships as elements of their environments. Data provided by such surveys can then be used to define simulation models' parameters of comprehensive sexual networks (Kretzschmar *et al.*, 1994).

Sex surveys ask individuals to describe some – two, three, more recent –
sexual relationships. It is possible to conceptualize sexual links as *interdependent* if they are reciprocally conditioned, for example, when an existing primary

relation influences the content of a secondary one, and when the latter allows – or in other cases endangers – the continuation of the former. The diverse rewards and costs of each link can be balanced. More generally, for different kinds of links, the resources provided and constraints imposed by relations are extremely varied, giving rise to myriad forms of interdependencies.

This chapter focuses on a small range of such interdependencies because the few available surveys that provide information on the relational environment of actors describe specific links and limited features of personal networks. Our aim is *not* to demonstrate that the number, content, and forms of sexual relations depend upon such or such interpersonal relations. This would call for complex multivariate statistical analysis. Through simple cross-tabulations we want to illustrate and to give some credibility to specific hypotheses by showing that basic trends in relational processes, structures, and interdependencies exist.

For the first issue, we assume that a change in sexual behaviour implies change in the definition of situations that is facilitated and supported by discussions about emotional and sex affairs. That depends upon the composition of the personal network: mainly, do actors speak of emotional and sexual affairs with someone in their environment? Here we take the direct functional effect of symbolic exchanges and supports as a given, but we examine major trends which define who can and cannot talk, and which indirectly affect the ability to transform sexual relations.

The second and third issues refer to the effect of the perception of personal networks' boundaries, that is, the effect of perceived relational proximity to 'the risk'. Most people perceive themselves as 'straight' and 'clean', since they conceive of their personal networks as 'straight' and 'clean', given the dominant representation which suggests that HIV risks are 'out there', in foreign, distant milieus. So, the chance of knowing a seropositive individual is first conceived of from a positivist point of view as a quasi mechanical effect of networks' sizes and compositions in communities with various HIV prevalences. We suppose that knowing a person with HIV/AIDS (PWHA) is important enough to increase information about, and fear of, the illness to the point where Ego may reconsider the network boundary between him/ herself and PWHAs. Our second hypothesis, therefore, is that the personal network definition influences Ego's sexual behaviour (use of condoms, or other changes) when he perceives HIV as a risk in his/her world. The third issue focuses more specifically on perceptions of possible chains of sexual relations. By definition, an exclusive sexual relation is the simplest, most bounded, sexual network. The question of reciprocal risk of HIV transmission can be managed by the dyad, mainly at the beginning of the relation. On the contrary, if one supposes that a simultaneous partner's partner exists, Ego can perceive the relation as a simple element in a more or less unbounded, potentially risky network.

The fourth issue relates to the social network's normative influence. Our hypothesis is that norms of close relationships influence Ego's norms and behaviour. The first question is to examine if these norms are homogeneous or not, and if there are one or several potential influences. The second is to describe the correspondence between the norms people perceive in their networks and their own norms and behaviour.

We shall present for each of these topics the principal social issues involved, the way each survey formulated questions and operationalized variables, the most interesting comparative analyses, and comments about these comparisons, especially convergent and divergent trends.

Unlike the approach developed in most of the other chapters, that is, one focusing on comparisons between countries, here we shall focus on the potential relevance of a number of research questions which will be explored using information from separate countries. Data from only three countries – Belgium (1993), France (ACSF 1992) and the Netherlands (1989) – are included.

The populations taken into account are all respondents between the ages of 18 and 49 in some cases, and all individuals between the ages of 18 and 49 who have already had sex over a specified period (in the course of the lifetime, over the past five years, or over the past 12 months) in other cases. In the questionnaires we are considering, some of the questions were asked of a random subsample only. As a result, the total reference population may vary from one question to the next and thus from one table to the next.

Several variables were chosen for cross-tabulation with dependent variables. We have selected those which are the more common in comparative studies but also the more pertinent regarding personal networks' properties: age, gender, and size of the community of residence, which are known to influence the composition of people's networks; and the number of sexual partners as a very rough indicator of sexual socialization.

The Network of Confidants

We assume that the possibility of talking about one's emotional and sex life with one or more confidants has an effect on the ability to control sexual behaviour (at both the cognitive and affective levels) and possibly to respond to HIV risk, even if these discussions do not explicitly concern HIV risk (Ferrand and Mounier, 1993b). First, these discussions produce new frames for apprehending daily life and organizing one's experiences, and, we suppose, in particular, for understanding HIV transmission risks and changing views about potential means of protection. Second, the disclosure of private life allows close relationships both to control and to support actors' sexual behaviours or opinions. In contrast, an inability to find confidants or a deliberate choice to avoid confiding one's secrets can make the self-assessment of behaviour more difficult and leave the individual without reference points.

If we accept these presuppositions, it is important to know which categories of people can talk in confidence about such subjects with a close friend or relative. We shall thus start by trying both to establish the profile of the kind of person who can count on confidants and to understand confidants' places within his or her social network. To do this, we shall focus on the link between the number of confidants and the size of the network of friends and relatives.

The question of confidants was tackled in a similar manner in only two surveys, the Belgian and French ones. The relevant questions, which did not refer explicitly to discussions about HIV risk, were 'There are some people with whom you can discuss personal matters. With how many people besides the person with whom you are living do you discuss love affairs, sexual problems or venereal disease or marital relations?' in the French survey and 'If you felt the need to talk about your emotional and sex life, could you count on someone other than your main partner in whom you could confide, a sort of confidant?' in the Belgian survey. The Belgian and French surveys' wordings of the question are analogous, even though some minor differences might partly explain differences in the response rates for the two countries, and differences in the degrees of association with other variables. While the word 'confidant' is stated explicitly in the Belgian question, this is not the case in the French question. The latter also draws a slightly different picture of 'confidant' involving a less intimate connotation through the use of the verb 'to discuss with' rather than 'to confide in'. The two surveys also make reference to different time frames. The French question considers current confidants, while the Belgian question enables one to group current and supposed potential confidants through the use of the conditional. Finally, the Belgian and French questions exclude different groups of people from their lists of confidants, namely, the partner of a one-partner interviewee and the main partner of a multiple-partner interviewee in the case of the Belgian survey, and the respondent's cohabitant in the case of the French survey. As a result, the confidant of the Belgian survey is not quite the confidant of the French survey. Still, we can nevertheless posit that the two notions overlap considerably.

Having set the stage, let us now look at the findings. Twenty-four and a half per cent of the French respondents declared they had a confidant and 45.0 per cent stated they had more than one confidant, compared with 45.8 and 30.6 per cent, respectively, of the Belgian respondents. The key finding is that roughly a quarter of the respondents in each country said they had no one with whom they could talk over emotional and sexual matters. The characteristics of this subpopulation can be deduced from Table 11.1.

In both the French and Belgian surveys, a higher percentage of women than men said they had one or more confidants. The number of people who said they had at least one confidant diminished with age. These percentages declined steadily from similar initial values. However, the decline was more marked in the French survey.

Table 11.1 *Proportions of individuals who have at least one confidant to talk over emotional and sexual matters*

	Belgium 1993		France 1992	
	%	N	%	N
All	76.4	1392	69.5	2049
Sex				
Men	70.0	653	61.4	1132
Women	82.1	739	77.9	917
Age				
18–19	90.6	101	92.5	146
20–24	87.5	229	79.9	508
25–29	82.6	220	75.9	435
30–39	73.2	449	68.6	589
40–49	67.7	393	54.9	371
No. of partners over last year				
Never had sex	89.4	88	82.0	65
0	69.0	50	78.6	120
1	74.5	1087	66.8	1153
>1	85.5	167	81.4	711

Likewise in both surveys more people with multiple partners than with single partners had at least one confidant. Talking about and having sexual relations thus seem to be two forms of interpersonal exchange that go hand in hand. Nevertheless, 14.5 per cent (in Belgium) and 18.6 per cent (in France) of the respondents who engaged in sex with more than one person in the course of the previous 12 months had no one with whom they could talk about sexual matters and possible HIV risk-related behaviour.

Inversely, we must also point out that many of the respondents who stated they had no sexual partner both over the previous 12 months and in general nevertheless had at least one confidant to talk to about emotional and sexual matters. The existence of at least one person with whom one can talk should doubtless be considered as the effect of both sociability and the particular need to exchange information and opinions about these matters. Similarly, despite an absence of sexual activity, many young people stated they had at least one confidant to talk to about emotions and sex.

The confidants generally form a subnetwork within a set of 'significant others', that is, people perceived as 'close' and important even if they do not meet very often. The more extensive the network of significant others, the greater the theoretical chances of having confidants. This link between the size of the network of significant others and number of confidants can be examined for the Belgian survey only, in which a variable embracing the size of the network of significant others (NSO = number of significant others) was constructed from the questions concerning the family, professional, and social (leisure-time) networks.[1] As hypothesized, the results show that the more extensive a network is, the greater the chances of finding at least one person with whom one can talk about one's emotional and sex life.[2] Still, some people do not have any confidants despite an extensive network, many close friends and relatives. Very contrasting reasons can explain such situations, for example, not needing to talk about one's private life, social taboos about sexual disclosure, or psychological inhibition.

This link between the size of the network of close friends and relatives and the number of confidants is influenced by the respondent's gender. As we have seen, women, as a rule, have more confidants than men. This is borne out in both the French and Belgian surveys. In contrast, the Belgian data show that men generally had more extensive social networks than women.[3] However, this difference may have resulted to a certain extent from the way the index was designed, as more women than men have no job and thus no colleagues with whom to achieve the maximum score of nine significant others.

These two surveys show that people without confidants tend to be men rather than women, older rather than young, have one partner rather than multiple partners, and have rather smaller social networks. Locality size does not seem to influence this characteristic. However, as bivariate rather than multivariate analyses were performed, we cannot assert that it is necessarily the same people who combine all these different characteristics, nor can we give a general profile of the confidant-less individual.

Even if we have identified only a few of the properties that characterize confidants' networks, without showing how networks influence representations, opinions, and behaviour, these results tell us something very important about the exposure of individuals to social pressure. If prevention messages are to be understood and applied, we have to seek explanations in individuals' characteristics as well as in the social network processes by which an important part of the information received is transformed into interpersonal knowledge and control.

Knowing Someone with HIV/AIDS and Sexual Behaviour

Many studies (for example, Pollak, 1988) have stressed the importance of knowing one or more PWHAs on a person's perception of the risk of HIV infection. Some authors (for example, Catania, Kegeles and Coates, 1990) have even considered this factor to be decisive in triggering behaviour change.

Table 11.2   *Proportions of people stating they know at least one PWHA*

	Belgium 1993		France 1992		Netherlands 1989	
	%	N	%	N	%	N
All	8.1	2810	14.8	2049	7.7	990
Place of residence						
Rural	5.8	85	11.3	421	2.5	40
Small towns	6.4	1405	14.4	438	5.9	699
Towns	9.0	410	15.5	755	13.5	251
Cities: Brussels/Paris	16.5	910	19.7	424		
No. of partners over last year						
Never had sex	2.6	172	11.8	71	4.3	47
0	7.5	94	12.0	120	7.1	70
1	7.9	2198	13.4	1149	7.7	759
>1	13.2	346	27.0	709	13.1	114

In this section we first approach this question by focusing on the conditions that lead someone to know a PWHA. We begin by a comparative description of the situation (Table 11.2). From a positivist point of view, various probabilities of knowing a PWHA can be analyzed as mechanical effects of the prevalence of cases and the differential social 'reachability' of the cases. This last point is dependent on networks' sizes, boundaries, structures, and overlapping in a large population. Even if we do not have indicators for these broad properties for large interpersonal or sexual networks, we can use the available personal network variables as local indicators of some characteristics of large networks to examine their effects. A second approach goes back to the hypothesis that knowing a PWHA reinforces safe sexual behaviour and examines simple comparative cross-tabulations on the potential influence of knowing one or more PWHAs on condom use. These research questions were not handled identically by the Belgian, French, and Dutch surveys. However, bipartite and often tripartite comparisons are possible.

The surveys used slightly different wordings in tackling the issue of acquaintance with PWHAs.[4] The Belgian survey took people with HIV, people with AIDS, and the deceased victims of AIDS into account; the French survey did not take the deceased into account; and the Dutch survey did not explicitly include people with HIV in the formulation. The percentage of respondents who stated they knew at least one PWHA in France (14.8 per cent) was higher than those recorded in the Netherlands (7.7 per cent) and in Belgium (8.1 per cent).

These differences doubtless are due in part to the three countries' respective HIV prevalences. The cumulative AIDS case rates at the times the surveys were conducted were 0.341 per thousand for France, 0.078 per thousand for the Netherlands, and 0.137 per thousand for Belgium.[5] The HIV prevalence rate was three to four times higher in France, where the proportion of people who knew a PWHA was about twice as high as in the other surveys. But, as suggested above, rates are only one of two combined conditions. Fairly similar prevalence rates can be associated with a) different virus dissemination patterns due to the relative closeness of the riskiest sexual milieus, and/or b) various social 'reachabilities' of PWHA due to the relative closeness of social milieus. A typical case here is Belgium where it is known that, unlike other countries, non-residents account for a large proportion of notified cases. If we assume that such individuals have fewer social contacts with the resident population, this can account for a lower rate of people knowing a PWHA at a given HIV prevalence rate.

A more precise analysis of these effects can take into account the size of the community of residence and the number of sexual partners over the previous 12 months. A clear link between the probability of knowing a PWHA and the size of the locality appears. Although the numbers of Belgian and Dutch respondents residing in rural localities of less than 5000 inhabitants are too small to draw statistically reliable conclusions concerning this relationship, the overall trend is clear and analogous in all three countries, namely, the probability of knowing one or more PWHAs increases with the size of the locality of residence (between the villages and capital it doubles in France and triples in Belgium). That can be interpreted as an effect of the higher prevalence of HIV in large cities, but also as an effect of different social norms: the moral contexts specific to small towns and villages may prevent people disclosing their seropositivity.

Having multiple sexual partners has virtually the same influence in all three countries. The proportion of people who reported knowing at least one PWHA practically doubles between the group of respondents who had no or one sexual partner over the previous 12 months and those who had two or more partners (the 'multiple-partner' group). In this simple cross-tabulation the number of sexual partners is a direct indicator of the size of the sexual network, which thereby increases the chances of meeting a PWHA and of belonging to networks where the proportions of PWHA are greater (because they are more numerous and disclosure of serological status is better tolerated), but it can also be interpreted as an indirect indicator of general types of sociability.

Indeed we can wonder if the first and more general condition for knowing a PWHA is not simply knowing a lot of people, *regardless of who they are*. That assumption can rest on the relative ambiguity of the term 'to know' combined with the effect of 'weak ties'. Through weak ties – typical of large networks – people are connected with people out of their social (and sexual) world. We tested the hypothesis that the more contacts an individual has, the greater the probability of his/her being informed that someone among them is seropositive. The data from the Belgian survey, which is the only one for which the influence of the size of the 'significant others' network could be verified, show that the proportion of respondents who know or have known at least one PWHA *does not* vary significantly with the size of the network of 'significant others'.

The real issue is the number of channels through which information about someone's serostatus can flow, and only particular relationships, such as those with confidants, can permit such disclosure. We therefore examined the influence of the number of confidants (people with whom one talks about one's emotional and sex life) in the French and Belgian surveys. In both surveys, respondents who had two or more confidants were more likely to know at least one PWHA than those who had only one confidant. The probabilities of knowing a PWHA depend on the number of confidants. Those who have no confidants, know a PWHA less often than those who have one confidant in France, but more often in Belgium. The greater the number of channels through which it is possible to speak about sexual affairs, the greater the chance of knowing a PWHA. However, this factor is far from being the only one involved, as the disparities among the Belgian data show.

Let us examine comparative cross-tabulations with the potential influence of knowing one or more PWHAs. Two kinds of influence can be analyzed in the surveys: a specific influence on condom use, and a more overall influence on sexual behaviour change. In interpreting the results one must bear in mind that many people (people who are not injecting drug users, do not have sex, or who have a steady, one-on-one relationship in which both partners are faithful to each other, and so on) have no objective reason to use condoms or to change their practices because of the HIV epidemic. If it were possible, the number of people who reported condom use or a behaviour change should thus be compared with the percentage of the population who formerly engaged in risky practices.

Table 11.3 summarizes condom use for the previous 12 months according to gender, number of stated sexual partners for the previous 12 months, and knowing or not knowing a PWHA. It shows that respondents who knew at least one PWHA used condoms slightly more often than those who had no HIV-infected acquaintances (some deviations are statistically insignificant). And it holds true for each gender, where stated condom use was highest for respondents who knew at least one PWHA. Knowing a PWHA did not have a statistically significant influence on condom use in the 'one-partner' group, but it increased condom use slightly in the 'multiple-partner' group.

We can also analyze the data in relation to our second point: whether knowing a PWHA leads one to change one's own behaviour. Only the French and Dutch surveys provide some elements of the answer to this question.[6] Table 11.4 summarizes the responses to these questions according to gender, stated number of sexual partners over the previous 12 months, and knowing or not knowing a PWHA.

The first row in Table 11.4 shows that the proportion of respondents in each survey who stated they had changed their behaviour was small, but we

Table 11.3 *Condom use by gender, number of sexual partners, and knowing a PWHA*

	Belgium 1993		France 1992		Netherlands 1989	
	%	N	%	N	%	N
All	23.9	2810	29.4	2049	23.7	990
Know PWHA	31.3	309	35.7	422	27.6	76
Gender						
Men	30.4	1329	33.3	1132	28.5	418
Men, know PWHA	39.9	142	39.2	227	32.4	37
Women	18.0	1481	25.3	917	20.3	572
Women, know PWHA	24.0	167	32.4	195	23.1	39
No. of partners over last year						
1	21.2	2198	27.7	1153	26.6	759
1, know PWHA	24.6	230	28.8	200	18.5	54
2+	62.0	346	62.8	711	55.3	114
2+, know PWHA	66.7	66	72.8	190	80.0	15

Table 11.4 *Proportions of respondents stating a behaviour change in response to HIV/AIDS*

	France 1992		Netherlands 1989	
	%	N	%	N
All	18.5	2049	11.0	990
Know PWHA	31.9	422	19.7	76
Gender				
Men	22.7	1132	17.2	418
Men, know PWHA	38.2	227	32.4	37
Women	15.0	917	6.5	572
Women, know PWHA	26.0	195	7.7	39
No. of partners over last year				
1	15.3	1153	8.7	759
1, know PWHA	28.4	200	18.5	54
2+	43.1	711	25.4	114
2+, know PWHA	46.8	190	40.0	15

can assume[7] that the proportion of people who have had to change was also relatively small. It shows also that these proportions are different in the two countries: roughly one out of ten respondents in the Dutch survey and one out of five in the French survey declared a behaviour change in response to HIV/AIDS. These differences are probably not unrelated to the year in which each survey was carried out (see Chapter 8). There was much more talk about AIDS in 1992, when the French survey was conducted, than in 1989, the year the Dutch survey was conducted. In an area such as AIDS, where the givens (course of the epidemic, advancement of research, public information, and so on) change quickly (Cohen and Hubert, 1997), the times at which the various surveys were conducted must be taken into account when interpreting differences in their findings.

Now, regarding our hypothesis, Table 11.4 shows the expected result: a higher proportion of the respondents who knew a PWHA changed their behaviour (and this effect was of the same order of magnitude for the two surveys). We have to analyze that general finding to take into account various kinds of sexual conduct linked to various levels of potential risk. If we use the number of partners for the last 12 months, we can see that, generally speaking, fewer one-partner than multiple-partner respondents changed their behaviour (this held true in both studies). The effect of knowing a PWHA is different for each population: it seems to increase the percentage of one-partner respondents who change but to have only a slight influence on the proportion of multipartner respondents who change their behaviour (some deviations are statistically insignificant).

These results confirm that knowing a PWHA or counting a PWHA in one's network of personal relations usually prompts people to take the risk of HIV transmission into account, either by using condoms or by making some other behaviour change. Usually this occurs, but not always. The difficulty lies in understanding why and why not. A number of good *ad hoc* reasons can be proposed. Let us try one to explain the stronger effect amongst the one-partner respondents. Most of them are long-term 'monopartners' living in a couple relationship and convinced of their partner's faithfulness (see the section on tolerating love affairs outside stable relationships below) and of the safety of their social and sexual milieu. For that large majority of monopartners, changing their behaviour in response to AIDS would not make any sense to them. But two subpopulations do exist. One is made of sequential monopartners: for them, knowing a PWHA can be important to increasing information on, and perhaps fear of, the illness. But, more importantly, it can also change their perception of the network boundary between themselves and persons with AIDS, their perception of the presence of HIV risk *in* their own social and sexual network; and that can produce a profound effect. The second group is composed of the people who react to knowing a PWHA by becoming faithful to one partner. For respondents with two or more sexual partners, the weak influence of knowing a PWHA might mean that knowing an infected person is a socially more frequent and less incredible event. That possibility is a characteristic of the kinds of milieu they belong to or occasionally frequent. One does not need a specific personal tie to be aware of HIV risks in one's surroundings. That interpretation stresses the specific effect of knowing a PWHA on the representation of the overall safety of one's social and sexual world. One person can be a symbol of the state of the whole personal network of an individual because the network is known as a more or less generalized exchange network.

The Steady Partner's Partners

From the standpoint of prevention, a key problem is a person's knowledge of his/her partners' sexual network. Although this question is important for everyone, it has special connotations for people with steady partners, for it brings up the issue of multiple partnership within a steady couple that is supposed to operate according to the model of faithfulness. In studying this particular question we shall look at only those individuals who had at least one steady partner for at least five years so as to omit specifically adolescent high partner turnover.

This question is tackled by all three surveys using almost identical terms.[8] There is one notable difference in that the Belgian question, unlike the other two, considers partners' affairs over an indeterminate period of time, not necessarily the entire length of the relationship. Table 11.5 shows the percentages of respondents, by gender, age, and number of partners over the previous year, who said they knew their steady partners had or had had other partners.[9]

The total percentages given in the first row of Table 11.5 show that, overall, a very small percentage of respondents said they knew that their partners had had, or were having, sex with someone else concurrently with their own relationship. At least 90 per cent of the respondents believed they were their steady partners' only partners and thus could 'trust them'. The relatively small number of 'don't knows' indicates that almost all of the respondents truly thought they knew how their partners behaved in this matter.

The age- and gender-dependent effects are quite different, though, in the three surveys. The strongest rise in the belief in one's partner's extra-couple sex was correlated with the increase in the number of the respondent's partners. This may be explained by several partly complementary hypotheses, to wit: a certain number of multipartner respondents most likely live in circles where such behaviour is common; the love affairs or concomitant relationships of one member of a couple may prompt his/her steady partner (often a spouse) to follow suit; some couples have a looser, more flexible relationship than the norm; a certain number of 'steady partners' are actually singles who nevertheless maintain a special relationship; and some multiple-partner respondents may project their 'philandering' onto their partners. The large percentages of 'don't knows' may indicate not only doubt but also, in some cases, the respondent's weak commitment to the relationship. Still, these findings and hypotheses should not mask the fact that a large majority of the respondents with multiple partners thought they knew, with certainty, that their steady partners did not have other partners.

We compared the multipartner respondents' answers with regard to the last partner with whom the respondent had sex (usually the main partner with whom the respondent was living, that is P1) and the penultimate sex partner

Table 11.5 *Respondents' assessments of their partners' infidelity*

	Belgium 1993			France 1992			Netherlands 1989		
	% yes	% don't know	N	% yes	% don't know	N	% yes	% don't know	N
All	4.2	5.9	1725	2.9	3.7	762	6.2	2.4	532
Gender									
Men	3.6	6.0	770	1.9	1.5	426	4.2	2.6	190
Women	4.6	5.9	955	3.9	6.0	336	7.3	2.3	342
Age									
20–24	0.6	3.0	52	3.8	6.3	39	17.4	0.0	23
25–29	3.0	3.5	229	2.0	2.6	141	6.8	1.4	73
30–39	4.1	6.2	715	2.0	4.5	333	5.0	2.9	242
40–49	4.9	6.6	729	3.9	3.2	249	6.2	2.6	194
No. of partners over last year									
1	3.3	5.4	1599	2.2	3.2	579	5.1	2.1	513
>1	17.8	15.1	126	13.4	12.9	183	36.8	10.5	19

(P2), for the French study only. While 13.4 per cent of the French multipartner respondents believed that their P1s had at least one other sexual partner, versus 12.9 per cent 'don't know', the figure rose to 60.6 per cent of the same population for their P2s (versus 15.2 per cent 'don't know'). In many cases P2 was known to be someone else's spouse, a multipartner single (engaged in serial or parallel relationships) or someone (such as a sex worker) well-known for multiple sexual encounters. However, aside from such purely objective interpretations, these figures seem to indicate that a person tends to segment his/her sexual world into the 'first circle' of the stable partner, where fidelity is the key norm and the partner is thus presumed not to have affairs outside the couple, even if the individual him/herself is not; and a 'second circle' of occasional, unofficial relationships where the partners are not presumed to limit themselves to an exclusive relationship. The result is an interweaving of objective and subjective reasoning characterized by the construction of a segmented universe in each person's mind whereby the individual manages a complex web of relations and organizes his/her ways of coping with the risk of HIV/AIDS (for example, not using a condom in the supposedly safe inner circle and using a condom, at least when one manages to, in the reputedly dangerous second circle), as Peto *et al.* (1992) have shown.

To sum up, these data show not only that people with multiple partners are more inclined than monopartners to consider their partners to have several partners as well, but that the various partners are also qualified and/or perceived differently according to whether they belong to the respondent's first or second circle of relations.

Tolerating Love Affairs outside Stable Relationships

Personal networks are complex worlds, and they allow various – sometime contradictory – forms of social conduct because the contexts of relations are segmented and their content differentiated. Each segment (family, friends, colleagues) exerts normative pressure over the partners. In studying this system of normative pressure, we shall make a distinction between ideal and practical norms. We shall assume that ideal norms – what people answer when questioned explicitly on 'what is good?' – consist basically of a general reference within a group, social circle, subgroup or context. Practical norms correspond in this study to how people perceive the actual behaviour of significant others. The effectiveness of these norms is explained by the fact that an individual seeks nothing more than the esteem of his/her significant others and fears nothing more than their disapproval. But, as personal networks are complex, so are normative pressures. They have neither the same direction nor the same weight for different relational contexts. In other words, the direction and force of normative pressures can vary depending on whether the individual is dealing with his/her family, friends, workmates, or fellow students. Then the question is to know how people *perceive* and manage the normative diversity of their various contexts of sociability, as well as the gap between ideal and practical norms, so as to build a sustainable compromise between expected rewards and punishments.

Of course, it is impossible to analyze all the types of norms involved in sexual life. Amongst the few normative dimensions that surveys enable one to compare, we have selected the topic of concomitant love affairs because this was the only aspect for which connections between the network's norms and the respondent's norms and behaviour could be envisaged in more than one survey. We have also selected a subsample of people who have had at least one steady sexual partner for at least five years, guided by the assumption that the issue of concomitant sex affairs may be more crucial for them, since their lives as couples can be centred upon the norm of fidelity in which having another sexual partner takes on more significance than for people who have simultaneous or rapidly changing sequential multiple partners. We shall gauge the social network's normative influence in three steps. First, we shall identify how respondents perceive their various social circles or contexts' norms of sexual relations. Second, we shall identify the respondents' own norms in this regard. Third, we shall study the links between the network's and respondent's norms.

Country-to-country comparisons with regard to this aim are likewise fraught with difficulty but highly worthwhile. If we consider the circles or contexts' norms, the French survey focused on ideal norms, while the Belgian one focused on practical norms and the Dutch survey did not consider the matter at all. In contrast, all three surveys tackled the issue of the respondent's norms, which we shall call 'Ego's norms' hereafter. As a result, the connections between the significant others' norms and those of Ego could be studied using the Belgian and French data only.

Perceived Norms

As mentioned above, the French survey examined the perception of ideal norms whereas the Belgian survey looked at the perception of actual norms. Separate tables were thus compiled to summarize perceived acceptance of infidelity in respondents' networks according to the French (Table 11.6) and Belgian (Table 11.7) surveys.[10]

The higher percentages recorded in the French survey are doubtless linked to the item chosen ('some agree and others don't'), which provided much more flexibility than the Belgian item. This forces us to comment on the comparative trends more than absolute levels of the phenomenon in the two countries.

Table 11.6 *Perceived acceptance of infidelity in various networks (French survey)*

	Friends %	Colleagues %	Family %	Total N
All	66.8	55.2	29.4	762
Gender				
Men	70.1	63.6	32.4	426
Women	63.2	46.1	26.3	336
Age				
20–24	66.6	60.5	33.3	38
25–29	72.6	63.9	29.9	141
30–39	68.6	54.8	25.3	333
40–49	63.0	52.8	32.9	249
Place of residence				
Rural	63.3	54.5	27.1	205
Small towns	65.2	53.6	26.4	194
Towns	69.7	53.6	32.1	228
Cities: Paris	71.5	62.4	34.7	135
No. of partners over last year				
1	65.7	54.3	29.0	579
>1	83.8	70.2	37.3	183

Table 11.7 *Perceived acceptance of infidelity in various networks (Belgian survey)*

	Friends %	Colleagues %	Family %	Total N
All	15.2	23.7	7.4	845
Gender				
Men	17.7	31.5	7.7	372
Women	13.1	17.4	7.1	473
Age				
20–24	20.4	8.8	5.9	25
25–29	8.5	22.6	4.9	128
30–39	16.3	23.7	6.9	364
40–49	16.1	24.9	8.9	328
Place of residence				
Rural	4.8	19.4	4.8	20
Small towns	15.1	20.3	7.8	488
Towns	12.0	33.6	3.5	102
Cities: Brussels	22.4	34.4	10.4	235
No. of partners over last year				
1	13.5	22.7	6.5	796
>1	52.1	22.1	26.3	49

Both tables show that the three circles examined here are not perceived as tolerant by equal proportions of the respondents. The family is perceived as being tolerant of extra-couple sex by the smallest number of people. This perception of family norms is probably grounded in the importance of the roles safeguarded by the family and the influence of gender. First of all, the family is the objective and symbolic stage *par excellence* for producing the sexual fidelity norm through the role of faithful spouse. Second, admitting concomitant sex affairs in the family circle implies admitting one's own parents' departure from the norm, and that opens a field of uncertainty concerning one's own patrilineal origin and identity. However, as the tables show, the roles of parent and spouse do not prevent the same people being perceived as more tolerant when filling the roles of friends, for example, in other social areas. This means that the perceived norms are less attached to the social images of individuals than to the different roles they play in different circles. This is a very well-known, classical sociological finding. But it is important for prevention: people perceive norms as applying to 'role takers' (Rose, 1962), to one facet of a person (with regard to specific roles and social contexts), not to a total, indivisible 'individual'.

While the average respondent perceives these circles differently, differences between respondents also exist. As Tables 11.6 and 11.7 likewise show, a greater percentage of men than women perceive their environments as being tolerant. This doubtless reflects a mixture of objective reality and mental constructs. On the one hand, male extra-relational affairs seem to be accepted more than female extra-relational affairs. On the other hand, the various perceptions of normative orientations can also partly be due to real differences in the kinds of people who belong to the circles and contexts. Indeed, male and female respondents' answers are closest when assessing family norms, but take fairly different stands when they evaluate the norms put across in the working world. The world of friends has an intermediate position. While women's families are also men's families, the same does not apply to friends and colleagues. Several studies (Fischer, 1982) have shown that workmates and friends are more often of the same gender, so that men and women are not evaluating the same workmates' and friends' norms.

There was no gender-based difference in the answers to such questions in the Belgian survey, which evaluated actual norms. In other words, men and women saw the same things. But in the French survey, in contrast, where ideal norms were being evaluated, the gender difference was admittedly smaller in the case of family norms than those of friends and colleagues, but was not negligible. So it seems that the more people are concerned by actual norms, the more dependent they are on the properties of the significant others who compose their social circles.

The age-related differences are rather small as a rule. So are the differences associated with residential community size, even though people who live in large cities apparently tend to perceive close contacts as being slightly more tolerant of having several sexual partners (F) or as having slightly more brief affairs or concomitant relationships (B) than those who live in small towns. However, the differences related to locality size were far from impressive and lead us to believe that the differences between large cities and small towns, even villages, are narrowing because of new lifestyles and means of communication. In addition, we must also point out that friends and colleagues and, to a lesser extent, family members commonly include both city-dwellers and people from the country.

Once again, 'multipartnership' appears to be the most decisive factor. In both the French and Belgian surveys, respondents with multiple partners systematically had the highest perception of tolerance to extra-relational sex affairs in the above-mentioned circles. As these respondents themselves have steady partners (for more than five years, by the selection of a subsample) and simultaneously one or several others, their own behaviour often is labelled 'infidelity' by society. Perhaps these respondents legitimate their behaviour by showing that they are not straying from the norms of the social circles to which they belong. Perhaps also they do meet more tolerant people in the contexts they frequent. But most important is the fact that the proportions of respondents who perceive friends as tolerant are in both surveys and for the two subpopulations (mono- and multipartnership) roughly twice the proportions who judge the family tolerant. Consequently, we can say that the normative differences between these two circles remain constant, whether we look at mono- or multipartner respondents. It then becomes impossible to think of norms as being specific to subpopulations of individuals only through the subcultures they have internalized. In the same subpopulation, they are specific to social roles and narrow social circles. Most often an individual faces various – possibly contradictory – normative pressures, depending on the circle in which he interacts at the time and the role relationship in which he is engaged. Finally, Ego's norms have to be understood as a kind of more or less stable compromise among these various pressures.

Ego's Norms

The wordings of the questions concerning Ego's norms with regard to love affairs vary greatly from one survey to the next, but overall tendencies can nevertheless be picked out. Table 11.8, which summarizes the rates of acceptance of concomitant sex affairs in the three survey populations by gender, age, locality, and number of stated sexual partners over the previous 12 months, shows that the model of fidelity dominates everywhere.[11] Stating that one of the members of a couple's departures is acceptable or approved remains rare. The degree of acceptance of extra-relational sex was clearly lower in the Dutch survey, doubtless because of the more 'black-and-white' wordings of the propositions on which the Dutch respondents were asked to make a pro-

Table 11.8 *Acceptance of infidelity*

	Belgium 1993		France 1992		Netherlands 1989	
	%	N	%	N	%	N
All	8.6	845	11.6	762	3.6	532
Gender						
Men	12.2	372	11.1	426	5.3	190
Women	5.7	473	12.1	336	2.6	342
Age						
20–24	2.9	25	6.1	39	0.0	23
25–29	5.8	128	11.3	141	5.5	73
30–39	8.7	364	11.2	333	4.1	242
40–49	10.0	328	12.5	249	2.6	194
Place of residence						
Rural	9.7	20	8.3	205	0.0	27
Small towns	8.4	488	11.8	194	2.6	389
Towns	6.2	102	12.4	228	7.8	116
Cities: Brussels/Paris	13.0	235	16.5	135		
No. of partners over last year						
1	6.5	796	9.6	579	3.1	513
>1	55.1	49	44.5	183	15.8	19

nouncement. This may also explain the relatively high 'no answer' rate (8.5 per cent) in the Dutch survey.

In the Belgian survey women were clearly less willing to accept departures than men. The pattern was similar in the Dutch survey, but not statistically significant. There was no gender-based difference in the French responses. The age effect was relatively weak in this area. Table 11.8 shows the very clear effect of the degree of urbanization in the three countries. This is in keeping with classic studies of the metropolis (Grafmeyer and Joseph, 1979) and studies of urban subcultures (Fischer, 1982), according to which extra-relational sex and marginal practices and values find specialized networks and niches in the segmented diversity of urban settings, where they become locally the rule and are protected from dominant outside pressures. Still, here yet again, having multiple partners led the pack by several lengths as the most decisive explanatory variable in all three surveys (with a slight reservation for the Dutch survey, given the very small sample size). Inversely, a small group of single-partner respondents accepted extra-relational sex affairs. Thus, between an overwhelming majority of single-partner respondents having adopted monogamy as their model and a small group of multipartner respondents condoning departures we find a small group of people who exhibited a gap between norms and behaviour at the time they were surveyed.

In the three surveys, respondents with multiple partners (and who, we must recall, were all involved in stable relationships lasting more than five years) were five to eight times more tolerant of extra-relational sex than one-partner respondents. Actually, for the former, there is a relative convergence between practices and norms, but a very interesting phenomenon is reflected by figures not shown in the table, namely, that about half of the respondents with multiple partners disapproved of extra-relational sex affairs. Are these people 'cheating' on their steady partners because they have 'succumbed to temptation'? Are their steady relationships punctuated by regular crises (we know that marital life is not calm) that prompt them occasionally to 'look elsewhere, albeit regretfully'? Or are they people whose lasting relationships are nevertheless unstable, consisting of a series of periods of monogamy alternating with temporary separations?

Correspondence between the Network of Significant Others' Norms and Those of Ego

The degree to which Ego's and significant others' norms correspond can be verified for the Belgian and French surveys only.[12] Overall, the data reflect a clear social network effect. Yet the individual is not a carbon copy of his or her networks, as most of the respondents who perceived their circles as being more favourably disposed to or practising extra-relational sex did *not* condone departures themselves.

Table 11.9 summarizes the percentages of respondents who accepted sexual contact with a third person outside a relationship (at least in part) versus their perceptions of the practical norms (Belgian survey) or ideal norms (French survey) assumed to prevail among their relatives, friends, and colleagues. However, the most salient revelations in this table are the large differences between the Belgian and French survey responses. This seems to confirm the hypothesis that the social network norms that influence individuals most strongly are practical norms (taken into account in the Belgian survey) rather than ideal norms (taken into account in the French survey).

The concordance between network norms and Ego's norms is maximal for the family network. Now, this is also the type of circle with regard to which individuals who dare to perceive it as being favourable to extra-relational sex are in the minority (29.4 and 7.4 per cent in the French and Belgian surveys, respectively, versus 66.8 and 15.2 per cent, respectively, with regard to the circle of friends and 55.2 and 23.7 per cent, respectively, with regard to colleagues). This may be the place to take up a hypothesis put forward elsewhere (Ferrand and Mounier, 1998), to wit, that the more a behaviour or norm is practised only by a social minority, the greater the effect of the

Table 11.9 *Acceptance of infidelity versus perceived practical (Belgium) and ideal (France) norms*

	Belgium 1993		France 1992	
	%	N	%	N
All	8.6	845	11.6	762
Family: do accept infidelity	47.7	69	18.6	231
Family: do not accept infidelity	5.3	768	8.6	531
Friends: do accept infidelity	29.4	144	14.0	545
Friends: do not accept infidelity	4.3	592	6.6	217
Colleagues: do accept infidelity	18.0	215	13.3	452
Colleagues: do not accept infidelity	4.4	453	9.4	310

network of significant others supposed to uphold it. Families that are per-ceived as tolerant are normative niches whose power is enhanced by their being a minority in an environment that massively conveys the fidelity norm.

Still, the weight of Ego's opinions and behaviour may still be decisive in the family itself, since Ego is a key member of the family. Ego thus gives the pitch, especially if he/she is an adult. In considering the family, one probably has to allow for Ego's influence even more than for other networks. What is more, the closer the link of the normative content under consideration with the circle's very functioning, the more the circle will be perceived to be in agreement with the member's own norms.

Conclusions

These few comparisons suffice to show the importance of taking network effects into account when examining HIV/AIDS risk-related attitudes and behaviour. Individuals do not face such risks as individuals, but as members of social circles who are engaged in various interpersonal relations. Most indi-viduals also have one or more confidants with whom they can talk about sexuality. Interpersonal knowledge and control are affected by what happens within these networks of confidants. The comparison also shows that behav-iour varies depending on whether or not one knows people with HIV/AIDS. Finally, the various circles of relatives, colleagues and friends exert different normative influences and exercise different social controls over individual attitudes and behaviour.

The effects of sociability must be taken more into account when design-ing prevention campaigns. In this connection, the comparisons that have been presented above suggest the following four main avenues of research that may be of interest for prevention.

First, the influence of each factor, such as having confidants or knowing PWHAs, on the phenomena studied here was considered separately for reasons of facility. We may hypothesize, however, that these factors are actually interrelated. Multivariate analysis would doubtless reveal a certain number of specific sociability types defined by a set of traits bound by 'elective affinity', as Max Weber would say (for example, a single-gender specific age group in an urban environment with a specific population density and linked by a particular socio-occupational culture in which ideal norms are partially contradicted by practical norms, partner's partners tend to ignore each other, and confidants are rather rare). Each of these types corresponds to normative frameworks, relational experiences, and social controls that react differently to prevention messages and thus expose their subjects to variable degrees of risk. Analyses such as the one presented here should be followed by attempts to identify these different types of sociability with a view to using them, if necessary, to design suitable preventive action.

Second, the comparisons have also shown that each individual is linked to several different networks. The norms that prevail in Ego's family may be contradicted by his colleagues, forcing him to play different roles in different settings. As a result, the concordance between an individual's norms and those of his/her social networks can never be total. Network theory calls attention to the fact that the search for the significant other's esteem is the most widespread motivation behind this process of individual adaptation. However, when Ego has different significant others who expect different, even contradictory, types of behaviour from him, he may be obliged to segment his social universe in practice and/or in his mind (Peto *et al.*, 1992). Analyzing social networks consequently also means examining the ways these various influences fit (or do not fit) together and individuals manage (or fail) to arbitrate among the diverse normative pressures with which they must cope. Indeed, this issue of how individuals cope with the tension between their networks merits further investigation, for vulnerability to risk is often linked to difficulties in this area.

Third, network analysis begins as soon as the researcher no longer limits the scope of his/her investigation to the relationship between two partners, but broadens it to include the 'absent third parties', in a word, with the shift from the dyad to the triad. These 'absent third parties' may be the other's other sexual partners. To have a satisfactory, lasting relationship with a steady partner, Ego may have a tendency to ignore the possibility that the steady partner may him/herself have other partners. Similarly, in the budding phase of a new relationship, Ego may not want to worry about the other's sexual partners and the risks they may represent. This matter of knowing one's partners' partners is a major problem for prevention that should be taken into account in surveys and the ways the data are analyzed.

Fourth, in several studies, Ferrand and Mounier (1990, 1993b, 1998) have shown the importance of confidants' networks in determining individuals' representations and behaviour. Indeed, it seems reasonable to posit that in many cases the transformation of representations and behaviour is more a collective than an individual process that occurs in interactions between confidants, and is subject to the reciprocal reinforcing effects that are characteristic of very close groups. Prevention should be able to rely on more extensive knowledge of what goes on in these networks of confidants and produce messages that these processes can assimilate.

Notes

1 The question was worded as follows: 'Do you have people you feel close to, that is to say, friends or at least very good chums, in the circles that I am going to read out? How many people / in your family (extended family) / at work or your place of study / whom you meet through leisure activities / would you say you are close to?' The score for each of these circles could be 0, 1, 2, or 3 (for three or more persons to whom the respondent felt close). Adding the scores for the three questions could give a maximum cumulative score of nine for respondents with at least three close friends/relatives in each circle. This index does not correspond strictly to the network's size, however. Rather, it expresses the network's structure. Thus, a person who had 10 confidants among his/her friends and family but not a single confidant among his/her workmates would have a score of only six.

2 Sixty-one per cent of the people who had NSO scores of from zero to three had at least one confidant, compared with 82.1 per cent of the respondents who scored nine.

3 Of the male respondents 45.6 per cent had a NSO score of nine (nine or more significant others) versus 37.5 per cent of the female respondents.

4 The questions are 'Do you personally know one or more people in your entourage, that is, family, friends, officemates, and neighbours, who are seropositive, ill with AIDS, or have died from AIDS?' for the Belgian survey; 'Do you personally know one or more individuals (family, friends, co-workers) who are seropositive or have AIDS?' for the French survey; and 'Have you ever personally known someone who has or had AIDS?' for the Dutch survey.

5 European Centre for the Epidemiological Monitoring of AIDS (1995), *AIDS Surveillance in Europe*, Quarterly Report, 47, Saint-Maurice.

6 The questions eliciting this information were worded as follows: 'Have you changed your sexual behaviour since people have started talking about AIDS?' in the French survey; and 'Did you do anything to prevent infection or do you just consider it impossible for you to have become infected? – did something to prevent infection – ran no risk at all' in the Dutch survey.

7　It cannot be demonstrated due to a lack of information about sexual behaviour before 1985 when sexual HIV transmission began to be a public issue.

8　The wordings are as follows: 'To your knowledge, has this person had or did this person have sexual relations with other persons during his/her sexual relationship with you?' (The partner with whom the relationship has lasted more than five years and the respondent last had sex) in the French survey; 'Do you currently believe that this person has sex with someone other than yourself?' in the Belgian survey; and 'Has your partner, during this relationship, ever had sexual contact with someone else?' in the Dutch survey.

9　'Yes' means that the partner knows the partner has/had another partner. 'I don't know' combines the 'I don't know' and 'no answer' categories in the French and Dutch surveys and 'you have no idea' and 'no answer' categories in the Belgian survey.

10　The question in the French survey was worded as follows: 'What do you believe your mates and close friends think about having love affairs or sexual relations outside a stable relationship? They are all in favour / some are in favour, others are not / they are all opposed' with the same question being asked with regard to colleagues and family members. The answers 'they all agree' and 'some of them agree, others don't' are grouped together in this table. The questions concerning this matter were included by A. Degenne, who has developed a theory of social circles (Degenne and Forsé, 1994). The question in the Belgian survey was worded as follows: 'What model of relationship dominates each of the various circles that I am going to list, that is to say, how do people actually behave? In your immediate family, is it the model of . . . ? faithfulness for life / faithfulness as long as one is with somebody / faithfulness with some rare departures / frequent brief affairs or concomitant relationships' with the same question being asked with regard to friends and colleagues. The answers 'faithfulness with some rare departures' and 'frequent brief affairs or concomitant relationships' are grouped together in Table 11.7.

11　The questions were worded as follows: 'Each of us has his or her own point of view about love and sexual desire. Do you, personally, agree fully, rather agree, rather disagree or disagree totally with the following ideas? – being faithful to each other is vital for the couple's happiness' (items grouped in this table: 'rather disagree' and 'disagree totally') in the French survey; 'What is your model for a conjugal relationship? Is it the model of . . . ? faithfulness for life / faithfulness as long as one is with somebody / faithfulness with some rare departures / frequent brief affairs or concomitant relationships' (items grouped in this table: 'faithfulness with some rare departures' and 'frequent brief affairs or concomitant relationships') in the Belgian survey; 'In a steady relationship you should allow each other to be free to have sexual contact with a third person. Do you / completely agree / basically agree / neutral (50/50) / basically disagree/ completely disagree?' (items grouped in this table: 'completely agree' and 'basically agree') in the Dutch survey.

12　The questions summarized in this table are the same as for Tables 11.6 and 11.7.

References

CATANIA, J.A., KEGELES, S.M. and COATES, T.J. (1990) 'Towards an understanding of risk behavior: an AIDS risk reduction model (ARRM)', *Health Education Quarterly*, **17**, pp. 53–72.

COHEN, M. and HUBERT, M. (1997) 'The place of time in understanding sexual behaviour and designing HIV/AIDS prevention programs', in VAN CAMPENHOUDT, L. *et al.* (Eds) *Sexual Interaction and HIV Risks. New Conceptual Perspectives in European Research*, London: Taylor & Francis.

DEGENNE, A. (1983) 'Sur les réseaux de sociabilité', *Revue Française de Sociologie*, **24**, 1, pp. 109–18.

DEGENNE, A. and FORSÉ, M. (1994) *Les réseaux sociaux*, Paris: Armand Colin.

FERRAND, A. and MOUNIER, L. (1990) *Relations sexuelles et relations de confidence – Analyse de réseaux*, Enquête méthodologique financée par l'ANRS, LASMAS-CNRS, Paris.

FERRAND, A. and MOUNIER, L. (1993a) 'Paroles sociales et influences normatives', in SPIRA, A., BAJOS, N. and LE GROUPE ACSF, *Les comportements sexuels en France*, Paris: La Documentation Française.

FERRAND, A. and MOUNIER, L. (1993b) 'L'échange de paroles sur la sexualité: une analyse des relations de confidence', *Population*, **5**, pp. 1451–76.

FERRAND, A. and MOUNIER, L. (1998) 'Influence des réseaux de confidence sur les relations sexvelles' in BAJOS, N. *et al.* (Eds), *La sexualité aux temps du sida*, Paris, PUF.

FERRAND, A. and SNIJDERS, T. (1997) 'Social networks and normative tensions', in VAN CAMPENHOUDT, L. *et al.* (Eds) *Sexual Interaction and HIV Risks. New Conceptual Perspectives in European Research*, London: Taylor & Francis.

FISCHER, C.S. (1982) *To Dwell Among Friends: Personal Network in Town and City*, Chicago: University Press.

GRAFMEYER, Y. and JOSEPH, I. (1979) *L'Ecole de Chicago* (Recueil de textes), Paris: Champ Urbain.

KRETZSCHMAR, M., REINKING, D.P., BROUWERS, H., VAN ZESSEN, G. and JAGER, J.C. (1994) 'Network models: from paradigm to mathematical tool', in KAPLAN and BRANDEAU (Eds) *Modeling the AIDS Epidemic: Planning, Policy and Prediction*, New York: Raven Press.

MARSDEN, P.V. (1990) 'Network data and measurement', *Annual Review of Sociology*, **16**, pp. 435–63.

PETO, D., REMY, J., VAN CAMPENHOUDT, L. and HUBERT, M. (1992) *Sida: l'amour face à peur*, Paris: L'Harmattan.

POLLAK, M. (1988) *Les homosexuels et le Sida. Sociologie d'une épidémie*, Paris: Métailié.

ROSE, A.M. (Ed.) (1962) *Human Behavior and Social Processes: an Interactionist Approach*, London: Houghton Mifflin.

WASSERMAN, S. and FAUST, K. (1994) *Social Network Analysis*, Cambridge: Cambridge University Press.

WELLMAN, B. and BERKOWITZ, S.D. (Eds) (1988) *Social Structures. A Network Approach*, Cambridge: Cambridge University Press.

Part 4

Representing AIDS

Chapter 12

Knowledge and Representations of HIV/AIDS

Jacques Marquet, Ester Zantedeschi and Philippe Huynen

Introduction

The issue covered in this chapter is the state of the population's knowledge of HIV transmission and means of protection.[1] In this respect, it is fruitless to isolate knowledge about a specific problem, such as knowing how HIV is or is not transmitted, from the complex process of apprehending the problem. As Schütz (1982, p. 5) writes, 'All our knowledge of the world, in common-sense as well as in scientific thinking, involves constructs, i.e., a set of abstractions, generalizations, formalizations, idealizations specific to the respective level of thought organization. Strictly speaking, there are no such things as facts, pure and simple. All facts are . . . always interpreted facts . . .'. Knowledge is part of a broader set of representations (Moscovici, 1983) comprising complex cognitive, affective, and cultural components that perform vital psychological and social functions for the individual. These include reassurance, the search for cohesion with close friends, and so on. Knowledge does not result from a purely rational approach and individuals do not necessarily accept the explanations given by the most qualified specialists, especially if they run counter to the convictions around which they tend to organize their lives and behaviour. Information uptake is selective and may be influenced by factors quite different from those influencing prevention guidelines.

While information remains crucial, some data nevertheless show that the knowledge acquisition process is not merely a question of having access to what is considered correct information. If one wants to change people's representations, it is not enough to identify 'poorly informed' or 'under-informed' groups and bombard them with messages containing information that is considered correct by specialists and policy-makers. The fact that a considerable proportion of the population has inappropriate representations of the risk of (in this case) HIV transmission is at least partly the result of more

Jacques Marquet, Ester Zantedeschi and Philippe Huynen

complex phenomena that we must try to elucidate. We have a duty to explore the reasons for, and significance of erroneous knowledge, which is just as much a social construction as knowledge and, like the latter, performs vital functions for the individual.

We shall begin by reviewing the state of adults' knowledge of HIV transmission and means of protection in Europe, country by country. The following country studies were used for this international comparison: Athens–PR (1990), Belgium (1993), Finland (1992), France–KABP (1992), East Germany (1990), East Germany (1993), West Germany (1993), the Netherlands (1989), Portugal (1991), Scotland (1992), Spain (1990), and Switzerland (1992). We shall also refer from time to time to the 'Eurobarometer' investigations.[2]

For reasons discussed later we shall not attach too much importance to variations between countries in the levels of knowledge. Instead, we shall focus on associations between variables. It can be hypothesized that two indicators that relate to a common variable will be sensitive to the same exogenous factor even if they do not exhibit the same degrees of sensitivity.[3] For example, for prevention purposes it is more important to know whether the degree of knowledge (the common variable) is correlated systematically with the level of education (exogenous factor) than to record variations in the rates of knowledge (measured by various questions) without knowing if the variations are 'real' or due to methodological particularities. In other words, we shall focus here more on the *structure* than on the *level* of knowledge.

In order to do so, knowledge indicators will be cross-tabulated against gender, age, and level of education. While these three variables are poor indicators of the complex knowledge acquisition process, they do make it possible to explore the issue. If the indicators of knowledge seem to be associated with the level of instruction alone, we cannot rule out the hypothesis that the degree of knowledge depends chiefly on access to and ability to understand accurate information. On the other hand, if specific indicators of knowledge appear to be correlated with factors such as age or gender, this initial hypothesis will have to be amended. On the basis of international comparisons, we shall show how knowledge of HIV's routes of transmission and means of protection is correlated with the individual's level of education first and foremost, but is also affected by other factors. This will lead us to distance ourselves from conceiving of prevention as being a simple problem of disseminating and receiving 'the right information'.

Methodology: Scope and Limits of the Comparison

The various investigations chosen for this international comparison vary greatly from a methodological point of view. The data collection periods (from 1989 to 1993), question and response wordings, questionnaire structures, sample structures with regard to gender, age, and so on, interview languages and associated nuances differ from one investigation to the next (see Chapter 1). For the purpose of our comparison we must wonder if these particular factors influence the degrees of knowledge that are registered.

While the respective weight of each methodological factor could not be measured, analysis shows that question wordings and types of responses are decisive. Let us take an example (Table 12.1).

First the results obtained for neighbouring countries are very different. Among other factors, the differences seem to be attributable in large part to the diversity of the questions and proposed standardized answers' wordings. More specifically, respondents' answers appear to be linked to the degree to which the disease is brought to the fore. The fact that the person being kissed is HIV positive is stressed strongly in the Portuguese and Dutch questions and much more weakly in the Spanish and Belgian questions. The latter two do make reference to the risk of HIV transmission, but when it comes time to answer the sub-question about kissing, respondents are not reminded of the partner's serological status with the same force. Rather, this serological status remains implied.

Second, responses are largely determined by the amplitude and structure of the answer scales. This factor seems to prevail over the preceding factor. To continue with the same examples, the Spanish and Belgian respondents were required to answer 'yes' or 'no', whereas the Portuguese were given a five-point scale (5 = very great risk, 4 = great risk, 3 = moderate risk, 2 = small risk, 1 = no risk) and the Dutch a scale with four possibilities (1 = quite possible, 2 = virtually impossible, 3 = totally impossible, 4 = don't know). The Belgian respondents could express hesitation – 'don't know' or 'no answer' –

Table 12.1 *Different question wordings on kissing as a way of transmitting HIV*

Spain 1990	'Which of the following do you believe can transmit the AIDS virus? . . . 4. By kissing'	'No': 93.4%
Portugal 1991	'Do you think a person can get AIDS by . . . giving a long kiss on the mouth to a person with AIDS or the AIDS virus?'	'No risk': 15.9%
Belgium 1993	'In your opinion, is transmission of the AIDS virus possible in each of the following circumstances? . . . by kissing someone on the mouth'	'No': 85.6%
The Netherlands 1989	'On these cards are various ways people think the AIDS virus is transmitted. With each card, please indicate if you think the virus can be transmitted that way: . . . from kissing someone who has AIDS?'	'Totally impossible': 38.9%

Table 12.2 *Different question wordings in the East German survey (1990) on the use of public toilets as a way of transmitting HIV*

'In your opinion, how great is the risk of catching AIDS[1] or the AIDS virus when carrying out one of the following social acts . . . using public toilets?	'Without risk': 43.5%
4 = extremely risky, 3 = very risky, 2 = risky, 1 = not very risky, 0 = without risk'	
'Here are some ways people believe AIDS can be transmitted to them. Please indicate what you think is true or false. . . . by using public toilets?'	'False': 68.7%

Note:
[1] Today, 'catching HIV' would be used in place of 'catching AIDS'; in this text, the questions in inverted commas are the original questions

or scepticism – 'they say it isn't possible, but I'm not sure' – but these categories of answer were not proposed to respondents immediately. As a result, their status is very different from those of the intermediate categories offered to Portuguese and Dutch respondents.

The examples in Table 12.2 enable one almost to 'measure' the impact of the differences in wording. The survey conducted in East Germany in 1990 included two questions about the risk of HIV transmission through the use of public toilets. The differences in the questions' wordings may be used to test the weights of the various answer scales. So, in this survey we find a 25-percentage-point difference in the attitude expressed to the same situation, depending on the wording that is chosen. This difference probably varies according to the daily living situations that are evaluated, the propositions' specific wordings, and the structure of the answer scale. Its magnitude, however, underlines the need to consider variations in question wordings as much more than simple 'background noise' likely to produce secondary variations.

The results presented in Figure 12.1 appear to be particularly eloquent in this respect. This graph displays the proportion of the population in each country that feels that each of the daily life situations that are studied – kissing, being bitten by a mosquito, drinking from someone's glass or eating off someone's plate, and using the toilet – does not carry any risk of infection. The dichotomous answer scales (true/false, yes/no, risk/no risk) are differentiated from the scales comprising at least three possible answers as follows: the former are represented by upper case letters (K, M, D, T), while the latter are represented by lower case letters (k, m, d, t).

The graph in Figure 12.1 shows that, regardless of the survey and subject studied, the dichotomous answer scales yield 'no risk' scores above 55 per cent, whereas the corresponding scores yielded by the at least three-point answer scales are all below this cutoff. The structure of the answer scale thus appears to be quite decisive in determining the response.

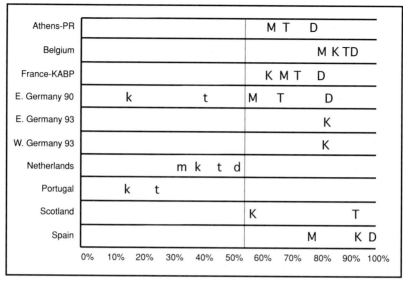

Key to Figure 12.1:
K/k = kissing   M/m = mosquito bites   D/d = drinking   T/t = toilet seats
Upper case letters are dichotomous answer scales; lower case letters are scales with at least three possible answers

Figure 12.1 *Proportions of respondents believing the specified situation carries no risk of HIV transmission*

We must also stress that the statements concerning kissing (Belgium, East Germany (1993), West Germany, Scotland, and Spain) and drinking from the same glass or eating off the same plate as someone else (Belgium and Spain) that do not state explicitly that the partner (of the kissing or meal) is seropositive or has AIDS yield higher scores than those in which the partner's seropositivity is expressly stated.[4]

Other factors can doubtless explain some of the inter-survey differences. We simply wanted to show that the indicators' heterogeneity prevented us offering a fine grained interpretation of the results. Thus, we shall not attach too much importance to inter-country differences in frequencies. Doing so would force us to use appreciably larger margins of error than the current ones, which are already considerable for some of the investigations, given the small sizes of their samples. Instead, we shall focus on factors that may be associated with knowledge.

However, we shall nevertheless refer from time to time to the Eurobarometer surveys (Huynen, Marquet and Hubert, 1995), as they have the advantage of having been conducted in all the countries over the same period of time, using comparable methods to obtain a picture of the levels of knowledge and differences between them, even though perfect homogeneity is impossible, if only because of language differences. These surveys also offer the advantage of being repeated at regular intervals, thus making diachronic analysis possible. The importance of this dimension with regard to knowledge is obvious.

Knowledge of Viral Transmission

Sexual Transmission, Transmission through Injection, and Vertical Transmission

Almost the entire population in each of the countries where these questions were asked was aware that HIV was transmissible by sexual relations and injecting drug use involving contaminated needles. In eight out of nine surveys, the proportion of the sample that recognized these two routes of viral transmission was systematically above 97 per cent. These overall encouraging results are virtually the same for men and women, different age classes and levels of education.[5]

Two surveys (France–KABP and the Netherlands) also included a question about vertical (mother–child) transmission of HIV during pregnancy. The results were very similar: 81.8 per cent of the French and 79.8 per cent of the Dutch respondents recognized the risk of vertical transmission. No significant gender-related differences were observed in these studies. In terms of age, differences were sometimes very large, with the middle age groups giving the highest and the youngest the lowest correct response rates. Differences in relation to level of education were moderate in the case of France (a 6.6 percentage-point difference between the 'high education' and 'low education' groups' correct response rates) and high in the Netherlands (27.6 percentage-point difference).

False Transmission Routes

Besides these very general indicators, a certain number of people were found to fear alleged 'transmission routes' despite specialists' and prevention officials' assurances to the contrary. Many surveys therefore included questions about what some call 'false transmission routes'. Depending on the survey, the respondents were asked how they perceived the risk of HIV transmission through such everyday activities and situations as kissing (on the mouth, on the cheek), drinking from someone else's glass or eating off someone else's plate, eating food prepared by a person with HIV/AIDS, sitting on a toilet seat, shaking someone's hand or touching someone, playing with a child with HIV, using someone's razor blade or electric shaver, using public toilets, being bitten by a mosquito or other insect, being bitten by someone, and so on. None of the surveys included all of these possibilities. For this comparative analysis we thus selected the most frequently studied situations, that is, kissing (or saliva) (K), mosquito bites (M), drinking from the glass or eating off the plate of a person with HIV/AIDS (D), and using public toilets (T).[6]

Figure 12.1 shows the proportion of respondents in each survey who answered that the above-mentioned daily life situations did not carry any risk of transmission. Beyond the foregoing methodological remarks, the results' great sensitivity to the answer scale structure also shows that each time the possibility of expressing a reservation, fear, or doubt, no matter how slight, was explicitly provided, the rate of 'no risk' responses declined. This tendency held true for each of the four situations studied. It seems that one need only legitimize the doubt or apprehension by providing an item that explicitly translates the feeling for the latter to be voiced. Moreover, for many people things are not understood in terms of 'true or false' or 'yes or no'. The situations to be evaluated may be more ambiguous than to allow such cut-and-dry responses. Be that as it may, we can note that besides those people whose answers frankly contradicted conventional preventive messages, there are others who try to express reservations and answer in a more nuanced fashion.

The graph in Figure 12.1 shows us that kissing (K) is the subject of maximum fear, followed by using public toilets (T), then drinking from someone else's glass or eating from someone else's plate (D). Mosquito bites are positioned in various places within this ranking, depending on the survey.

However, the K > T > D order seen in all the surveys emerges from respondents' aggregate responses. It may not necessarily correspond to an individual assessment. Overall, it can nevertheless be seen that wherever the potential for HIV transmission is seen as direct, for example through the exchange of saliva and perhaps contact with blood during a kiss, it seems to trigger more fear or doubt than when it is seen as indirect, for example, mediated by a toilet seat or bowl, by a plate or cooking utensil. Second, in both the situations where infection would occur indirectly (T and D), fear is heightened when the situation involves parts of the body, such as the genital and anal region, that prevention messages highlight as HIV's main ports of entry.

Kissing and drinking from someone else's glass bring two fearful HIV vectors into play, namely, saliva and, via sores in the mouth, blood. The problem of using toilets is related primarily to the body fluids that may be found on the toilet seat, that is, blood, semen, and urine. The mosquito is a blood-sucking insect. The transmission routes being evaluated above thus are not seen as equivalent by the man or woman in the street, by research scientists and by prevention officials.

It may be difficult for a part of the public to understand the subtleties of scientific discourse which suggest that while HIV antibodies can be found in the blood, saliva, and urine (Chamaret, 1992; Reboulot, 1994), HIV itself cannot be transmitted this way (CDC, 1985; Friedland *et al.*, 1986). This difficulty is compounded by the fact that official prevention messages may be distorted by parallel representations and messages that stray from scientific knowledge (Morin, 1994), nevermind revisionist theories that deny the causal relationship between HIV and AIDS (Closel, 1994).[7]

Three of the four situations, namely, kissing, drinking, and sitting on toilet seats, were also studied in several Eurobarometer surveys conducted between 1989 and 1995 (Huynen, Marquet and Hubert, 1995). These three activities were considered at risk by 16 per cent, 9 per cent, and 11 per cent, respectively, of the European Union's population in 1995, compared with the slightly higher figures of 21 per cent, 11 per cent, and 13 per cent, respectively, in 1989. However, these overall trends hide some important disparities between countries.[8]

Kissing

As shown in Figure 12.2, kissing a person with HIV/AIDS was judged risk-free by similar proportions of men and women. Differences between the various age classes and levels of education were nevertheless evident. Three of the surveys (France, East Germany (1993) and Spain) yielded a bell-jar curve, with a maximum percentage of people believing kissing to be risk-free in the intermediate age group (20–39 years of age) and smaller percentages sharing this view at the two extremes (under 20 and over 40 years of age). The curves in the six other surveys generally tended to decline with increasing age.

The surveys yielded three patterns of distribution with respect to level of education. The correctness of response with regard to prevention messages rose with increasing level of education in five surveys, namely, West Germany

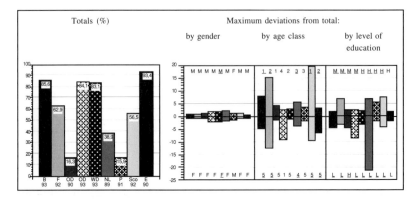

Figure 12.2 *Proportions of respondents believing that kissing carries no risk of HIV transmission*

Key to Figures 12.2, 12.3, 12.4, 12.5, 12.7, 12.8, 12.9 and 12.10:

Symbols	*Surveys:* Ath90 = Athens 1990, B93 = Belgium 1993, F92 = France–KABP 1992, OD90 = East Germany 1990, OD93 = East Germany 1993, WD93 = West Germany 1993, NL89 = the Netherlands 1989, P91 = Portugal 1991, Sco92 = Scotland 1992, E90 = Spain 1990
	Variables. Gender: M = male, F = female. *Age:* 1 = 18–19, 2 = 20–24, 3 = 25–29, 4 = 30–39, 5 = 40–49, except for Spain, where 1 = 19–21, 2 = 22–28, 4 = 29–38 and 5 = 39–50. *Level of education:* L = low, M = intermediate, H = high.
Items represented	The deviations from the totals for each survey are calculated for each item. The '0' on the right-hand graph thus represents the total (in percent) shown on the left-hand graph. The negative values (values below the axis) correspond to the items for which the percentages measured are below the total percentage and the positive ones those for which the percentages measured are above the total percentage. For the variables 'age' and 'level of education', which have more than two items, only the extreme items are represented. An equal sign ('=') instead of an item's symbol signifies no deviation for the variable considered.
Magnitude of deviations	Besides the magnitude of each deviation, which is proportionate to the column height, there is the issue of its statistical significance. If the deviation between extreme scores is statistically significant at the 0.05 threshold (homogeneity of frequencies test, Spiegel (1993)), the symbols corresponding to these scores are underlined.
Example: the Belgian results in Figure 12.2	In the Belgian survey 85.6% of all the respondents but 86.5% of the men versus 84.8% of the women, 93.5% of the 18–19-year-olds versus 80.9% of the 40–49-year-olds and 87.3% of the medium educated versus 81.0% of the low educated believed that kissing carries no risk of HIV transmission. For the Belgian survey, the '0' on the right-hand graph thus represents 85.6%; for each variable, the highest percentage – 86.5% (male), 93.5% (18–19) and 87.3% (medium) – is represented above the axis, and the lowest one below the axis. The deviation between men and women's scores (only 1.7%) is not statistically significant at the 0.05 threshold, consequently the 'M' and 'F' symbols are not underlined.

(1993), the Netherlands, Portugal, Scotland, and Spain. In three other surveys (Belgium, France–KABP, and East Germany (1993)), this general trend is also observed, except that the 'medium education' groups contained the same percentage (even a little higher but the deviation is not statistically significant) of people who believed kissing to be risk-free than the 'high education' groups. Finally, the 1990 East German survey was distinguished by the fact that its highly educated group contained the smallest percentage of people who believed kissing was risk-free.

Mosquito Bites

In three out of six surveys, there were no significant gender-related differences with regard to the perceived risk of mosquito bites. In contrast, significantly fewer women in the Athens–PR and Netherlands surveys felt the risk of contamination was nil, whereas the France–KABP survey gave the opposite

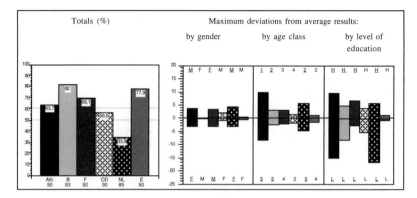

Figure 12.3 *Proportions of respondents believing that mosquito bites carry no risk of HIV transmission*

result. The Athenian survey was characterized by a large proportion of young people who thought the risk of HIV infection from mosquito bites was nil and a marked smaller proportion of older subjects who shared this opinion. In the Dutch and (to a lesser extent) French surveys, both young and old had smaller proportions of people who felt the risk of infection was nil than the middle group did. Age-specific differences in the other surveys were small. All of the surveys showed a positive correlation between the percentage of respondents who felt the risk of infection to be nil and level of education.

Drinking and Eating

Only in the Dutch survey was the gender-specific difference in answers greater than three percentage points. Age-class distributions showed little variations in the Spanish survey. In contrast, in the other surveys the percentage of respondents who believed these practices were risk-free was noticeably lower among the oldest groups. All of the surveys showed a positive correlation between the percentage of respondents who considered the risk of HIV transmission from drinking or eating from a person with HIV/AIDS's glass or plate to be nil and level of education.[9]

Toilet Seats

The breakdown by gender showed very similar patterns among the Belgian, French, and Scottish respondents. In contrast, in four other surveys significantly fewer women than men felt that the risk of infection was nil.[10] With the

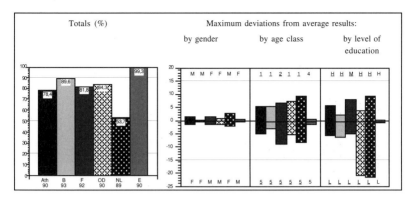

Figure 12.4 *Proportions of respondents believing that drinking from someone else's glass carries no risk of HIV transmission*

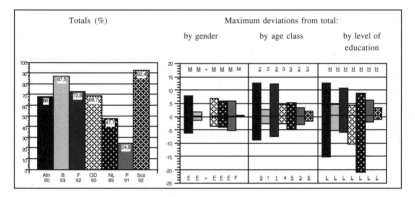

Figure 12.5 *Proportions of respondents believing that using public toilets carries no risk of HIV transmission*

exception of Portugal, the middle age groups seem more inclined to feel that public toilets carried no risk of HIV transmission. The picture with regard to level of education is practically the same across the board. With the exception of one of the two indicators (not shown in Figure 12.5) studied in the 1991 East German study, level of education was consistently positively correlated with the proportion of respondents who felt using public toilets to be risk-free.

Giving Blood

From a technical standpoint the question of possible infection through receiving infected blood and blood products is close to that of injecting drug use given the role of the needle. However, from the standpoint of social

Table 12.3 *Proportions of respondents believing there is no risk in giving blood*

	Athens 1990	Belgium 1993	France 1992	Germany East 1990	Portugal 1991	Scotland 1992
Total	75.9	63.7	50.7	37.8	39.4	76.7
Gender						
Men	78.9	64.5	50.6	40.8	43.9	74.9
Women	73.2	62.9	50.7	35.8	35.1	78.1
Age						
18–19	73.4	66.1	34.3*	42.9*	29.5	72.2
20–24	79.5	73.2	46.8	37.4	38.8	76.6
25–29	80.0	64.2	51.6	40.5	41.9	78.2
30–39	74.9	63.0	53.2	37.3	42.8	79.5
40–49	73.0	58.6	51.5	35.4	38.4	73.0
Education						
Low	61.1	45.3	43.3	18.8	31.0	71.0
Medium	75.9	62.8	56.2	38.9	43.5	79.5
High	85.2	75.0	68.7	40.7	47.3	88.1

Note:
*The denominator of the cell is between 21 and 50

representations, blood transfusions and injecting drug use are two distinct issues. The subject of blood transfusions, which is very directly linked to the issue of contaminated blood, requires specific analysis. Consequently, we decided not to study blood transfusions but to focus on blood donations. While prevention statements do not rule out the possibility (although it is presented as very slight) of being infected by HIV from blood transfusions, giving blood is presented as being without risk to donors in all the Western European countries.

Table 12.3 gives the breakdown by gender, age class, and level of education of the percentage of the population in each survey which considered giving blood to be risk-free. A general remark is in order before we go on to examine specific data. In Belgium and France, giving blood elicits more fear than the 'false routes of transmission' studied above. It is not impossible that this reflects social anxieties triggered by the repercussions of France's contaminated blood scandal, which also spread to France's closest neighbours. However, a similar situation pertained in East Germany in 1990. The 1995 Eurobarometer study (Huynen, Marquet and Hubert, 1995), in which it appeared that overall 67 per cent of the European Union's population thought giving blood carried no risk of infection, provides no clues as to the French and Belgian populations' fears of giving blood.[11] Beyond the question of the possible spread of a feeling of fear, it is important to note that recent debates about the quality of blood for transfusion may have cast a shadow on the entire blood collection–processing–storage process, including the blood donation stage.

In the three surveys where gender-specific difference in answers was five percentage points or more, fewer women than men considered giving blood to be risk-free. The patterns by age are variable, even though the largest proportion of respondents to consider the risk of transmission nil was systematically found in the intermediate age class. With respect to education, all surveys showed that the more educated respondents were, the more likely they were to consider the risk of infection through giving blood to be nil.

Knowledge of Means of Protecting against HIV Transmission

Condoms, HIV Testing and Fidelity

When means of protection from the risk of HIV infection are mentioned, one of the first things that comes to mind is the condom, even though other protective strategies exist. As far as knowledge is concerned, this tendency to give priority to one means of protection to the detriment of others is found in the questionnaires as well. Six surveys (Belgium, France–KABP, East Germany (1993), West Germany, the Netherlands, and Switzerland) (Table 12.4) contain at least one question about the condom's effectiveness as a barrier to HIV. Two surveys (Belgium and France–KABP) contain a question about the efficacy of HIV testing as a tool to reduce the risk of HIV transmission when two partners take the test and wait for the result before having unprotected sex together, but with very different question wordings. The Belgian survey also contains a question about being faithful as a means of protecting oneself from HIV infection. None of the surveys asks about the efficacy of abstinence. Given these differences, large-scale comparison of the findings is possible in the case of condom use only.

In the four surveys that yielded a gender-specific divergence of five percentage points or more, fewer women than men were found to believe in the efficacy of condoms as a means of protecting against HIV. It also appears that the oldest age groups systematically showed the smallest percentages of respondents who believe in the condom's effectiveness.[12] The results show a positive association between the percentages of respondents agreeing that the 'condom is effective' and the level of education.[13]

Table 12.4 *Proportions of respondents believing that the condom is an effective means of protection against HIV*

	Belgium 1993	France 1992	Germany East 1993	Germany West 1993	Netherlands 1989	Switzerland 1992
Total	56.5	72.6	59.9	76.9	86.3	52.7
Gender						
Men	59.1	76.0	69.9	79.7	84.0	52.2
Women	54.1	69.2	49.8	73.9	87.9	53.2
Age						
18–19	60.3	62.8*	65.5*	78.5	85.5	54.7
20–24	59.4	75.0	71.8	79.6	86.8	53.6
25–29	56.5	78.5	59.7	81.0	88.4	51.1
30–39	54.6	72.7	57.9	74.7	87.2	53.3
40–49	56.2	69.4	55.2	75.1	83.3	51.1
Education						
Low	58.1	72.1	41.0	70.4	80.4*	48.8
Medium	57.7	72.5	61.6	77.8	85.8	52.9
High	54.4	72.9	64.1	83.6	89.2	54.5

Note:
*The denominator of the cell is between 21 and 50

The 1995 Eurobarometer survey (Huynen, Marquet and Hubert, 1995) also contained a question about the condom's effectiveness in preventing HIV transmission. According to this, 93 per cent of European Union inhabitants think that the condom is an effective means of protection. The country-to-country differences spread over 14 percentage points.[14] This same survey also studied abstinence, which was considered effective in preventing HIV transmission by only 67 per cent of Europeans. However, the range between the highest and lowest country scores was 51 percentage points.[15] Ireland is the only country in the European Union where more people consider abstinence to be effective than the condom. This encourages us to interpret answers concerning the relative efficacies of the various means of protection in reference to local representations and acceptance of these practices, rather than simply in relation to the boundaries of their theoretical effectiveness.

While it is rather hard to imagine proposing abstinence as a solution to the entire population, the relative absence of questions about the effectiveness of fidelity and HIV testing in the surveys doubtless reflects two phenomena: first, the difficulty of assessing practices, the effectiveness of which depends on what is going on beyond sexual intercourse *per se*; and second, the 'banking on the condom' and 'zero risk' ideologies – which adapt poorly to the subtlety of human communication – that are espoused by many researchers.

False Protective Measures

In addition to the protective measures that specialists acknowledge as having some efficacy, there exists a string of practices that experts strongly condemn but a segment of the population considers effective in protecting against HIV transmission. Four of these practices were examined by at least two of the surveys, namely, coitus interruptus (C), washing after sex (W), taking the pill (P), and belief in the existence of a vaccine or therapy that can cure a person of AIDS (T).[16] Figure 12.6 gives the country-by-country breakdown of the percentages of the population that judge each of these four measures (when they were studied by the survey) to be totally ineffectual in protecting a person against HIV.

Figure 12.6 shows that a large proportion of the adult population in each country understands the effectiveness of the practices under study. Still, the number of people who do not reject out of hand such practices as coitus interruptus, washing after sexual intercourse, and taking the pill, as affording protection from HIV, and those who believe that an AIDS vaccine exists, is far from negligible. These figures temper somewhat the optimism that might result from the observation that almost everyone knows that the virus can be transmitted during sexual intercourse.

We must note that the four types of 'protection' considered above are not equivalent from a scientific and prevention point of view. Currently, even though what have been called 'encouraging' trials have been conducted (Girard, 1993; Kieny, 1993), there is no vaccine for HIV or treatment capable of curing AIDS. Work on the subject has shown the inefficacy of the pill as a means of protecting against HIV (Stein, 1993). The effectiveness of washing the genital region (douching) after sexual intercourse is little discussed in the scientific literature. On the other hand, recent investigations have revealed, after a long line of investigations with sometimes contradictory results

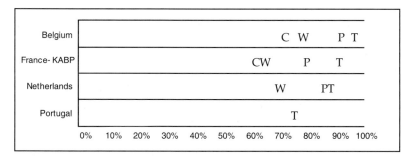

Figure 12.6 *Proportions of respondents believing that coitus interruptus (C), washing after sexual intercourse (W), using the pill (P), vaccine or treatment to cure AIDS patients or HIV carriers (T) are totally ineffective in preventing HIV*

(Musicco, 1992; European Study Group, 1992), an at least partial efficacy of coitus interruptus as a means of protecting against HIV transmission (De Vincenzi *et al.*, 1994), despite the fact that coitus interruptus has never been presented as a possible means of prevention in this area.

Respondents' assessments of the (in)efficacy of these 'means of protection' may reflect in part debates within the scientific community. Aggregating individual responses reveals that belief in their effectiveness systematically follows the order 'coitus interruptus' > 'washing' > 'pill' > 'treatment'. Most important, however, we find a 14- to 15-percentage point difference between the first two and last two practices. A considerable proportion of the population ascribes relative, albeit weak, effectiveness to washing and coitus interruptus. Some respondents' answers here may have been guided by the controversy that exists within scientific circles (a controversy which remains relatively confidential). Nevertheless, these attitudes are more likely due to the reactivation of knowledge and representations of two practices that have been used as means of contraception, with variable success, or as an ineffective and perhaps even harmful means of preventing STDs, for centuries.

Let us now look at findings for each 'protective measure' taken separately.

Coitus Interruptus

In the two surveys that contained a question on this subject, namely, Belgium and France–KABP, more men than women thought coitus interruptus was ineffective as a means of protecting against HIV transmission. Such a gender-based difference can be explained by the unequal risks of HIV transmission connected to coitus interruptus for men and women and the overall assessment of the practice. With regard to the first hypothesis, if a seronegative woman has unprotected sexual intercourse with a man with HIV/AIDS, the perceived benefit of his not ejaculating inside her body, besides being partly confirmed by scientific study, is easy to imagine, since it boils down to transposing knowledge concerning reproduction to the area of prevention.[17] The benefits for the male partner in the case of a seronegative man who has intercourse with a woman with HIV/AIDS are less obvious. With regard to the second hypothesis, we must doubtless allow as well for the fact that coitus interruptus is often perceived by men as frustrating. This could lead them to judge the practice negatively, regardless of its purpose. If we look at respondents' ages, the proportion of respondents thinking that coitus interruptus is totally ineffective against HIV is significantly smaller in the '18–19-year-old' class than in the '20–24-year-old' class and all the other age classes combined. The most highly educated respondents also have the highest percentage of 'absolutely no effectiveness' responses, but the differences remain small.

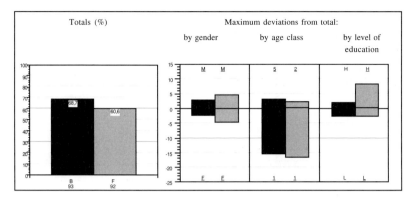

Figure 12.7 *Proportions of respondents believing that coitus interruptus is totally ineffective in preventing HIV*

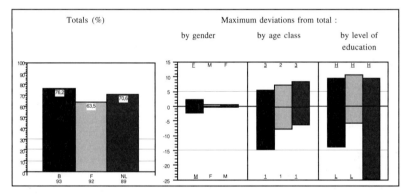

Figure 12.8 *Proportions of respondents believing that washing after sex is totally ineffective in preventing HIV*

Washing after Sexual Intercourse

In France and the Netherlands there were no gender-based differences in opinions on this practice. In Belgium, slightly more women than men considered douching after sexual intercourse to be totally ineffective as a means of protection. Age-specific differences were sometimes very large, with the youngest group systematically having the smallest proportion of respondents who rejected all notions of efficacy of this practice (this position was closer to that of the 'over 40s' than to those of the other groups). The opinion that washing after sex was totally ineffective appeared to be correlated with level of education in all three surveys. The proportion of the more educated respondents who deemed this practice totally ineffective was systematically higher.

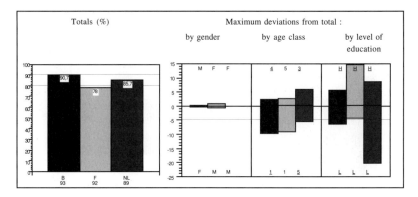

Figure 12.9 *Proportions of respondents believing that taking the pill is totally ineffective in preventing HIV*

Using the Pill

The three surveys do not exhibit any differences in the perceived efficacy of using the pill to protect against HIV as judged by men and women. In contrast, the age-related differences are sometimes very large, with the highest percentages of 'not effective' responses being found in the intermediate age groups. The evaluation of the pill as a means of protecting against HIV is correlated with level of education in all three studies. The most highly educated respondents were the most likely to consider the pill totally ineffective for this purpose. According to the 1995 Eurobarometer survey (Huynen, Marquet and Hubert, 1995), which also included a question about the efficacy of the pill in protecting against HIV, substantial differences are observed between countries.[18]

Treatment

Four surveys contained a question on the existence of either an AIDS vaccine (Belgium and France–KABP) or a treatment to cure AIDS (the Netherlands and Portugal). Although these two questions are different, they both suggest that medicine offers at least a partial solution for the problem of AIDS. The gender-specific differences in the answers never exceeded 2 per cent. With the exception of the French survey, the results of which are very uniform, breakdowns by age show relatively large divergences without, however, any clear trend. The breakdown by level of education shows a correlation between knowledge of the non-existence of a vaccine or treatment and level of education, with the 'highly educated' being the most likely to answer that there was no treatment or vaccine.

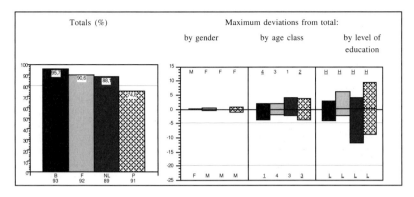

Figure 12.10   *Proportions of respondents stating there is no effective treatment for HIV*

Choosing Partners

Rather than being managed at the moment of sexual intercourse, the risk of HIV transmission can be taken into account beforehand. Abstinence is the most radical form of this type of risk management. A weaker form involves choosing seronegative partners. The certainty that they are seronegative can be had, however, only by a test and/or through dialogue in a climate of trust. The complexity of the approach notwithstanding, three surveys (Belgium, France–KABP, and the Netherlands) tried to measure how the population evaluated partner selection as a means of protection. The France–KABP survey speaks of 'choosing one's partner correctly' while the Dutch one speaks of 'being careful with whom you have sex'. These attitudes are deemed 'not at all effective' by 17.6 per cent of the French respondents and 'not effective' by 16.1 per cent of the Dutch respondents. The even more restrictive wording used in the Belgian survey – 'Is choosing partners who appear to be in good health totally effective, rather effective, rather ineffective, or not at all effective as a means of protection against AIDS?' – netted a much higher negative response rate ('not at all effective') of 57.1 per cent. Given the small number of surveys concerned and the lack of uniformity in the wordings used, we shall not examine this point in greater depth except to stress that considerable proportions of respondents in all three countries seemed willing to accept a 'relational' rather than 'technical' risk management approach (for the implemented practices see Chapter 8 in this book).

HIV and Symptoms of AIDS

The problem implicitly raised by the Belgian survey's question on the effectiveness of choosing one's partners is that of the visibility of HIV or AIDS. In

Table 12.5 *Proportions of respondents believing a person can be a symptomless carrier of HIV*

	Athens 1990	Belgium 1993	France 1992–1	France 1992–2	Netherlands 1989–1	Netherlands 1989–2	Portugal 1991
Total	70.1	86.3	72.5	94.5	83.0	85.8	76.9
Gender							
Men	71.7	87.3	73.9	93.9	81.3	88.8	77.6
Women	68.8	85.4	71.2	95.1	84.3	83.6	76.2
Age							
18–19	68.3	78.6	76.3*	100*	73.7	84.2	74.9
20–24	77.1	84.2	71.2	96.6	77.8	89.8	79.6
25–29	77.3	88.9	66.3	93.2	89.0	87.2	81.5
30–39	70.7	86.7	74.1	94.1	83.9	85.4	78.0
40–49	61.2	87.2	74.3	93.9	84.1	82.8	72.2
Education							
Low	46.1	86.3	77.3	94.3	67.4*	67.4*	61.9
Medium	71.7	86.4	72.4	96.2	82.0	83.4	84.1
High	83.9	86.1	59.3	93.4	88.5	94.6	90.9

Note:
*The denominator of the cell is between 21 and 50

other words, can one say that a person is seronegative or positive or has AIDS, based on his or her external appearance? Several surveys tackle this subject directly. Two main wordings, with minor variations, are found. The first one asks the respondent whether he feels he can recognize a person with HIV (Belgium, France–KABP (second question), and the Netherlands (first question)) or an AIDS patient (France–KABP (first question)). The second one asks whether it is possible for a person with HIV not to show any symptoms (Athens–PR, the Netherlands (second question), and Portugal). The responses to all of these questions are summarized in Table 12.5. The percentages given in this table express for each population considered either the percentage who feel it is impossible to recognize a person with HIV/AIDS by external signs alone or the percentage who answered that a person with HIV could very well be asymptomatic. Although they are not identical, these indicators do point to one and the same problem, that of the existence of signs of HIV on the body. The Dutch example, in which both wordings were chosen, shows that the positions elicited by the two questions are relatively close.

The percentage of the population who said HIV disease was not necessarily manifested by visible symptoms ranged from 70.1 per cent in the Athens–PR survey to 94.5 per cent in the France–KABP (second question) survey. The French example shows the importance of differentiating healthy people with HIV from AIDS patients, for the overall difference in the answers to these two questions exceeds 20 percentage points.

The gender-specific differences in answers are slight. Only for the second Dutch indicator does it exceed 5 per cent. There is no clear pattern with regard to age. However, except for France the highest percentages are seen in the intermediate age classes. Some questions (Belgium, France–KABP (second question)) do not show correlations with level of education, others (Athens–PR, the Netherlands (first and second questions), and Portugal) are positively correlated with level of education, and a last survey (France–KABP (first question)) shows a negative correlation with this parameter. This negative correlation prompts us to recognize once again the specificity of this indicator, which refers to the case of AIDS patients rather than people with HIV. The more highly educated respondents are more inclined than the rest to think they can detect the signs of the disease.

Knowledge is More than Just Knowledge

Areas of Inaccurate Knowledge

A considerable amount of the total population's knowledge of AIDS, HIV's routes of transmission, and means of protecting against it is insufficient, even frankly incorrect, in light of what is commonly accepted by specialists in the field. What is more, those with misconceptions about transmission do not necessarily hold such misconceptions about means of protection, and vice versa (Marquet, Hubert and Van Campenhoudt, 1995).

A higher level of information is necessary because while improved knowledge about disease does not lead automatically to the adoption of risk-reducing behaviour, ignorance is even less a guarantee of low-risk behaviour. Moreover, the role of people who serve as vectors of incorrect representations of the disease in communication chains must not be neglected (see Lazarsfeld and Katz's (1955) 'two-step flow' theory). The continued broad dissemination of incorrect knowledge doubtless means that, to reach adequate information levels, messages aimed at the entire population continue to be necessary, even though the effectiveness of prevention messages depends for a good part on their appropriateness to the targeted group. The fact that misconceptions about transmission routes overlap only partially with those about means of protection also means, as Morin (1994) points out, that ' "making a mistake" in identifying transmission routes and "making a mistake" in choosing the means of protection do not necessarily derive from the same logic'.

The degree of knowledge both of how the virus is transmitted and means of protection is tied to level of education. Regardless of the survey and topic involved, the systematic trend is for the least educated to have lower rates of answers complying with prevention messages than people with intermediate and high levels of education. The key element here is the level of education and what it covers, that is, the individual's cultural environment, critical attitude towards common prejudices, degree of proximity to scientific discourse and to prevention messages generally conceived of for the middle and upper classes by people who belong to higher educated social subgroups, and so on. The school itself is part of this broader context. Still, it is no less true that the school may have a decisive role, particularly with regard to certain categories of young people, for whom it is one of the rare entities to transmit reliable knowledge. The problem of informing people who have dropped out of school at an early age or young people who are truant or refractory to the school's influence thus becomes crucial.

The frequency of what are considered incorrect representations is also linked to age. The two classes at the far ends of the age scale are characterized by smaller proportions of people whose remarks match official prevention messages in respect of many of the topics investigated. This finding tends to show that age is above all an indicator of a position in the life cycle which in turn influences the degree of concern about, and experience in, the areas of sexual relations and prevention. Many 18- and 19-year-olds have not yet had sex. They thus resemble older respondents who also have relatively fewer partners.

These two groups, that is, the oldest and youngest groups, nevertheless pose different problems. Elders stand out notably by the fact that they believe various situations of daily life carry a potential risk of transmitting HIV despite specialists' reassurances. They thus overestimate the risks of HIV transmission. This singularity could well lead to 'excessive' mistrust of other people and of people who are considered, rightly or wrongly, to be likely to transmit HIV. For young people, their knowledge of how HIV is transmitted is relatively good, sometimes better than that of other age groups. But, on the other hand, many young people are inclined to believe in the relative effectiveness of 'protective' strategies that are rarely recommended (coitus interruptus), even cautioned against (washing oneself after sex, taking the pill) by prevention campaigns.

Young people's relatively poorer knowledge might also be explained by the fact that although the process of assimilating prevention messages encountered in the course of their studies starts very early, it does not produce its full effects until this knowledge is objectivized by actual sexual experience. However, it remains to be understood why their misconceptions concern ways of protecting themselves against the virus in particular.

Gender appears to be a discriminating variable less often than age and level of education. However, three different types of situations stand out clearly with regard to HIV transmission: the medically correct response rate is statistically lower for women when the risks of transmission via mosquito bites, using public toilets, and giving blood are mentioned. Of all three situations the case of public toilets yields the clearest trend. Differences in the responses of men versus women are likewise seen with regard to the effectiveness of the condom, coitus interruptus, and washing after sex as a means of protecting against HIV transmission. So, as we can see, the issues for which the greatest gender-specific differences emerge refer to either blood (mosquito bites, giving blood) or anatomical differences between the sexes (condom, coitus interruptus, washing). Using public toilets ties to both domains, since the female urogenital tract is also concerned with menstrual blood flow.

In the case of a heterosexual relationship, the real and imagined risks of infection are not the same for the man and the woman. Coitus interruptus may appear to protect the woman because it spares her direct contact with potentially infective semen, whereas washing after sex may seem easier and thus more effective in the view of the male partner, given that his genital organs are external. Many studies have shown gender-specific differences in people's relationships to blood and the key position of menstruation in women's relationships to their bodies in general.[19] Toilets, which are places for defecation but also the elimination of urine and menstrual blood, symbolize these sexually differentiated relationships to the body and blood. The female genital region has closer ties to the realm of blood than the male genitals, and combines fears linked to sexuality and blood.

Overall, the international comparisons based on the Eurobarometer survey results show that Europe is split into two parts, a northern part with higher medically correct response rates, and a southern part with lower medically correct response rates. However, Ireland joins the southern group of Greece, Portugal, Spain, and, to a lesser extent, Italy, in overestimating the risks of infection via kissing, drinking, and using toilets, and expressing greater reservations with regard to condom use.

Questioning Knowledge

The preceding analysis shows that one cannot content oneself with explaining inadequate knowledge by a lack of information. Several indices plead in favour of taking additional hypotheses into account.

First, as we have just shown, knowledge, or rather, representations of HIV/AIDS are correlated with level of education, but also other factors. The differences in men's and women's answers seem to be explained at least in part by the existence of stores of 'preprogrammed' representations that are partially gender-dependent rather than by the specificity of information channels reaching one or the other gender. These ways of apprehending reality work like specific receivers for the information that is carried by prevention messages. In our opinion, a similar mechanism is instrumental in explaining the specific evaluations of abstinence and condom use as means of protection against HIV that were recorded in Ireland. In a similar way, the life cycle measured by the age scale influences the degree of concern about, and experience in, sexual relations and seems to select prevention messages. These correlations between specific indicators of knowledge, and factors other than level of education, lend strength in turn to our reading of the level of education as being a complex mosaic of interconnected elements – cultural environment, attitudes towards popular prejudices, scientific discourse, prevention messages – rather than merely reflecting the person's access to, and ability to comprehend accurate information.

Second, we have shown that each time respondents were explicitly given the possibility of expressing a reservation or doubt, the rate of responses excluding all risks of HIV transmission in situations that prevention officials present as being risk-free nevertheless declined. As soon as expressing such scepticism becomes legitimate, people take advantage of the opportunity, sometimes in considerable numbers. In other words, many people do not see things as being either black or white, true or false, transmission or no transmission. Some situations and questions would definitely benefit from being defined more precisely. The main lesson is that some people want to express reservations with regard to official medical discourse.

Third, current prevention messages are squeezed between the inherent limitations of preventing both the HIV epidemic's spread and discrimination against people with HIV/AIDS. They are also torn between a scientific approach which consists of specific analyses of complex findings and for which there is no 'zero risk', and a public health approach which strives to disseminate practical, pragmatic advice that can be understood by the largest number of people possible and sometimes gives the impression of subscribing to the 'zero risk' utopia.[20] How is it possible to say that kissing is risk-free yet concomitantly advise dentists to wear gloves when working on their patients? How does one mention the risk presented by potential sores in the mouth without triggering a tidal wave of panic? And so on. The responses collected in these population surveys may reflect in part the hesitations, even contradictions (or what is perceived as being contradictory) in prevention messages. In some cases, what may have been interpreted as being ignorance may simply reflect 'vigilant mistrust'.

In conclusion, if one aims at improving the level of the population's knowledge of HIV transmission and means of protection, the preceding analyses encourage us to abandon perspectives that see prevention as being a simple problem of disseminating and receiving 'the right information'. Instead, they lead us to question the concept of knowledge itself. The problem is no longer one of measuring who knows or does not know something, but rather one of questioning the logic and rationales that are specific to the stock of representations surrounding knowledge. Those taken-for-granted representations are not in need of further analysis but are reactivated from time to time and constitute the receivers for new information, which depends on age, gender, level of education, but also a great many other factors that future analysis should uncover.

Notes

1 See the final section 'Knowledge is More than Just Knowledge' of this chapter for a summarized discussion of this issue.

2 The Eurobarometer investigations are opinion surveys carried out on European Commission initiative in the twelve European Community countries before 1994 and the fifteen European Union countries since 1994. Among the various topics tackled, the questionnaires contained some questions on AIDS in 1989, 1990, 1994 and 1995.

3 That is, the slopes of the plots of their least squares are different.

4 The only exception to this rule concerns the Scottish survey, where the 'don't know' rate was nevertheless 19.3 per cent.

5 The male/female difference was always less than 3 per cent. The variations between age classes were less than 4 per cent everywhere except in Spain. In the countries where the differences between the 'low' and the 'high education' groups were greater than 3 per cent, that is Belgium, East Germany (1990 and 1993), the Netherlands, and Spain, the more highly educated respondents had higher levels of knowledge than the others.

6 An index which summarizes the results for the four situations (KMDT) will be provided in Chapter 14.

7   The French journal *Le journal du sida* (issue No. 35, p. 2, and the supplement to issue No. 43–44, p. 2) mentions two cases of discordant messages concerning kissing, one in Italy, the other in the United States. Issue No. 34 (p. 2) likewise reported some rather worrying remarks by a French scientist concerning the mosquito's ability to transmit HIV.

8   Kissing and drinking seemed to elicit special fear in Greece (30 and 15 per cent, respectively), Portugal (27 and 13 per cent, respectively), Ireland (25 and 13 per cent, respectively), and Spain (20 and 11 per cent, respectively). Sitting on a public toilet seat was considered particularly dangerous in three of these countries, namely, Greece (25 per cent), Portugal (17 per cent), and Ireland (17 per cent).

9   One notes a slight particularity for the French survey, where the percentage in the 'high education' group was the same, even slightly lower (–1 per cent), but the deviation is not statistically significant than that in the 'medium education' group.

10 Although this factor alone cannot explain the observed divergences, we should like to underline the advantage of giving priority to 'gender-neutral' wordings. From this standpoint, the expression 'using public toilets' that was used in most of the surveys can refer to different uses for men and women, whereas 'sitting on a toilet seat' (the wording used in the Belgium survey) seems less ambiguous.

11 The difference between the most extreme national figures was 45 percentage points. Former East Germany and Portugal registered scores less than or equal to 50 per cent while Denmark, Sweden, and the Netherlands had scores greater than or equal to 82 per cent.

12 It should be pointed out, however, that 18–19-year-olds in France are more sceptical than their elders about the condom's effectiveness.

13 If we look at the figures presented in Table 12.4, this does not hold true for Belgium and France. Still, the breakdown of 'fairly effective' answers by level of education shows a similar correlation with increasing level of education. This is the case in France and even more so in Belgium, where the 'fairly effective' rate rises from 19.5 per cent for the 'low education' group to 42.0 per cent for the 'high education' group. The highly educated respondents had more problems dealing with the 'totally' than the 'effective' component of the answer. The questions asked in the other surveys did not contain the idea of '*total* effectiveness'.

14 Five countries (Ireland, Italy, Portugal, Belgium, and Spain) had scores less than or equal to 91 per cent, while five other countries (Sweden, Denmark, France, former East Germany, and the Netherlands) had scores greater than or equal to 95 per cent.

15 Four countries (Greece, Portugal, former East Germany, and Italy) had scores less than or equal to 57 per cent, while five countries (Sweden, Finland, Denmark, Ireland, Great Britain, and the Netherlands) had scores greater than or equal to 77 per cent.

16 A summary index for three out of the four situations (WPT) will be provided in Chapter 14.

17 Coitus interruptus aims to prevent contact with semen; it might also prevent contact with potentially infective semen.

18 According to this survey, 82 per cent of the European Union's population considers the pill to be ineffective in protecting against HIV. The range between the high and low country scores is 29 percentage points. Three countries (Portugal, Spain, and Greece) had scores less than or equal to 72 per cent, while two countries (Denmark and Sweden) had scores greater than or equal to 94 per cent.

19 See M. Cros (1990) *Anthropologie du sang en Afrique*, Paris: L'Harmattan; M. Douglas (1971) *De la souillure*, Paris: Maspero; J.-P. Roux (1988) *Le sang: mythes, symboles et réalités*, Paris: Fayard; Y. Verdier (1979) *Façons de dire, façons de faire*, Paris: Gallimard.

20 This is notably the case when reference is made to *safe* rather than *safer* sex and also each time the condom is presented as being the only truly safe means of protection. See also Edelmann (1994).

References

BECKER, M. and JOSEPH, J. (1988) 'AIDS and behavioral change to reduce risk: a review', *American Journal of Public Health*, **778**, 4, pp. 394–410.

CDC (1985) 'Education and foster care of children infected with lymphoadenopathy-associated virus human T-lymphotropic virus type III', *MMWR*, **34**, pp. 517–21.

CHAMARET, S. (1992) 'La recherche d'anticorps dans la salive et les urines', *Transcriptase*, **8**, p. 23.

CLOSEL, H. (1994) 'Révisionnisme à la une', *Journal du sida*, **60**, pp. 17–18.

DE VINCENZI, I., for the EUROPEAN STUDY GROUP ON HETEROSEXUAL TRANSMISSION OF HIV (1994) 'A longitudinal study of HIV transmission by heterosexual partners', *New England Journal of Medicine*, **331**, 6, pp. 341–6.

EDELMANN, F. (1994) 'La prévention au fil de la vie', *Journal du sida*, **62**, p. 3 and p. 51.

EUROPEAN STUDY GROUP, (1992) 'Comparison of female to male and male to female transmission of HIV in 563 stable couples', *British Medical Journal*, **304**, pp. 809–13.

FRIEDLAND, G.H. *et al.* (1986) 'Lack of transmission of HTLV III/LAV infection to household contacts of patients with AIDS or AIDS-related complex with oral candidiasis conditions', *New England Journal of Medicine*, **314**, pp. 344–9.

GIRARD, M. (1993) 'Essais de candidats vaccins anti-VIH encourageants', *Transcriptase*, **16**, pp. 6–7.

HUBERT, M. and MARQUET, J. (Eds) (1993) *Comportements sexuels et réactions au risque du SIDA en Belgique*, rapport à la Commission des communautés européennes (DG V), Brussels: Centre d'études sociologiques, Facultés universitaires Saint-Louis.

HUYNEN, PH., MARQUET, J. and HUBERT, M. (1995) 'Les Européens et le SIDA: situation actuelle et tendances', in INRA (Eds) *Les Européens et la santé publique*, Rapport pour la Commission Européenne, Brussels.

KIENY, M.-P. (1993) 'Vaccin anti-VIH: passage à la vitesse supérieure', *Transcriptase*, **17**, pp. 4–5.

LAZARSFELD, P. and KATZ, R. (1955) *The Personal Influence*, Glencoe: The Free Press.

MARQUET, J., HUBERT, M. and PETO, D. (1994) *Comportements sexuels et réactions au risque du SIDA en Belgique: spécificités bruxelloises*, rapport à la Région de Bruxelles-Capitale, Brussels: Centre d'études sociologiques, Facultés universitaires Saint-Louis.

MARQUET, J., HUBERT, M. and VAN CAMPENHOUDT, L. (1995) 'Public awareness of AIDS: discrimination and the effects of mistrust', in FITZSIMONS, D., HARDY, V. and TOLLEY, K. (Eds) *The Economic and Social Impact of AIDS in Europe*, London: Cassell.

MOATTI, J.-P., DAB, W. and POLLAK, M. (1992) 'Les Français et le SIDA', *La Recherche*, **23**, 247, pp. 1202–11.

MOATTI, J.-P., DAB, W., POLLAK, M., QUESNEL, P. and ANES, A. (1990) 'Les attitudes et comportements des français face au Sida', *La Recherche*, **23**, pp. 888–95.

MORIN, M. (1994) 'Les espaces d'évolution des représentations sociales du sida', in ANRS, *Connaissances, représentations, comportements. Sciences sociales et prévention du SIDA*, November 1994, pp. 47–53.

MOSCOVICI, S. (1983) 'The phenomenon of social representations', in FARR, R.M. and MOSCOVICI, S. (Eds) *Social representations*, Cambridge: Cambridge University Press.

MUSICCO, M. (1992) 'Quali comportamenti sessuali possono modificare il rischio di trasmissione?', in CONSIGLIO NAZIONALE DELLE RICERCHE, *Atti Prima giornata italiana di studio sulla trasmissione eterosessuale del virus HIV-1*, December 1992, pp. 48–59.

POLLAK, M. and MOATTI, J.-P. (1990) 'HIV risk perception and determinants of sexual behaviour', in HUBERT, M. (Ed.) *Sexual Behaviour and Risks of HIV Infection. Proceedings of an international workshop supported by the European Communities*, Brussels: Publications des Facultés universitaires Saint-Louis.

REBOULOT, B. (1994) 'Quid des tests salivaires?', *Journal du sida /Transcriptase*, Special issue, Autumn 1994, p. 47.

SCHÜTZ, A. (1982) *Collected papers I*, The Hague: Martinus Nijhoff (first edition 1966).

SPIEGEL, M.R. (1993) *Statistique. Cours et problèmes*, Série Schaum, Paris: McGraw-Hill (2nd edition).

SPIRA, A., BAJOS, N. and GROUPE ACSF (1993) *Les comportements sexuels en France*, Paris: La Documentation Française, Collection des rapports officiels.

STEIN, Z. (1993) 'HIV prevention: an update on the status of methods women can use', *American Journal of Public Health*, **83**, 10, pp. 1379–81.

Chapter 13

Attitudes towards People with HIV/AIDS

Elizabeth Ioannidi and Michael Haeder

Introduction

Discrimination against people with HIV/AIDS (PWHAs) has been registered widely in all parts of the world. HIV infected people have lost jobs and homes, children with AIDS have been denied access to public schools, and funeral directors have refused to handle the corpses of people who have died from AIDS (Fineberg, 1988). These 'rituals of decontamination' were rampant mainly between 1982 to 1985, the period of moral panic (Weeks, 1989). Subsequently, while earlier fears and loathing have perhaps diminished, prejudice and discrimination against PWHAs continue to be widespread (Weeks, 1989). Such tendencies persist not only among the public at large, but also among health workers, which is a much more alarming phenomenon (Hornung, Lert and Moatti, 1995). Today, as we deal with the second decade of the AIDS epidemic and the disease is continuing to spread around the world, it seems appropriate to discuss attitudes towards those who are infected, as they were expressed in various European countries.

Illness is defined by sociologists in terms 'of social situation and social behaviour, as well as in terms of biological reality' (Herzlich and Graham, 1973). As society is considered a system of social relationships and inter-actions, sickness from the social behavioural standpoint refers to a state of social dysfunction that affects the individual's relation with others. According to Parsons (1951), who first conceptualized the notion of the sick role, sickness can be classified as a form of deviant behaviour that requires legitimization and social control (Turner, 1987). Illness is considered an unnatural state of the human body, causing both physical and social dysfunction and, according to classic functionalist theorists, may be interpreted as a potential state of social 'deviance', that is, failure to conform to societal expectations and norms in some way (Lupton, 1994).

In the sociological sense, deviance is a social behaviour since it involves other people's reactions to an individual's behaviour with some kind of sanction such as social disapproval, ostracism, imprisonment or execution. Becker (1963) and Lemert (1951), who first formulated labelling theory, and Goffman (1963), who analyzed the stigma attached to various forms of deviance, agree that deviant activity leads to a re-evaluation of one's identity whereby, in being labelled as a certain 'kind' of person, a person becomes viewed and treated by others in the light of this label (Giddens, 1981).

Societies have different responses to sickness. While they have devised different forms of support – symbolic and material – that aid their members during periodic crises, with illness being one kind of crisis (Susser, Watson and Hopper, 1985), there is often a simultaneous tendency to isolate the victims of infectious and incurable diseases. The histories of leprosy, mental illness, syphilis and tuberculosis remind us of the ways in which people have behaved towards the infected members of their society (Grmek, 1983; Herzlich and Pierret, 1984). How people interpret and respond to sickness is in great part an expression of culture. This implies that in order to understand people's reactions towards sickness and the sick, one has to place them in their comparative social and historical context.

The issue of discriminatory attitudes towards PWHAs should be examined within the above theoretical framework, taking also into consideration the complexity of the syndrome itself. The concept of sickness as described above and the human response to those suffering from infectious diseases need to be linked to the multidimensionality of this disease. First, AIDS, unlike other infectious diseases that are transmitted through insects or animals or even needing special climatic requirements, is carried and transmitted by the human host. This classifies AIDS as belonging in the group of those contagious fatal diseases such as leprosy and syphilis where the sick person can also be blamed by society's members for his/her state of health, since he/she is considered responsible for spreading the disease. Second, the first people with AIDS at the start of the epidemic in Western countries were mostly homosexuals, injecting drug users and members of ethnic minorities, that is, already stigmatized social groups. According to Goffman (1963), one may talk of multiple stigmatization. Existing prejudices against these groups combined with the fear of a lethal transmissible disease lead to discriminatory practices (Hornung, Lert and Moatti, 1995; Hattich, Helminger and Hornung, 1995).

From the moment it was identified, AIDS elicited human fears and inhibitions that are linked to infectious, incurable diseases. The overwhelming fear is that of death, especially today in modern societies which try, by all means, to prolong life. As Schulman (1991) says, 'As society's response to death becomes increasingly phobic, so, too, is the response to those infected with an incurable, invariably fatal disease. They force, after all, an unwelcome recognition of one's own mortality, with its anticipation of a comfortless death.' In the case of AIDS, infected people, who are already labelled as 'dangerous', are given the additional label of 'high risk' – and this is followed by the stigmas that such diseases carry, resulting in discriminatory actions expressed against them.

Another important factor that should be taken into consideration in the case of AIDS is the false information that was spread about the origin of the disease. It is evident that from the start the public was alarmed and eager to learn more about this new epidemic. The media with its constant flow of information (indeed, AIDS has become known as the 'first media disease' (Street, 1988)) on the one hand provided useful information, but on the other hand stimulated many false ideas and unnecessary fears, attributing something mysterious to it.

It can be argued that mystery is linked to fear. As Susan Sontag wrote, in *Illness as a Metaphor* (1979), 'Any disease that is treated as a mystery and acutely enough feared will be felt morally, if not literally, contagious. Contact with someone afflicted with a disease regarded as a mysterious malevolency inevitably feels like a trespass; worse like the violation of a taboo.' Moreover, AIDS is an illness in which the symptoms are not visible initially, in contrast, for example, to leprosy. The fact that an infected person can keep his or her situation secret from others can create additional fear and is a matter that has led to public discussion concerning the right of infected people to remain anonymous.

All these factors lead to the development of highly variable attitudes against infected people which are not stable over time. In the 16 years since AIDS was first recognized, people's attitudes have changed from 'hysterical', as exhibited in such behaviour as refusing to serve lesbians and gay men in restaurants and theatre personnel refusing to work with gay actors, to more tolerant attitudes by the late 1980s with the formation of many organized bodies willing to aid and support PWHAs (Weeks, 1989).

In this chapter an effort is made to present some of the main trends in discriminatory attitudes which might contribute to discriminatory behaviour in the European countries examined. First we will describe people's attitudes towards PWHAs as recorded in four European surveys. An attempt is then made to discuss these attitudes, although the limited data do not permit wider cross-national comparison and thus interpretations within the theoretical framework described above can be only partially attempted.

Methods

The European data examined in order to study the similarities and differences in attitudes towards people with HIV and AIDS reflect not only the situation of each country at the moment the research was undertaken, but also the variety of ways in which discriminatory attitudes can be assessed. The range of

Table 13.1 *Complete question wordings: Attitudes towards PWHAs*

Belgium 1993	France 1992	Germany East 1990
People with AIDS must be isolated from the rest of the population: 'agree totally', 'agree somewhat'	People with AIDS must be isolated from the rest of the population: 'agree completely', 'agree more than disagree'	If you learned that one of your friends was infected with the virus, what would your reaction be? 'turn away from him'
An employer must be able to sack a person who has AIDS: 'agree totally', 'agree somewhat'	Sacking a person with AIDS is legitimate: 'agree completely', 'agree more than disagree'	
Would you accept to work or study in the company of a seropositive person? 'no'	If you knew that someone was seropositive, would you accept to work with him/her? 'no'	
Would you accept to have an AIDS patient centre open next door to you? 'no'	If an association wanted to open a centre for AIDS patients in your building or a neighbouring house, would you: 'more disagree than agree', 'disagree completely'	
Would you leave your children or grandchildren in the company of a seropositive person? 'no'	If you knew that someone was seropositive, would you accept to leave your children or grandchildren with him/her? 'no'	
Medical staff must be able to refuse to take care of people with AIDS: 'agree totally', 'agree somewhat'	The medical profession (nurses and doctors) must be able to refuse to care for AIDS patients: 'agree completely', 'agree more than disagree'	
To avoid being rejected, a seropositive person has the right to keep his or her diagnosis a secret: 'disagree more or less', 'disagree totally'	A seropositive individual is right to keep the diagnosis secret in order to avoid discrimination: 'more disagree than agree', 'disagree completely'	
People who know that they are seropositives and have unprotected sex without warning their partners should be prosecuted: 'agree totally', 'agree somewhat'	People who know that they are seropositives and have sex without informing their partners should be prosecuted: 'agree completely'; 'agree more than disagree'	
	I am going to read you a number of proposals. Please tell me if they do, might, or do not apply to you: a friend who gets AIDS will continue to be my friend: 'no'	

different indicators used in these studies also shows the range of ways in which discrimination can manifest itself. The data available for cross-national comparisons of discriminatory attitudes in Europe are limited, which contrasts with the abundance of data available concerning knowledge of HIV/AIDS. Because of the various kinds of discriminatory attitudes and the limited availability of data for our analysis, only selected aspects are indicated in the findings. The tendency to want to segregate people with HIV and AIDS, the right of infected people to keep their situation secret, the attitudes of people towards medical professionals and AIDS transmission, and the possibility of prosecuting infected people who do not warn their partners are some of the aspects that were examined by the four European surveys, namely Athens–KABP (1989), Belgium (1993), France–KABP (1992) and East Germany (1990), that we selected for comparison.

It has to be emphasized that the selection of indicators from the different surveys was not systematic or guided by any given theory. Although the surveys include similar questions on discriminatory attitudes, differences in the wording of the questions (see Tables 13.1, 13.2), the different years that surveys were conducted, and the variety of study designs permit only minimal discussion of the trends in each country. It should be noted also that the Greek survey was carried out in Athens only. Moreover, questions on discriminatory attitudes were incomplete and did not cover the whole spectrum of issues relating to discrimination. The methodological constraints imposed by this diversity do not permit us to compute a European index of discriminatory attitudes for cross-cultural analysis.

Despite this major obstacle, we were able to obtain an overall impression from the data provided from the four European surveys. An effort has also been made to present some conclusions based on the discrimination indicators from the national surveys and some common variables built the same way

Table 13.2 *Complete question wordings: Attitudes towards medical professionals with AIDS*

Athens 1989	France 1992
Would you continue visiting a doctor or dentist who accepts in his office AIDS carriers/patients? 'no'	If you learnt that your doctor was treating a number of AIDS patients, would you continue to go to him? 'no'
	If you learnt that your dentist was treating a number of AIDS patients, would you continue to go to him? 'no'
Would you visit a doctor or dentist that you know is an AIDS carrier? Tell me first about the doctor, then about the dentist: 'no'	If you learnt that your (family) doctor was himself/herself contaminated with the AIDS virus, would you continue to go to him/her? 'no'
	If you learnt that your dentist was himself/herself contaminated with the AIDS virus, would you continue to go to him/her? 'no'

into all surveys. In this way some trends concerning the relationship between certain demographic characteristics on the one hand and the phenomenon of discrimination on the other can be detected.

Cross-national Comparisons of Discriminatory Attitudes in Europe

There are many different ways in which PWHAs may be disadvantaged or discriminated against. Such kinds of discrimination are clustered particularly in the fields of employment, housing, everyday social contacts and interactions, and care for AIDS patients. It is not possible to cover all potential kinds of discrimination with the help of only a few indicators, as our analysis of the indicators which are included in the surveys on AIDS in Europe shows. Moreover, only four of the surveys selected actually contain questions on discriminatory attitudes, with the focus being on very different aspects of discrimination. This permits a cross-national comparison of limited dimensions only.

This section therefore investigates differences and similarities in discriminatory attitudes in relation to four topics, namely, a) segregation, b) AIDS transmission and medical professionals, c) management of information about seropositivity, and d) prosecution of infected person for not warning a partner. Belgium and France are the only two countries where data are available on all these topics. References to Athens and East Germany survey findings will be made when possible.

The discriminatory indicators in each national survey were cross-tabulated against the following common variables: 1) age, 2) gender, 3) educational level, and 4) occupation. The indicators presented in the following tables were chosen from the Belgian and French surveys. The differences in the levels of agreement between the segregation indicators and the indicators of other forms of discrimination appear clearly in Tables 13.3 and 13.4.

Segregation

Only a small number of people in Belgium and France (where similar questions were asked) seem to fear proximity to seropositive persons. Only 7.8 per cent of the Belgian survey respondents stated that they would not accept working or studying with a seropositive person and an even lower percentage (2.8 per cent) of French survey respondents said that they would not accept

Table 13.3 *Segregation of PWHAs in Belgium and France*

		'agree to isolate AIDS patients'		'agree to sack AIDS patients'		'disagree to work with a seropositive person'		'don't accept an AIDS patient centre next door to him/her'		'don't accept to leave the children in the company of a seropositive person'	
		B93	F92	B93	F92	B93	F92	B93	F92	B93	F92
Total	%	4.7	5.6	6.5	3.7	7.8	2.8	17.0	9.2	33.0	20.7
	N	1404	1321	1400	1324	1397	1321	1324	1304	1409	1319
Gender											
Men	%	5.2	6.8	7.0	2.6	8.8	3.1	18.9	11.4	35.4	22.6
	N	673	632	686	654	682	677	683	667	681	664
Women	%	4.3	4.7	5.9	4.8	6.8	2.5	13.3	6.8	31.0	18.7
	N	721	681	729	646	721	680	722	662	723	658
Age											
18–19	%	0.4	15.7	0.0	10.3	3.7	5.6	15.4	8.8	16.5	17.4
	N	250	51	–	49	81	54	91	45	85	46
20–24	%	3.7	4.1	6.8	3.1	7.8	0.2	13.0	6.0	29.9	15.1
	N	243	220	235	226	231	500	231	217	231	219
25–29	%	5.7	5.2	8.9	3.3	9.2	3.6	14.9	10.0	38.1	17.9
	N	211	212	202	212	207	222	208	210	207	212

Table 13.3 *(cont.)*

		'agree to isolate AIDS patients'		'agree to sack AIDS patients'		'disagree to work with a seropositive person'		'don't accept an AIDS patient centre next door to him/her'		'don't accept to leave the children in the company of a seropositive person'	
		B93	F92	B93	F92	B93	F92	B93	F92	B93	F92
30–39	%	2.8	3.9	4.4	2.9	6.9	2.9	16.7	9.1	31.7	17.4
	N	464	436	455	448	449	448	449	440	451	443
40–49	%	7.6	7.3	8.5	4.2	8.8	3.5	17.4	10.5	37.2	29.4
	N	434	397	424	405	432	400	431	400	430	398
Education											
Low	%	8.4	8.0	11.0	4.7	9.5	3.8	16.5	12.0	39.4	25.8
	N	321	812	327	808	326	816	327	808	325	810
Medium	%	5.4	1.5	6.3	1.0	10.2	1.2	18.8	4.8	35.3	11.3
	N	519	267	524	200	520	250	521	229	521	230
High	%	2.0	2.0	4.0	2.2	4.5	1.5	13.2	4.7	27.6	14.1
	N	500	350	550	273	555	267	2068	277	558	270
Place of residence											
Rural	%	5.1	–	3.1	–	7.0	–	5.7	–	33.7	–
	N	59	–	65	–	57	–	53	–	50	–
Small towns	%	4.9	–	6.9	–	8.4	–	18.8	–	34.0	–
	N	898	–	899	–	893	–	899	–	900	–
Towns	%	4.1	–	6.2	–	7.1	–	12.6	–	31.3	–
	N	293	–	290	–	282	–	286	–	281	–
Cities	%	4.9	–	5.8	–	6.0	–	10.0	–	31.4	–
	N	184	–	172	–	167	–	170	–	175	–

Table 13.4   *Other opinions on PWHAs in Belgium and France*

		'do accept the refusal of medical staff to care for AIDS patients'		'disagree with the seropositive person who keeps the diagnosis secret'		'agree to prosecute seropositive person who has sex without warning partner'	
		B93	F92	B93	F92	B93	F92
Total	%	14.0	11.2	64.4	30.5	81.6	66.6
	N	1379	1321	1404	1321	1404	1320
Gender							
Men	%	16.1	11.5	60.5	30.9	84.9	71.1
	N	677	670	679	663	680	664
Women	%	11.5	10.9	68.1	30.1	78.6	61.9
	N	722	661	724	658	724	658
Age							
18–19	%	17.9	13.2	60.8	30.1	75.3	71.4
	N	84	45	86	50	85	48
20–24	%	12.9	10.6	57.3	30.0	86.8	67.3
	N	217	217	232	220	233	218
25–29	%	12.0	13.4	64.0	29.8	80.5	70.5
	N	208	209	206	208	206	210
30–39	%	12.9	9.9	66.9	31.4	81.2	66.8
	N	450	444	451	446	451	445
40–49	%	15.5	11.7	66.6	30.2	81.1	63.2
	N	426	402	428	401	428	399
Education							
Low	%	15.2	10.9	70.0	32.1	87.6	70.1
	N	322	807	324	785	324	810
Medium	%	16.3	8.8	66.0	34.3	80.3	65.5
	N	521	227	521	227	522	227
High	%	10.5	14.4	59.5	26.3	79.5	57.9
	N	552	264	556	266	557	266
Place of residence							
Rural	%	11.5	–	59.8	–	82.8	–
	N	52	–	50	–	51	–
Small towns	%	15.9	–	68.4	–	81.1	–
	N	899	–	898	–	899	–
Towns	%	9.4	–	62.1	–	83.4	–
	N	277	–	282	–	162	–
Cities	%	10.0	–	49.1	–	81.2	–
	N	170	–	173	–	174	–

Table 13.5 *Athenian and East German results*

		'would turn away from a friend if found out that he or she was infected with HIV' Germany East 1990	'would not continue visiting a doctor or dentist who accepts AIDS patients' Athens 1989	'would not continue visiting a doctor or dentist who is AIDS carrier' Athens 1989
Total	%	8.1	60.1	69.4
	N	1024	953	952
Gender				
Men	%	10.1	56.9	68.1
	N	386	844	480
Women	%	6.8	63.4	70.6
	N	632	744	472
Age				
18–19	%	10.4	71.2	68.5
	N	48	73	73
20–24	%	6.8	57.0	58.1
	N	162	172	172
25–29	%	9.0	38.18	69.1
	N	189	265	262
30–39	%	6.2	56.6	72.7
	N	387	362	362
40–49	%	11.1	68.0	73.8
	N	234	172	172
Education				
Low	%	17.5	69.5	79.2
	N	80	197	197
Medium	%	8.7	60.3	65.9
	N	644	355	355
High	%	4.3	50.5	63.3
	N	302	305	305
Place of residence				
Rural	%	11.3	–	–
	N	204	–	–
Small towns	%	8.7	–	–
	N	506	–	–
Towns	%	6.1	–	–
	N	230	–	–
Cities	%	2.6	–	–
	N	77	–	–

working with a seropositive person. However, when respondents were asked about leaving their children or grandchildren in the company of a seropositive person, the percentages of those who disagreed were much higher (33.0 per cent in Belgium and 20.7 per cent in France).

When asked, few people were in favour of denying certain rights to PWHAs. Only 6.5 per cent of the respondents in Belgium agreed 'completely' or 'somewhat' that an employer should be able to sack a person who has AIDS. A slightly lower percentage of French survey respondents held similar attitudes, with only 3.7 per cent believing ('agree completely' or 'agree more than disagree') that sacking a person with AIDS is legitimate (the question was basically the same, albeit phrased somewhat differently). The desire to isolate infected people is not shared by many people. In the Belgian survey, 4.7 per cent of the respondents agreed 'completely' or 'somewhat' that people with AIDS must be isolated from the rest of the population, while 5.6 per cent of the French survey respondents agreed ('agree completely' or 'agree more than disagree') to the statement that people with AIDS must be isolated from the rest of the population. Once again, these figures are very close.

The tendency to segregate infected people was also examined indirectly by asking if respondents would accept having an AIDS patient centre open next door to them. The negative response rates to this question were 17.0 per cent in the Belgian study and 9.2 per cent in the France–KABP study.

The East German survey tackled the segregation of HIV positive people differently by looking at solidarity among friends when one becomes seropositive. In this survey 10.4 per cent of respondents said that they would turn away from a friend if they found out that he or she was infected with HIV, whereas 17.1 per cent declared that they would spend time with him or her more intensively if they found out about the situation. These two answers illustrate the human response to the sick as presented in the theoretical framework. AIDS, as an incurable, infectious disease, elicits different feelings in human beings. On the one hand it stresses the need for support that a sick person should be offered, while on the other hand the fear of the fatal disease along with the blame attached to the infected person turn a number of people away, even from a friend. Only 0.6 per cent of the French sample answered 'no' to the following proposition: 'A friend who gets AIDS will continue to be my friend.'

AIDS Transmission and Medical Professionals

At the end of the 1980s, when instances of people who had been infected by dentists or during surgery had been reported by the media, people were asked whether they would visit their doctors under certain circumstances. In the Athenian survey 60 per cent of the people said that they would not continue visiting a doctor or dentist who accepted carriers/AIDS patients in his office (12 per cent said that they were not sure or did not know). By contrast, in the French survey, only 4.6 per cent reported that they would not continue to go to their (family) doctor if they knew that he/she was treating AIDS patients, and 30.9 per cent would not visit a dentist who accepted AIDS patients. The French survey refers specifically to the family doctor, while in the Athenian survey reference is made to doctors of all kinds in general, including dentists. In Athens 69.4 per cent of people would not continue visiting a doctor or dentist if they knew that he was HIV positive (6.6 per cent said that they were not sure or did not know). Older respondents tend to be more hesitant. In the French survey 18.7 per cent would not continue to go to their doctor if they knew that he/she was infected and 39.8 per cent would not visit their dentist. In the Athenian survey, the question referred to doctors and dentists together.

Management of Information about Seropositivity

As mentioned earlier, AIDS differs from other infectious diseases in that its symptoms are not visible from the moment a person is infected. Infected people have the choice of keeping their situation secret if they wish to. But does the public agree that people should have this right? In Belgium 64.4 per cent of the respondents stated that they 'did not really agree' or 'disagreed completely' with the proposition that a seropositive person had the right to keep his or her diagnosis a secret in order to avoid being rejected. In the French survey 30.5 per cent of the respondents ('more disagree than agree' and 'disagree completely') believed that a person did not have the right to keep his or her diagnosis secret.

Prosecution of Infected People for Not Warning Partner

In the Belgian survey 81.6 per cent of the respondents ('agree completely' or 'agree somewhat') contended that people who know that they are seropositive and have unprotected sex without warning their partners should be prosecuted. The French survey respondents' position on this issue appears to be more liberal. Of the French respondents, only 66.6 per cent agreed ('agree completely' or 'agree more than disagree') that a seropositive person should be prosecuted if he or she had sex without warning his or her partner. But here we must bear in mind that the Belgian question introduced the notion of *unprotected* sex, whereas the French question drew no distinction between protected and unprotected sex.

Summarizing responses concerning the attitudes examined, we can argue that statements that included drastic forms of discrimination, and more specifically the idea of segregation, met with low agreement. The rates of agreement with the statements about punishing a seropositive person who had sex without warning the partner and allowing an HIV seropositive person to keep his or her diagnosis secret are higher. There consequently appears to be a general tendency for most people to be tolerant and not seek to promote drastic solutions for the HIV-infected. For example, only a small number of people believe that those infected must be isolated from the rest of the population, and only a few would not accept working or studying alongside a seropositive person.

The degree of discrimination depends on both the relationship between the respondent and the infected person and the way in which questions are asked. Thus a question referring directly to the interviewee's actions and an impersonal question referring to other people's actions trigger different answers. For example, sacking a person from work has no consequences for the person being asked – unless he or she is an employer or is HIV seropositive – since it refers to an action that a third party should take. As a result, people can express liberal attitudes. In contrast, when people were asked about leaving their children or grandchildren in the company of a PWHA, their personal involvement made them more hesitant and they gave negative answers at higher rates. The close contact that hypothetically exists between an HIV-infected doctor or dentist and the interviewee refers to a situation with possible personal consequences; here people are more careful in their responses. It is evident that when people feel they are not in a situation where they could be infected, that is when they are expressing their views about people who are HIV-positive in general or are merely spatially close to an HIV-positive person (studying or working together), then they appear very liberal. On the other hand, in the topics concerning medical professionals, the management of information about seropositivity, and prosecution of infected people for not warning their partners, respondents felt more involved in the sense that they could become infected themselves or that they would not have access to information concerning the seropositivity of someone around them. In this case, the personal involvement in a situation provokes discriminatory attitudes to a much greater degree.

Conclusions

As a result of this analysis it is possible to describe the main trends in the four European surveys under study that seem to be connected with discriminatory attitudes towards people with HIV/AIDS. The social response to AIDS, even though unique from several perspectives, is little different from other life-threatening, incurable diseases of the past. The way we interpret illness organizes the ways in which we respond. Diseases which have become the bearers of sexual meaning 'have been shaped by a host of moral assumptions about the sexual behavior of those they affected. These assumptions insensibly infiltrate medical theories and responses, and in turn shape and reshape popular attitudes' (Weeks, 1989, referring to Mort, 1987).

When seen in this light, attitudes towards PWHAs expressed by the Europeans who participated in the four surveys examined in this chapter appear to indicate that there is greater tolerance of, and less overall negativeness towards, infected persons than reported in the first years of the epidemic, which were characterized by a kind of mass hysteria (Weeks, 1989). According to Weeks (1989), the major reason for this change 'was the increasing evidence that AIDS was not just a disease of execrated minorities but a health threat on a global scale, and one which in world terms, largely affected heterosexuals. This initiated the period in which we now live, one in which the dominant response has been crisis management.' However, fear of a fatal contagious disease is not easily overcome, as is evident when people are posited as being in closer contact with seropositive persons. Then, as in the case of the infected doctor/dentist, people are more reluctant to express positive views, preferring to keep a distance between themselves and the medical professionals.

However, to be able to interpret such attitudes towards medical professionals, one must also consider that doctor–patient relationships are cultural experiences. Anthropology has revealed the cultural variations in medical myths, beliefs and practices that exist, and the ways they are related to the overall pattern of values in each culture (Herzlich and Graham, 1973; Lupton, 1994).

While people do not desire to isolate PWHAs, on the other hand they disagree with the statement that infected persons have the right to keep their diagnosis secret. With this response, indirectly, people might be expressing their desire to know about the HIV positive people with whom they are in close contact. But why do people want to know who is infected? Perhaps this response reflects the tendency to 'label' and treat the sick person in the light of this label.

As the surveys reviewed here show, age seems not to influence discriminatory attitudes and there are few gender-related differences in discrimination. Occupation also seems not to have a clear influence on discriminatory attitudes. However, educational level plays an important role in attitudes towards HIV infected persons. A higher level of education is related to a lower level of expressed discriminatory attitudes while a lower level of education is related to higher levels of discrimination. It can be argued that two factors influence the degree of tolerance for infected people. First, there is the nature of the relationship posited between the interviewee and a seropositive person. People appear to be very liberal when expressing attitudes in general towards other people's behaviour with regard to infected people, whereas when the posited relationship is more personal and more direct, discriminatory attitudes reach their highest rates. Second, there is the educational level, with the less educated being more likely to have discriminatory attitudes and to search for drastic solutions.

In conclusion, it can be said that although people currently appear to be tolerant and liberal in their attitudes towards PWHAs, discriminatory attitudes still exist. AIDS as a disease, some forms of behaviour, and some individuals are seen as health threats for people and society. Personal threats to oneself and one's family provoke the greatest intolerance, while higher educational levels seem to diminish negative and discriminatory attitudes.

References

BECKER, H., (1963) *The Outsiders*, Glencoe, Ill.: Free Press.

FINEBERG, H. (1988) 'The social dimensions of AIDS', *Scientific American*, October, pp. 128–34.

GIDDENS, A. (Ed.) (1981) *Contemporary Social Theory*, London: Macmillan Press.

GOFFMAN, E. (1963) *Stigma Notes on the Management of the Spoiled Identity*, Englewood Cliffs, NJ: Prentice Hall.

GRMEK, M.D. (1983) *Les maladies à l'aube de la civilisation occidentale: recherches sur la réalité pathologique dans le monde grec, préhistorique, archaïque et classique*, Paris: Payot.

HATTICH, A., HELMINGER, A. and HORNUNG, R. (1995) 'Predictors of discrimination against AIDS patients and cancer patients: a multivariate comparison', in FRIEDRICH, D. and HECKMANN, W. (Eds) *AIDS in Europe – The Behavioural Aspect, Vol. 5: Cure and Care*, Berlin: Editions Sigma.

HERZLICH, C. and GRAHAM, D. (1973) *Health and Illness*, London: Academic Press.

HERZLICH, C. and PIERRET, J. (1984) *Malades d'hier, malades d'aujourd'hui: de la mort collective au devoir de guérison*, Paris: Payot.

HORNUNG, R., LERT, F. and MOATTI, J.P. (1995) 'Health services: perception, communication and discrimination', in FRIEDRICH, D. and HECKMANN, W. (Eds) *AIDS in Europe – The Behavioral Aspect, Vol. 5: Cure and Care*, Berlin: Editions Sigma.

LEMERT, E.M. (1951) *Social Pathology*, New York: McGraw-Hill.

LUPTON, D., (1994) *Medicine as Culture, Illness, Disease and the Body in Western Societies*, London: Sage.

MORT, F. (1987) *Dangerous Sexualities: medico-moral politics in England since 1830*, London: Routledge and Kegan Paul.

PARSONS, T. (1951) *The Social System*, London: Routledge and Kegan Paul.

SCHULMAN, D. (1991) 'AIDS discrimination: its nature, meaning and function', in McKENZIE, N. (Ed.) *AIDS: Social, Political, Ethical Issues*, New York: Meridian.

SONTAG, S. (1979) *Illness as a Metaphor*, London: Lane.

Elizabeth Ioannidi and Michael Haeder

STREET, J. (1988) 'British Government policies in the UK', *Parliamentary Affairs*, **41**, pp. 490–508.

SUSSER, M., WATSON, W. and HOPPER, K. (1985) *Sociology in Medicine*, New York: Oxford University Press.

TURNER, B.(1987) *Medical Power and Social Knowledge*, London: Sage.

WEEKS, J. (1989) 'AIDS: the intellectual agenda', in AGGLETON, P., HART, G. and DAVIES, P. (Eds) *AIDS: Social Representations, Social Practices*, London: The Farmer Press.

Chapter 14

Knowledge and Discrimination: What Kind of Relationship?

Jacques Marquet and Nathalie Beltzer

Introduction

Common sense tells us that discriminatory attitudes towards people who are HIV seropositive are a consequence of inaccurate knowledge about HIV transmission and means of protection. In this chapter we shall first examine whether there is a relationship between knowledge and discrimination. We shall also explore the possible existence of factors influencing both the level of knowledge about the disease and the degree of tolerance of persons with HIV or AIDS (PWHAs).

Such factors seem to exist. Preceding analyses (Chapters 12 and 13) have already shown that level of education is correlated both with knowledge of the disease and discriminatory attitudes towards PWHAs. As a rule, people who are relatively unknowledgeable about HIV and AIDS and those with feelings of discrimination were over-represented among the least educated respondents. Here, we shall explore the possible influences of three other factors, namely, mistrust, subjective perception of risk, and knowing a PWHA, on both knowledge of HIV/AIDS and discriminatory attitudes.

Mistrust

It has been shown elsewhere in Chapter 12 that a sizeable number of people express reservations and doubts about the validity of official medical discourse. Here, we should like to test whether what might be interpreted as ignorance of the disease might not reflect mistrust of prevention messages rather than a lack of information. First, respondents with very little or no

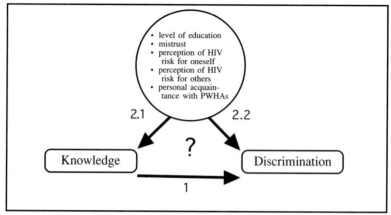

Notes:
1. Hypothesis: The level of knowledge explains the discriminatory attitudes.
2.1 Hypothesis: Some external factors influence knowledge.
2.2 Hypothesis: Some external factors influence the discriminatory attitudes.

Figure 14.1 *Knowledge and discrimination: what kind of relationship?*

inaccurate knowledge express scepticism of specific prevention messages related to HIV transmission routes. Second, there seems to be a mistrust of
experts that distances the subject from scientific discourse and from prevention messages, unless social distance from experts explains the mistrust.
This also leads us to wonder about the possibility of a relationship between
mistrust of prevention messages and discriminatory attitudes, Conklin (1975)
has shown in his work on criminality that mistrust of neighbours and foreigners can engender the desire to distance oneself from the community as a
whole.

Subjective Perception of Risk

Moatti, Beltzer and Dab (1993) have shown that information-based HIV
transmission prevention measures have improved knowledge of the disease,
fostered solidarity with PWHAs, and raised awareness of the existence of
risk. Ekstrand and her colleagues (Ekstrand and Coates, 1990; Ekstrand
et al., 1992) have shown improved knowledge of the disease to be one of the
factors lessening perceived personal risk of HIV infection. One may hypothesize that access to accurate technical information enables each person to
evaluate more adequately his or her own risk. Accordingly, the degree of
knowledge would influence the subjective perception of risk. While it is
difficult to imagine that perception of a phenomenon of whatever nature does

not involve elements of knowledge, the relationship between the two phenomena is obviously much more complex. First of all, knowledge of the disease comes into play as only one element in the person's stock of representations of the disease. What is more, this element is sometimes hard to isolate from other factors tied to risk perception, such as attitudes towards disease and opinions about PWHAs. Next, one must consider the possibility that knowledge and risk perception interact with each other over time. A certain knowledge influences perception of the risk, but a certain perception of the risk may also determine how motivated a person is to seek (or accept) additional information, and thus ultimately impinges on levels of knowledge.

Regarding discrimination, risk awareness can lead to the stigmatization of PWHAs through heightened fear. Heightened risk perception, or the fact that individuals perceive a higher risk of being infected now than previously, can heighten apprehensiveness and trigger rejection or stigmatization of PWHAs. Allard (1989), for example, has shown that subscribing to coercive policies and attitudes of intolerance appear to be governed by a clear perception of individual risk of infection and society's vulnerability to the epidemic.

Knowing a PWHA

The question is whether the respondents who know PWHAs were more or less likely than other respondents to overestimate transmission risks associated with such casual actions as kissing or drinking, and the degree of protection of such ineffective practices as washing after sex or taking the pill, the hypothesis being that individuals who know a PWHA will have improved knowledge of the illness. A related question is whether proximity to the disease influences attitudes towards PWHAs. On the one hand, the tendency to reject PWHAs could be strengthened by making HIV and AIDS more real. On the other hand, such proximity could breed familiarity and thus reduce rejection. Knowing a PWHA probably has an effect on risk perception, so we can expect these two factors to be intertwined. Knowing a PWHA seems to trigger more frequent thoughts about the possibility of one being infected oneself and makes the impact of the disease on society as a whole more worrying. Analysis of the data shows that respondents who reported knowing one or more PWHAs generally perceived greater risks to themselves as well as expressing heightened overall fear of the risk.[1] These correlations must be taken with caution, however, for if we look at a finer measurement of proximity to the disease by separating respondents who know a close friend or relative with AIDS from those who have a more distant relationship, perceptions of risk seem to be highest among the latter. This suggests that while risk perception and proximity to the disease – defined as knowing or not knowing one or more PWHAs – have much in common, they also differ in several respects. Consequently, the specific influence of proximity to the disease on knowledge about HIV transmission routes, means of protection and discriminatory attitudes towards PWHAs must be taken into account.

To clarify the concepts we use in this chapter, we shall first describe the main indicators. We shall then investigate the existence of possible connections between knowledge and discrimination, and explore possible common factors. More specifically, we shall study to what extent mistrust, awareness of HIV/AIDS risk, and proximity to the disease are related both to knowledge of the disease and to attitudes (solidarity/discrimination) towards those effected. In assessing these relationships, it will of course not be possible to establish causes and effects. Unlike other chapters, we shall not focus on comparisons between countries, but use data from the various studies to explore the dynamic relationship between knowledge and discrimination.

Method

Our conclusions derive from the study of bivariate cross-tabulations, although multivariate analyses would have been helpful to account for each factor's importance and how the various factors are associated. Unfortunately, multivariate analyses were not possible because data files were not available and many of the investigations under consideration studied only one or the other of the factors covered by these hypotheses. Consequently, this chapter remains largely exploratory.

Knowledge

As shown in Chapter 12, almost the entire population in each of the countries under study knows about HIV transmission routes, that is, sexual transmission, transmission through injection and vertical transmission. So it is not possible to discriminate – in a statistical sense – between people on the basis of responses to these questions. However, besides these very general indicators, a certain number of people are found to fear alleged 'transmission routes' despite prevention messages to the contrary. Many surveys therefore include questions about these so-called 'false transmission routes'. Similarly, a large majority of the populations under study was found to believe in the efficacy of condoms as a means of protecting against HIV. However, there also exists a string of practices that specialists strongly condemn but a segment of the population considers effective in protecting against HIV transmission.

In this chapter, we look at knowledge by means of two aggregate indices, one of which refers to erroneous knowledge of HIV transmission routes and the other to erroneous knowledge of means of protection. If we consider that the genuine modes of transmission, that is unprotected sex, sharing needles, and vertical transmission, and the effective means of protection, such as abstinence, mutual faithfulness and condom use, are not taken into account, these two aggregate indices measure knowledge (or inaccurate knowledge) 'on the margins'. The indices have the merit of underlining common trends and smoothing scatter. They reflect the variations in the questions upon which they were built. Some methodological remarks concerning variations in question wordings that were discussed earlier (Chapter 12) likewise apply to the indicators' construction. To avoid repetition, the reader is referred to that chapter for a more detailed discussion of this matter.

Risk of HIV Transmission

The comparative analyses described earlier in Chapter 12 focused on the most frequently studied 'false transmission routes', that is, kissing (or saliva) (K), mosquito bites (M), drinking from the glass or eating off the plate of an HIV seropositive person or a person with AIDS (D), and using public toilets (T). Taking the official position that these situations carry no risk of infection as our starting point, we then built an aggregate KMDT index that could be applied to all the surveys that included at least three of the above-mentioned four items. Strictly speaking, the KMDT index was constructed only for the Belgian, Dutch, French–KABP and East German 1990 surveys. We should talk about a KMD indicator for the Spanish survey and an MDT indicator for the Athens–PR survey.

The index varied on a scale of 0 to 12, depending on the number of 'inaccurate' responses (not complying with the messages of preventive medicine) given by the respondents. As 12 is the least common multiple of three and four, a scale that varies from 0 to 12 enables one to compare the results of surveys that include either three or four of the items of interest. A minimum score of 0 means that the respondent correctly felt none of the situations under study carried a risk of HIV transmission.

Means of Protection

The comparative analysis presented in Chapter 12 focused on four inaccurate means of protection, namely, coitus interruptus (C), washing after sex (W), taking the pill (P), and belief in the existence of a vaccine or therapy that can cure a person of AIDS (T). The official stand in prevention is that it is very dangerous to present these practices as being even slightly effective in protecting against HIV transmission. However, since the partial efficacy of coitus interruptus is currently recognized, we constructed an aggregate WPT index that varied on a scale from 0 to 12, depending on the number of 'inaccurate' responses (not aligned with the messages of preventive medicine). The scale from 0 to 12 was chosen to allow comparability with the KMDT scale. A medically incorrect response with regard to one of the three indicators yielded a score of 4; incorrect responses to two of the indicators yielded a score of 8; and incorrect responses to three of the indicators yielded the maximum of 12. A minimum score of 0 means that the respondent felt that in accordance with medical messages all the practices under study were totally ineffective.

Discrimination

To respect the complexity of the subject of discrimination (Chapter 13; Hubert and Marquet, 1993, pp. 108–14), we shall break it down into two subdimensions, namely, segregation and the management of information about seropositivity. For the purposes of our analysis we define segregation as the manifest will of an individual to distance him/herself and possibly relatives from PWHAs and/or people who are regularly in contact with the latter. The analyses concerning discrimination focus on the data culled from the Belgian and French surveys, as they examined this topic in greatest detail. The four other surveys that considered this topic will be referred to where appiopriate.

The items with fairly similar wordings in the Belgian and French surveys that carry this idea of distancing oneself either directly or indirectly are:

1) 'People with AIDS must be isolated from the rest of the population' (B/F);
2) 'An employer must be able to sack a person who has AIDS' (B), 'Sacking a person with AIDS is legitimate' (F);
3) 'Would you accept working or studying with a seropositive person?' (B), 'If you knew that someone was seropositive, would you accept working with him/her?' (F);
4) 'Would you accept having an AIDS patient centre open next door to you?' (B), 'If an association wanted to open a centre for AIDS patients in your building or a neighbouring house, would you agree completely, more agree than disagree, more disagree than agree or disagree completely?' (F);
5) 'Would you leave your children or grandchildren with a seropositive person?' (B), 'If you knew that someone was seropositive, would you accept leaving your children or grandchildren with him/her?' (F).

Until now, the management of information about serological status has been studied basically from two angles, the HIV test's applicability (should testing without consent be allowed or not?) and the communication of test results (should partners be informed of each others' serological status?). The items with fairly similar wordings in the Belgian and French surveys are:

1) 'Getting the person's consent before performing a (HIV) test should be mandatory' (B), 'Should getting the person's consent be indispensable before testing for AIDS?' (F);
2) 'If your partner were seropositive, you should be informed even without his/her consent' (B), 'When a doctor knows that a patient is seropositive or ill, he should inform the patient's spouse' (F);
3) 'People who know that they are seropositive and have unprotected sex without warning their partners should be prosecuted' (B), 'People who know that they are seropositive and have sex without informing their partners should be prosecuted' (F).

Mistrust

The Belgian and Dutch surveys were the only ones to include the idea of mistrust. With regard to the Belgian survey, we shall distinguish two different types of mistrust: vigilant mistrust and retreating mistrust. The Belgian survey's pre-test (see Hubert and Marquet, 1993) showed that some respondents tried to say they knew but were sceptical of the 'official' position concerning various transmission routes. Their hesitations were recorded in an additional category called 'they say it is not possible, but I am sceptical'. To avoid soliciting such answers, however, the respondent was not aware of the possibility given to the investigator to note his or her scepticism. Such attitudes are called 'vigilant mistrust'. The term 'retreating mistrust' was coined to sum up the 'feeling of vague, general mistrust' or 'retreating from the scene'. This type of mistrust appeared to be totally independent of what we have called 'vigilant mistrust' (sceptical knowledge of the official line). 'Retreating mistrust' was measured by total agreement with the proposition: 'You can't trust anyone anymore'. (For a fuller discussion of this concept, see Marquet, Hubert and Van Campenhoudt, 1995.)

The Dutch survey contained the following two propositions concerning the faith respondents placed in AIDS prevention messages:

1) 'I get the impression that experts don't exactly know how one can prevent AIDS';
2) 'The information about how you can prevent getting infected with the AIDS virus is usually reliable'.

Table 14.1 *Individual risk perception by age*[1]

	Age of respondents			
	18–24	25–29	30–39	40–49
Athens 89–KABP				
What are the chances that you yourself might catch AIDS? Would you say that it is	(n = 244)	(n = 174)	(n = 362)	(n = 172)
Nil	56.6%	51.7%	56.6%	61%
Minor	32.3%	31.6%	28.2%	24.4%
Moderate or great	9.1%	10.9%	11.6%	11%
Belgium 93				
With what frequency have you ever wondered if you yourself have been contaminated by the AIDS virus?	(n = 666)	(n = 432)	(n = 894)	(n = 838)
Never wondered about that	60.2%	58.8%	63.7%	71.7%
Wondered about that in the past, but no longer	19.3%	23.4%	19.7%	16.8%
Sometimes or often	20.6%	17.8%	16.5%	11.3%
France–KABP 92				
Do you ever wonder if you have already been infected with the AIDS virus?	(n = 267)	(n = 210)	(n = 445)	(n = 399)
I never wonder	63.6%	64.1%	65.6%	85%
I sometimes or often wonder	36.4%	35.9%	31.8%	12.8%

East Germany 90

What are the possibilities, in your opinion, of being infected by the virus that causes AIDS?	(n = 212)	(n = 190)	(n = 391)	(n = 237)
Out of the question	26.9%	23.2%	27.1%	30.4%
Not likely	53.3%	58.9%	52.4%	48.9%
Could happen	11.8%	12.1%	15.9%	13.9%
Absolutely possible, fairly sure or sure	8%	5.2%	4.6%	5.5%

Netherlands 89

That I'm already infected with the AIDS virus	(n = 243)	(n = 172)	(n = 336)	(n = 239)
Never worry about	80%	84%	89%	93%
Rarely worry about	17%	13%	8%	6%
Occasionally, often, almost always worry about	3%	3%	3%	1%

West Germany 93

Have you ever worried that you might yourself contract AIDS or has it never worried you?	(n = 309)	(n = 312)	(n = 560)	(n = 449)
Yes	38.5%	37.5%	34.6%	25.5%
No	61.5%	62.5%	65.4%	74.5%

Note:

[1] To simplify the presentation, the 'no answer' and 'don't know' lines are not shown here. Given the small number of 18- and 19-year-olds, we combined them with the 20–24-year-olds

Subjective Perception of Risk

Five surveys (Athens–PR, Belgium, the Netherlands, East Germany (1990), and France–KABP) contained at least one question evaluating personal and/or collective risk perception. This relative scarcity of material was compounded by extremely heterogeneous wordings, making it difficult to compare the findings. Nevertheless, we can study subjective risk perception along two major axes. First, we shall analyze personal subjective risk of infection, that is: Where does the person place him- or herself with regard to potential infection and what are his or her own fears? Second, we can study the threat that HIV represents for the individual's environment: Is such a threat perceived and is this potential threat seen as a source of fear or apprehension for the city, society, or more immediate environment of family and friends?

To identify, quantify, and interpret risk factors, the epidemiologist divides the population into specific groups: the healthy versus the ill, those who are exposed to a risk versus those who are not, and so on. Our approach is closer to one in which risk is defined primarily by the individual's experience and social identity (Bajos and Ludwig, 1995). The measured risk is subjective, to the extent that we ask individuals if they consider themselves or others to be (or to have been) in a risky situation. Table 14.1 shows the questions' diversity, but also the unity of the prospect.

Knowing a PWHA

The proportion of respondents who reported knowing one or more PWHAs differed greatly from one survey to the next.[2] The different survey dates and real prevalence rates of infection in the various countries are some of the many factors that led to such deviations. Variations in question wordings might also explain some deviations.[3]

Knowledge and Discrimination: Is there a Connection?

Knowledge and Segregation

Figure 14.2 shows the responses to questions that include the idea of segregation in terms of the KMDT and WPT scores.[4]

The data presented in Figure 14.2 as well as additional Belgian, French and German (1993) data not shown here suggest that, as a rule, segregationist

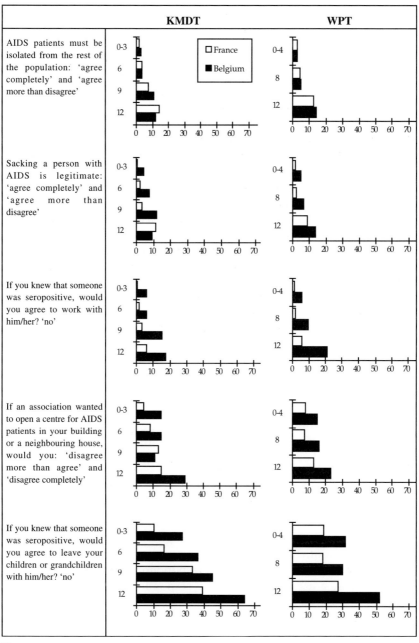

Note:
Abscissa = percentage expressing the attitude/*Ordinate* = aggregate index score categories

Figure 14.2 *Segregation of PWHAs: Breakdown by KMDT (knowledge of transmission routes) and WPT (knowledge of protective means) aggregate index scores in Belgium and France*

attitudes towards PWHAs are especially well developed in persons who have more inaccurate knowledge about the virus's transmission routes and means of protection.

As Ioannidi and Haeder showed in Chapter 13, attitudes towards seropositive physicians and dentists are something of a case apart. Distancing attitudes with regard to these groups are much stronger than more general ones. In the French survey, for example, close to 40 per cent of respondents were reluctant to be treated by an HIV-infected dentist or physician, while 12 per cent would refuse or hesitate to work with a seropositive person. This difference suggests that segregation is at least to some extent fuelled by the fear of being infected.

The fear of being infected seems to be all the more acute when the risk of casual transmission (infection through kissing, drinking, and so on) is overestimated. As a rule, the respondents who overestimated the risk of casual transmission (higher KMDT scores) had more discriminatory attitudes towards seropositive doctors and dentists and AIDS patients. In the same way, respondents who overestimated the efficacy of inaccurate means of protection (higher WPT scores) also had more discriminatory attitudes towards physicians but not towards dentists.

Knowledge and Management of Information about Seropositivity

Should testing without consent be allowed or not? The German surveys of 1993 revealed that significantly higher proportions of respondents who felt kissing was risky or believed that the condom did not afford sufficient protection were in favour of compulsory testing. In the Belgian survey, the proportion of respondents with less inaccurate knowledge of protective means (lower WPT scores) who thought that the person's consent was not necessary before conducting a test was significantly higher than for the rest of the respondents. It was as if these persons felt that protecting the doctor prevailed over the patient's freedom of choice. So, this result appears to be in conflict with the German one: the highest proportion of respondents who would accept testing without consent are found among the respondents with more inaccurate knowledge in Germany, and those with less inaccurate knowledge in Belgium.[5]

Once serological status is known, there arises for individuals and for physicians the question of revealing or keeping this information secret. As Ioannidi and Haeder showed in Chapter 13, the majority of respondents in both the Belgian and French surveys felt that they should be informed of their partner's seropositivity, even without the latter's consent, and a seropositive person who did not inform his or her sexual partner or partners of the situation should be prosecuted. In France the proportion of respondents who felt they should be informed of their partner's seropositivity is smaller among respondents with less inaccurate knowledge. This was, however, not the case for the Belgian survey, where the differences were not statistically significant.[6] The response to the question about prosecuting a PWHA who did not inform his or her sexual partner or partners of the situation did not appear to be correlated with the KMDT score. Such a correlation did exist with regard to the WPT score, but only in Belgium, where the question explicitly mentioned unprotected sex: the more informed respondents were even more in favour of prosecuting such people. It was as if not informing one's sexual partner was all the more unacceptable if sex practices were unprotected and for the respondents who knew that practices like washing after sex were ineffective.

There does not seem to be a single inter-survey tendency with regard to a possible association between the population's knowledge about HIV transmission routes and means of protection on the one hand and the population's attitudes towards the conditions of applicability of the HIV test and management of information about seropositivity on the other hand. This may be due to the great diversity of controversies surrounding these issues in the various countries. Consequently, we shall focus on segregationist attitudes instead of on discrimination in the broad sense. The hypothesis of there being two risk management approaches, as suggested by the Belgian data, bears mentioning, however. The distancing approach may prevail in underprivileged groups where the proportion of less knowledgeable respondents is higher, whereas the technical approach (testing, prosecution, and so on) cuts across socio-economic boundaries. Both are doubtless painful experiences for their victims, however.

Knowledge and Discrimination: Possible Common Factors

The group of respondents in each survey who had the most inaccurate knowledge of both the virus's transmission routes and protective means systematically held more segregationist attitudes towards PWHAs. How should this correspondence between inaccurate representations and segregationist attitudes be interpreted? The fear of being infected that ensues from inaccurate knowledge might explain these attitudes to a great extent. However, why do people who believe in the relative efficacy of ineffective measures and, as Marquet, Hubert and Campenhoudt (1995) have shown, overlap only partially with the group of people who overestimate the risks of casual activities hold more discriminatory attitudes than everyone else? A second, not necessarily contradictory, interpretation posits the existence of common factors –

mistrust, risk perception, and proximity – influencing both level of knowledge and segregationist attitudes.

Mistrust

Mistrust and Knowledge

The Belgian and the Dutch data show that people who express more mistrust also have more inaccurate knowledge. With regard to knowledge about HIV transmission routes, the Belgian survey[7] showed that besides the 53.8 per cent of the respondents who felt the virus could be transmitted via a blood transfusion performed in Belgium (in 1993), 7.6 per cent stated spontaneously that they were wary of specialists' reassuring declarations. Moreover, 12.8 per cent of the respondents voiced the same scepticism with regard to at least one of the six questions concerning HIV transmission routes, that is, receiving blood, giving blood, kissing, mosquito bites, using toilets, and drinking from someone else's glass. Here, what could at first be interpreted as ignorance may simply reflect 'vigilant mistrust'. This kind of mistrust seemed to add a measure of caution to prevention messages. The Belgian survey showed that respondents who voiced a feeling of vague, general mistrust – what we called retreating mistrust – also had relatively higher rates of inaccurate knowledge of HIV transmission routes than the rest of the population.

While the degree of generalized mistrust was directly correlated to the degree of inaccurate knowledge of protective means, vigilant mistrust was inversely correlated to the rate of inaccurate knowledge.[8] Retreating mistrust appeared to be inversely correlated with level of education, occurring primarily in the least educated group of adults, whereas vigilant mistrust seemed to be fairly independent of the level of education.

The main flaw in the reasoning subtending the correlation between mistrust and knowledge is that no single item in the Belgian survey explicitly measured mistrust of prevention officials. Provided that we accept the idea that the results of one survey can complement and enrich those of another survey, the Dutch survey enables us to delve deeper into the above vein of thought. In this survey, the answers to the two questions concerning the faith the respondents placed in prevention messages appeared to correlate with the answers to the question about the efficacy of condom use. Significantly higher percentages of the respondents who believed in the experts and prevention messages considered the condom to be very effective as a means of protecting against HIV. Moreover, the correlation appears to be stronger if the idea of mistrust is really in the core of the question. So, the correlation with the proposition 'The information about how you can prevent getting infected with AIDS is usually reliable' was especially strong.[9] In our opinion, this question expresses trust/mistrust, that is, prevention messages are perceived as being believable or unbelievable *as a rule*, whereas the other question ('I get the impression that experts don't exactly know how one can prevent AIDS') measures the population's perception of a certain feeling of being at a loss or the limits of science's ability to deal with AIDS as well as mistrust. In other words, prevention messages are imperfect because they are provisional but are disseminated 'for lack of something better'.

Mistrust and Segregation

The Belgian data show that while segregationist feelings are completely independent of vigilant mistrust, they are partly linked to the attitude of retreating mistrust. Indeed, a clearly higher percentage of the respondents who subscribed totally to the proposition 'You can't trust anyone anymore' than in the other groups accepted certain forms of segregation: 10.8 per cent of them felt AIDS patients should be isolated from the rest of the population, 10.2 per cent thought it was normal for an employer to fire a PWHA, 14.5 per cent stated they would refuse to work or study with an HIV carrier, 19.4 per cent were opposed to opening a treatment centre for AIDS patients in their neighbourhoods, and 44.5 per cent said they would not leave their children or grandchildren in the company of an HIV carrier. These percentages were 2.3, 3.1, 6.0, 14.5 and 22.1 per cent, respectively, for the respondents who rejected categorically ('completely disagree') the idea that you could no longer trust anyone.

Subjective Risk (Risk Perception)

Subjective Risk and Knowledge of the Disease

Subjective risk of infection and knowledge of the disease were relatively independent. However, some trends did seem to emerge. Respondents who perceived the risk at an intermediate level (neither zero risk or very high risk), those who attributed their risk to their sexual activity and those who reported intermediate fears of infection had less inaccurate knowledge of the disease.

It has already been mentioned that we cannot apprehend knowledge without referring to perception and we cannot apprehend perception without involving some elements of knowledge. Nevertheless, the analysis showed first of all that inaccurate knowledge of both transmission modes and means of protection is largely independent of personal subjective risk of infection, that is, the individual's personal evaluation of the possibility of finding or having found him- or herself in a risky situation. When the knowledge people had about genuine modes of transmission and means of protection was lower, the question was discriminant and a correlation between this knowledge and the perceived personal risk perhaps did exist. But as our surveys have shown, the level of knowledge about this question is currently very high everywhere. The observed lack of association might be explained in part by the fact that the aggregate indices measured knowledge (or inaccurate knowledge) 'in the margins', that is, knowledge of 'false transmission routes' and ineffective means of protection rather than knowledge of genuine modes of transmission and effective means of protection.

We shall now discuss the trends which have been mentioned before. First, having less inaccurate knowledge of the modes of transmission and means of protection seemed to go hand in hand with setting the risk of infection at an intermediate level. In the Athenian survey, large proportions of the respondents who claimed not to be able to assess their own risk of contracting the virus (68.2 per cent), who felt the risk was nil (53.9 per cent), and who thought it was very great (66.0 per cent) had inaccurate knowledge of HIV transmission (KMDT > 0). These figures have to be compared with 48.9 and 40.9 per cent, respectively, for those who judged the risk very slight or moderate. In the French survey, 62.5 per cent of the respondents who never wondered if they might have been infected and 81.3 per cent of the few respondents (n $=$ 25) who said they often wondered about the possibility versus 55.5 per cent of those who sometimes wondered if they might have been infected had inaccurate knowledge of HIV transmission. For this question, the Belgian survey proposed an additional answer mode that enabled one to indicate whether the doubt about possible infection belonged to the past or was current. Fewer of the respondents who situated the doubt in the past had inaccurate knowledge of HIV modes of transmission (29.4 per cent) and of means of protection (19.6 per cent) than did those who expressed sometimes (38.1 per cent for transmission modes and 28.2 per cent for means of protection) or often (36.3 per cent and 37.9 per cent) a current concern and those in whom the doubt had never arisen (34.4 per cent and 28.9 per cent).

Despite the differences in the question wordings, the results of these surveys seem to point to the same conclusion: better knowledge of the means of protection and, above all, modes of transmission seemed to go hand in hand with setting the risk of infection at an intermediate level. However, it is important to take into account the fact that the question wordings refer to different time frames. One might well wonder if the people who considered the possibility of being infected in the past and now gave proof of better knowledge of the modes of transmission and means of protection already had such knowledge at the time of their doubts or if their knowledge had improved in the interim.

Second, respondents who perceived a personal risk of infection and attributed it to their sexual activity had less inaccurate knowledge of HIV's modes of transmission and means of protection than the rest of the respondents. Specifically, wondering in the past or present about the potentially hazardous nature of one's own sexual behaviour seemed to be correlated with less inaccurate knowledge of transmission modes and means of protection. In the Belgian survey 29.1 per cent of the respondents who had current or past doubts as a consequence of their sex lives versus 35.2 per cent of the rest of the respondents had inaccurate knowledge of HIV transmission. These percentages were 52.1 and 61.4 per cent, respectively, for the French survey and 80.0 and 88.8 per cent for the Dutch survey. In the Belgian survey 20.4 per cent of the respondents who linked their (past or current) doubts to sexual activity versus 28.8 per cent of the rest of the respondents had inaccurate knowledge of means of protection. These percentages were 39.9 and 48.1 per cent, respectively, for the French survey and 26.8 and 40.4 per cent for the Dutch survey.

People who were worried about the consequences of their sexual behaviour had less inaccurate knowledge of transmission modes than people whose worries stemmed from other reasons. This is quite understandable to the extent that some of these other reasons concern situations – such as surgery and blood transfusions – taken into account in the KMDT index with regard to which specialists have offered reassurances. However, we also found that those who were worried about the consequences of their sexual behaviour had less inaccurate knowledge of ineffective means of protection. This set them apart from respondents who never wondered if they had been infected and who had more inaccurate knowledge of transmission modes and means of protection. Consequently, we may well ask whether being personally affected by AIDS, meaning that the virus's existence causes one to think about one's own behaviour, might not eventually lead to better knowledge of the disease, its transmission, and ways to protect against it, unless it is the level of knowledge that leads to the differentiated perception of the risks carried by sexual relations.

Third, it appears that respondents who reported intermediate-level fears of acquiring HIV (neither zero fear nor very great fear) had less inaccurate knowledge of the virus's modes of transmission and means of protection. With regard to transmission, the link between intermediate fear of contracting HIV and less inaccurate knowledge was borne out in all of the surveys in which an indicator that 'measured' fear of infection existed, even though the inter-group percent differences between surveys could be more or less great. So, 49.0 per cent of the respondents in the Athens–PR survey who said they were 'somewhat afraid' of contracting HIV had inaccurate knowledge of the virus's modes of transmission versus 65.1 per cent of those who were 'very afraid' of this possibility and 52.3 per cent of those who had 'never feared' such a possibility. The percentages in the French–KABP survey were 56.1 per cent of the 'quite afraid' respondents, 69.1 per cent of 'very afraid' respondents, and

59.5 per cent of the 'but little afraid' respondents. In the Dutch survey the percentages were 82.7 per cent of the 'seldom concerned by the fear of being infected' category, 91.3 per cent of the 'sometimes, very often and almost always' respondents, who were combined in one group (n = 23), and 87.5 per cent of the 'never' category. With regard to the means of protection, this trend was borne out above all in the Dutch survey, where 28.2 per cent of the 'seldom concerned by the fear of being infected' category, 39.1 per cent of the 'sometimes, very often and almost always' respondents and 38.8 per cent of the 'never' category had inaccurate knowledge of the means of protection.

Knowledge of HIV transmission modes and protective means seemed to be partly linked to the fear of acquiring HIV. Making a clear distinction between the fear of infection and the perceived risk of infection appears to be very difficult. This fear is incontestably fuelled by assessment of the risk, but on the other hand, the filtering of information that occurs in the assessment process is more or less influenced by various personal and social factors, notably fear and/or the need to be reassured. This may explain why fear of infection and perceived risk of infection were both related to knowledge of HIV transmission modes and protective means.

Based on the indicators at our disposal, the perceived risk of HIV infection for society as a whole is to a large extent independent of knowledge of the virus's modes of transmission and ways of protecting against it. Here, too, we hypothesize that the observed lack of association might be explained in part by the fact that the aggregate indices measured knowledge (or inaccurate knowledge) 'in the margins' of a high degree of current knowledge.

Subjective Risk and Segregation

The question is whether people who perceive a greater risk for themselves or for society have less tolerant attitudes. According to our data, 'perceived risk to society' did not trigger a stronger tendency to segregate. Regarding the personal axis, the results differ from one indicator to the other; fearing the disease and perceiving oneself as being at risk do not lead to the same attitude. Stated very simply, it appears that when the fear of infection is high, individuals show segregationist opinions a little more often. These remarks also apply to individuals who think of AIDS as a highly contagious disease. For example, in the France–KABP survey, 8.7 per cent of the respondents who were very much afraid of the personal risk of AIDS agreed completely or agreed more than disagreed with the item 'AIDS patients must be isolated from the rest of the population' versus 5.0 per cent of the respondents who had little fear of a personal risk. Similarly, 10 per cent of the respondents who said that AIDS is caught more easily than the flu agreed (totally or rather in agreement) with the idea of isolating people with HIV versus 5.2 per cent of

Table 14.2 *Influence of doubts about serological status on agreement (complete or more or less) with various propositions (Belgium 93 and France–KABP 92 surveys)*

Wonder about having been infected:	Belgium 1993		France 1992	
	often or sometimes	never	often or sometimes	never
People who know that they are seropositive and have – unprotected (B) – sex without warning their partners of their serological status should be prosecuted	80.1%	81.5%	64.3%	67.8%
To avoid being rejected – discrimination (F) – a seropositive person has the right to keep his/her diagnosis secret	37.5%	32.5%	65.9%*	58.5%*
If your partner were seropositive, you should be informed even without his or her consent (B). When a doctor knows that a patient is seropositive or ill, he should inform the patient's spouse (F)	80.9%*	89.3%*	72.2%*	78.8%*

Note:
*The difference is significant at p < 0.05

the rest of the French sample. In contrast, a perception of a high personal risk of infection as reflected in doubts about one's own serological status seems to make individuals a little more sensitive to the problems that may arise because of the stigmatization that can follow it becoming known that an individual is HIV seropositive and to make them more tolerant of PWHAs. So in the France–KABP survey, 97.2 per cent of respondents who felt they ran a high risk refused to isolate infected individuals versus 92.1 per cent of those who claimed a zero or below-average risk of infection.

Table 14.2 also shows that if people report that they wonder about possible infection more frequently, their attitudes are less intolerant. However, the differences are small. It should also be recognized that some items presented in this table do not refer directly to what we called segregationist attitudes in the strict sense of the word. In the same way, 6.5 per cent of the French survey respondents who never wondered about the possibility of having been infected were completely or rather in agreement with isolating people with AIDS, versus 3.9 per cent of those who wondered about the possibility occasionally or often. In the Belgian survey, the difference between these two groups of respondents' answers on this point was not significant.

Imagining oneself as (possibly) being infected fosters less segregationist attitudes. It thus seems that when one has doubts about one's serological status, assessing the consequences of such an infection for oneself, one's relationships with others, and so on, makes one more sensitive to the PWHA's situation.

Personal Acquaintance with a Person with HIV or AIDS

Knowing a PWHA and Knowledge of the Illness

Most of the analyses we carried out did not show any significant differences between respondents who knew and those who did not know PWHAs as regards knowledge of HIV's transmission modes and means of protecting against infection. In the French survey, which was the only one of the four surveys that could be analyzed from this perspective, respondents who knew a PWHA had a markedly lower rate of inaccurate knowledge of transmission routes (–11.5 percentage point). Two trends nevertheless did seem to support the hypothesized link between personal experience and knowledge. First, in the surveys that asked about the degree of proximity to the PWHA, respondents who said they were very close (Belgium) or specified it was a friend or colleague (France) had markedly less inaccurate knowledge of modes of transmission than other respondents.[10] The Belgian respondents who had close acquaintances with AIDS were also less inclined to believe in the efficacy of such practices as taking the pill or washing after sex as a means of protecting against HIV.[11] The Belgian data that differentiated respondents according to whether they knew one or several PWHAs showed that those who knew several PWHAs had a lower level of inaccurate knowledge, whereas such a difference did not emerge from the French data.

Knowing a PWHA and Segregation

In the European surveys as a whole, non-segregationist attitudes towards PWHAs seemed to be correlated to knowing one or more PWHAs. Thus, 94.7 per cent of the Belgian respondents who stated they knew a PWHA compared with 85.7 per cent of the rest of the sample said they would accept an AIDS treatment centre in their neighbourhood. This group also had a higher rate of acceptance for leaving their children or grandchildren in the company of a PWHA (78.7 per cent versus 64.2 per cent of the rest of the sample). Such trends could also be found in the France–KABP 1992 survey in which 97.8 per cent of the respondents who reported they knew one or more seropositive individuals were amenable to continuing to see (be friends with) a seropositive person, 98.7 per cent to working with a seropositive colleague, 94.7 per cent to eating at a seropositive person's house, 93.9 per cent to going on holiday with a seropositive person, and 82.9 per cent to leaving their children or grandchildren in the company of a PWHA, and only 3.3 per cent felt that people with AIDS should be isolated from the rest of the population. These percentages were 93.5, 94.8, 85.5, 81.9, 69.6 and 8 per cent, respectively, for the rest of the respondents.

Discussion

Here we should like to discuss the findings from the perspective of social representations (Moscovici, 1984; Doise and Palmonari, 1986). Social representations of AIDS serve as landmarks and guidelines for individuals coping with the HIV epidemic. Ideas circulating about AIDS are socially and culturally loaded and do not result merely from the dissemination of sufficient or insufficient, correct or incorrect information. Ignorance of disease and discriminatory attitudes do not necessarily reflect ignorance of prevention messages or resistance to, or even the absence of, change. They are not the monopoly of a few recalcitrant individuals who refuse all new ideas. Rather, they seem to be socially constructed, shared, and transmitted answers developed to try to comprehend situations that as a rule largely extend beyond the confines of AIDS *per se*.

The preceding analyses have shown that segregationist attitudes towards people with AIDS are especially frequent in people with poorer knowledge of HIV's routes of transmission and means of protection. Instead of following the common belief that discrimination is a direct consequence of lack of knowledge, we explored how both phenomena are related to various common factors. In doing so, we attempted to identify factors that affect knowledge and discrimination and must also be taken into account in understanding better the dynamics behind the relationship between knowledge and discrimination.

The preceding analyses (Chapters 12 and 13) showed that level of education was correlated with the two phenomena as follows: respondents who had a relatively poor understanding of the disease and those who expressed segregationist feelings were over-represented in the 'low level of education' category. These results may thus support in part the cause-and-effect hypothesis. Nevertheless, level of education is not just an indicator of knowledge reflecting the person's access to and ability to comprehend accurate information. It also refers to other phenomena such as the individual's cultural environment, critical attitude towards prejudices and proximity to scientific discourse and prevention messages.

From the foregoing analyses we can detect the outlines of a group that is socially 'withdrawn' from various points of view (older,[12] less educated, who think it useful to be wary of others, who seem fairly unable to assess the risk of exposure to the virus), has poorer knowledge of the virus's transmission routes and of the means of protecting against the virus, and adopts segregationist attitudes towards PWHAs. This combination of elements seems to validate the hypothesized distancing- and repulsion-based structuring of the subject's personal and social identities. We believe that rejecting people with HIV and AIDS as a whole occurs in one fell swoop. Indeed, it is as if retreating and segregation or 'out-grouping' were general characteristics of this group. Ignorance (or inaccurate knowledge) and segregation feed off one another without it being possible to determine which comes first. Constructing one's identity by distancing oneself from others against a backdrop of segregation explains the ignorance or inaccurate knowledge which, in turn, reinforces the possibility of stigmatizing and demonizing the other even more, the more the other himself is poorly known. According to this interpretation, segregationist attitudes towards PWHAs are not so much a consequence of a specific lack of knowledge of AIDS as the sign of a way of consolidating one's identity and sense of belonging to a group of significant others that consists in distancing oneself from other groups. Given some of the characteristics of this group (older, less educated, and so on), we might even wonder if it is not characterized as well by a vague feeling of insecurity and fear of everything that upsets one's usual social framework.

This distancing strategy, be it conscious or unconscious, seems to be a key to interpreting the opinions that certain social groups hold concerning HIV and the people who, rightly or wrongly, are perceived as being the virus's main carriers. Such a strategy goes beyond the specific bounds of the issue of the AIDS/HIV epidemic. This strategy and the issue of the epidemic feed off each other. Consequently, it would be naïve to believe one could put an end to such an identity-building process by means of a few prevention messages or calls for solidarity.

The preceding analysis also enables us to understand how the idea of a 'risk group' has a strong likelihood of becoming a reference notion to apprehend reality for certain social groups. Triggering feelings of invulnerability could appear to be a public health response to the problem, while placing the risk on the socially stigmatized groups' side of the scoreboard could appear to be a social response. Such a conceptual tool would align with the thinking of insecure groups that see relationships with 'outsiders' as essentially dangerous. Representations of AIDS that are based on the idea of risk groups have no effect on people's definitions of their own and others' identities; the other remains dangerous and the only one to display the features of the disease and thus the signs of social reprobation.

People's representations of HIV's transmission routes and means of protecting themselves from infection, opinions about people with HIV and AIDS, perceptions of personal risk of infection, and mistrust of others seem to be correlated. Reckoning with the intertwined nature of these phenomena allows us to grasp the social dimensions of representations surrounding AIDS. The reference systems are multiple and complex, and while a technical approach (testing, prosecution, and so on) to HIV/AIDS risk management shows that distancing is not the sole type of logic to organize the field of social responses to the epidemic, there is perhaps nothing surprising about the fact that it appears to be one of the most powerful.

As a phenomenon (an idea, knowledge, behaviour, representation, disease, and so on) spreads, it acquires the social image of those with whom it is associated, whether rightly or wrongly. Attempts to change representations and behaviour connected to the AIDS epidemic will succeed only if they take account of prior social structuring, which creates a relative socio-cultural balance that all changes are likely to upset and that some groups more than others will try to maintain at all cost. The issue of information cannot be raised in isolation from that of identity and identification with subgroups of society.

Notes

1 So, for example, 50.8 per cent of the respondents in the France–KABP survey who knew PWHAs wondered sometimes or often if they had already been infected with HIV versus 30.4 per cent of the rest of the sample. On the other hand, 86.8 per cent of the respondents in the Scottish survey who knew PWHAs thought that AIDS would spread in the general population and 89 per cent thought that AIDS was a problem in their city, compared with 77 per cent and 77 per cent, respectively, of the respondents who did not know anyone with AIDS.

2 The figures are 1.2 per cent of the respondents aged 18 to 49 in the East Germany 1990 survey, 4.0 per cent in the Athens–KABP 1989 survey, 8.0 per cent in the Belgium 1993 survey, 8.7 per cent in the Athens–PR 1990 survey, 10.5 per cent in the Portugal 1992 survey, 11.5 per cent in the West Germany 1993 survey, 13.5 per cent in the Scotland 1992 survey, and 15.4 per cent in the France–KABP 1992 survey.

3 For example, the Belgian question was 'Do you personally know one or more people in your entourage, that is, family, friends, officemates, and neighbours, who are seropositive, ill with AIDS, or have died from AIDS?', and the French (KABP) was 'Do you personally know one or more seropositives or AIDS patients amongst your friends, family or colleagues?'

4 For this comparison we allowed for the fact that the French answer scales always included a median position – 'neither agree nor disagree (neutral)' for scales measuring the degree of agreement; 'perhaps' for the 'yes-no' scales – whereas the Belgian answer scales never did, which could only increase the scores of the remaining categories. The scores of the French median category were 2.1, 2.1, 9.2, 9.1 and 15.3 per cent, respectively, for the five situations covered in Figure 14.2.

5 However, the Belgian respondents identified two distinct ways for physicians to manage the risk. A higher proportion of the respondents with more inaccurate knowledge (especially as determined by their WPT scores) accepted the idea that a physician could refuse to treat an AIDS patient, but a smaller proportion of this group accepted the idea of carrying out the test without the patient's consent. Inversely, a smaller proportion of the respondents with less inaccurate knowledge accepted the idea that a physician could refuse to treat an HIV-infected person, but a higher proportion of this group accepted the idea of carrying out the test without the patient's consent. So, in one case the risk was managed by a distancing strategy and in the other case by technical measures. This pattern was not seen, however, in the French survey data.

6 The references to the physician and spouse that occur in the French question but not in the Belgian one may explain this difference. The Belgian and French question wordings were as follows: 'If your partner were seropositive, you should be informed even without his/her consent' (B) and 'When a doctor knows that a patient is seropositive or ill he should inform the patient's spouse' (F).

7 The Belgian survey results covered in this section were published in Marquet, Hubert and Van Campenhoudt (1995). Unlike the preceding international comparisons, the population considered by this survey ranged from 15 to 59 years of age, not 18 to 49.

8 In other words, respondents who were aware of the 'official' line with regard to transmission routes, but expressed scepticism of such positions, also had a lower percentage of answers stressing the efficacy of the protective means that these same official messages advised against. The more you feel you cannot trust others, the more you recognize the effectiveness of taking the pill or washing after sex as a means of protecting against HIV.

9 Of the respondents who were completely or basically in agreement with this proposition 89.4 per cent felt the condom was 'very effective', compared with only 65.9 per cent of the other respondents.

10 Of the Belgian respondents 65.9 per cent scored the minimum of 0 on the KMDT index. This percentage rose to 80.3 per cent for the subgroup of people who stated they were close to a PWHA. Of the French respondents 39.4 per cent scored the minimum of 0 versus 69.2 per cent of the subgroup who knew a colleague with AIDS and 43.6 per cent of the subgroup who had a friend with AIDS ('with AIDS' meaning either seropositive or with serious illness).

11 Of the Belgian respondents 72.7 per cent scored the minimum of 0 on the WPT index (an aggregate index of inaccurate knowledge about means of protection). This percentage rose to 88.1 per cent for the subgroup who stated they were close to a person with HIV. In the French survey, the percentages were 53.2 per cent for the overall sample, 69.5 per cent for the subgroup who knew a colleague with AIDS and 62.7 per cent who had a friend with AIDS.

12 The Belgian survey showed that the 50–59-year-olds also had the highest percentage of acceptance of certain forms of segregation (Marquet, Hubert and Van Campenhoudt, 1995).

References

ALLARD, A.R. (1989) 'Beliefs about AIDS as determinants of preventive practices and of support for coercive measures', *American Journal of Public Health*, **79**, pp. 448–52.

BAJOS, N. and LUDWIG, D. (1995) 'Risque construit et objectivation du risque: deux approches des modes d'adaptation au risque de transmission sexuelle du Sida', in BAJOS, N., BOZON, M., GIAMI, A., SOUTEYRAND, Y. and DORÉ, V. (Eds) *Sexualité et Sida*, Paris: ANRS Publications.

COATES, T.J. (1990) 'Strategies for modifying sexual behavior for primary and secondary prevention of HIV disease', *Journal of Consulting and Clinical Psychology*, **58**, pp. 57–69.

COATES, T.J. and GREENBLATT, R.M. (1989) 'Behavioral change using community-level interventions', in HOLMES, K. (Ed.) *Sexually Transmitted Diseases*, New York: McGraw-Hill.

CONKLIN, J.E. (1975) *The Impact of Crime*, New York: Macmillan.

DE VROMME, E.M.M., PAALMAN, M.E.M. and SANDFORT, T.G.M. (1990) 'AIDS in the Netherlands: the effects of several years of campaigning', *International Journal of Sexually Transmitted Diseases and AIDS*, **1**, pp. 268–75.

DOISE, W. and PALMONARI, A. (Dir.) (1986) *L'étude des représentations sociales*, Neuchâtel: Delachaux et Niestlé.

EKSTRAND, M. and COATES, T. (1990) 'Maintenance of safer sexual behaviors and predictors of risky sex: the San Fransisco's Men's Health Study', *American Journal of Public Health*, **80**, pp. 973–7.

EKSTRAND, M. *et al.* (1992) 'Frequent and infrequent relapsers need different AIDS prevention programs', Communication at the VIIIth International Conference on AIDS, Amsterdam, July 1992 (POD 5126).

HUBERT, M. and MARQUET, J. (coordinator) (1993) *Comportements sexuels et réactions au risque du SIDA en Belgique*, rapport à la Commission des communautés européennes, Brussels: Centre d'études sociologiques, Facultés universitaires Saint-Louis.

HUYNEN, P., MARQUET, J. and HUBERT, M. (1995) 'Les Européens et le SIDA: situation actuelle et tendances', in INRA (Eds), *Les Européens et la santé publique*, Rapport pour la Commission Européenne, Brussels.

MANN, J. and KAY, K. (1988) 'Sida, discrimination et santé publique', Presentation at the IVth International Conference on AIDS, Stockholm, Sweden.

MARQUET, J., HUBERT, M. and VAN CAMPENHOUDT, L. (1995) 'Public awareness of AIDS: discrimination and the effects of mistrust', in FITZSIMONS, D., HARDY, V. and TOLLEY, K. (Eds) *The Economic and Social Impact of AIDS in Europe*, London: Cassell.

MARQUET, J., HUBERT, M. and PETO, D. (1994) *Comportements sexuels et réactions au risque du SIDA en Belgique: spécificités bruxelloises*, rapport à la Région de Bruxelles-Capitale, Brussels: Centre d'études sociologiques, Facultés universitaires Saint-Louis.

MOATTI, J.-P. and SERRAND, C. (1989) 'Les sciences sociales face au Sida: entre silence et trop parler?', *Cahiers de Sociologie et de Démographie Médicales*, **3**, pp. 231–62.

MOATTI, J.-P., DAB, W., LOUNDOU, A. *et al.* (1992) 'Impact on the general public of media campaigns against AIDS: a French evaluation', *Health Policy*, **21**, pp. 233–47.

MOATTI, J.-P., BELTZER, N. and DAB, W. (1993) 'Les modèles d'analyse des comportements à risque face à l'infection à VIH: une conception trop étroite de la rationalité', *Population*, **5**, pp. 1505–34.

MOSCOVICI, S. (1984) 'The phenomenon of social representations', in FARR, R.M. and MOSCOVICI, S. (Eds) *Social Representations*, Cambridge: Cambridge University Press.

Conclusions

Chapter 15

Sexual Behaviour and HIV Risk: Common Patterns and Differences between European Countries

Theo Sandfort, Michel Hubert, Nathalie Bajos and Henny Bos*

The AIDS epidemic that took the world by surprise brought social scientists across Europe up sharp against the limits of their knowledge and understanding of human sexuality. In most countries, one of the first responses after various studies focusing on gay men was to carry out general population surveys, each with its own priorities and theoretical perspectives, using a variety of data collection methods. Bringing the findings from the various European studies together offers us the opportunity to look at each country against the backdrop of other countries and to explore how differences are related to particularities in socio-cultural contexts and policies. This adds to an understanding of our own national sexual behaviour patterns, but also to a deeper understanding of sexuality in general. While these broader insights can be viewed from various theoretical perspectives, they also enable policy-makers to improve their health policies. Finally, the findings of the cross-national comparisons might be helpful in understanding the differences in the HIV/AIDS epidemic.

The major outcome of the cross-national comparisons is to have revealed several similarities in the ways sexuality is expressed in different countries. The comparisons also highlight the ways in which sexuality is structured by factors such as gender, personal development, historical aspects, education and place of residence, and people's relationship status. Of course, the similarities observed between countries do not signify that sexuality is expressed

*We would like to thank the participants in the concluding workshop of the European Union Concerted Action on Sexual Behaviour and Risks of HIV Infection (of which this book is a product), held in Brussels on 16–17 January 1997, for their comments on a first draft of this chapter, and Françoise Dubois-Arber and Michel Bozon for their additional comments.

and structured identically in each country; some differences have been observed as well.

In this chapter we shall summarize and discuss the major findings and the ways in which a number of key factors affect the expression of sexuality. After exploring the potential effect that AIDS has had on sexuality, we shall discuss the relevance of these findings from the perspective of HIV prevention and the lessons that can be drawn for the further design of prevention policies. We shall end by identifying new research areas and presenting suggestions for future cross-national research in the field of sexuality and AIDS. Before summarizing the results, we shall describe the major methodological characteristics of this European project and its limitations.

The Cross-national Project: Main Characteristics and Limitations

Bringing the data from the various national studies together, and preparing them for cross-national comparison, has been a challenging task. The complexity of the project resulted first of all from the decision to analyze and present the data for each topic instead of having chapters describing each country's findings separately. This complexity was compounded by diverging national research interests and priorities; the varying disciplinary backgrounds of the principal investigators; the different research protocols applied, including sampling strategies and data collection methods; and lack of international coordination at the outset (for an extensive overview see Chapter 1 in this volume). The abiding willingness of all of the researchers involved in the project to share experiences and data and their belief in the benefits of developing a cross-national perspective have contributed decisively to the project's success.

On a very concrete and practical level, since not all surveys contained all the relevant information, the number of countries which could be compared varied, depending on the issue under consideration. The situation was further complicated by the fact that there was probably not a single question common to all surveys. Since the answer formats varied enormously as well, various adaptations had to be made in order to achieve inter-survey comparability. As long as questions aimed conceptually to assess the same variable, it was possible to establish functional equivalence, which allowed valid comparison. On the other hand, these adjustments diminished variance, which may have obscured actual differences between countries. On a few occasions less comparable indicators also had to be accepted. Finally, for some topics, even establishing functional equivalence was not possible. The ways these problems were solved have been discussed extensively in the foregoing chapters.

As mentioned above, the involvement of scholars from various disciplinary backgrounds and nationalities has contributed to the project's success. This international and interdisciplinary collaboration also raised several challenges. Researchers had to abstract data from unfamiliar data sets, entailing considerable 'getting acquainted' periods. Since most data files were managed in the country of origin, extensive data exchange procedures had to be set up. Consequently, it was practically impossible to conduct multivariate analyses to control for confounding effects. Furthermore, the international co-authorship of the various contributions required adjustments in the various research perspectives.

This international project was established after most of the surveys had been carried out. All contributors tried to make optimal use of the data available. In general, no one theoretical perspective guided the entire project. Although a particular theoretical approach was adopted in a few chapters, the main perspective throughout the project has been exploratory. This was the case with respect to explaining potential differences between the countries, but also with respect to potential differences in relation to variables such as gender, age and the socio-demographic factors that most of the surveys had in common.

Working on this cross-national project taught us various methodological lessons, some of which might seem obvious. We think, however, that it is important to describe them here. First of all, to improve the quality of the comparisons between countries, sampling procedures should be harmonized as much as possible with respect to both sample composition and weighting. Furthermore, common definitions of major concepts, such as sexual experience and intercourse, should be developed and adopted uniformly in the various surveys. The ways in which specific socio-demographic variables are measured should be improved as well.

Although from the perspective of functional equivalence the wordings of the questions used in each questionnaire do not have to be identical, more can be done to promote functional equivalence. Each survey should ask questions on the same level of generality or specificity. The time frames to which people are asked to relate their reported behaviour must be standardized. Furthermore, the adoption of identical answer formats will prevent having to lump categories together in order to make data from different studies comparable, thereby preventing a loss of variance in the data that may obscure potential differences. If filters are used in the questionnaire, care should be taken to ensure that the same subpopulation is being questioned in each survey.

Adopting a common protocol in a cross-national study would yield a database with greater possibilities for analysis.[1] It would, for instance, permit statements to be made about sexuality in Europe as a whole and analysis of units other than nations, such as regions or cities. Furthermore, multivariate analysis would become more feasible, as would the analysis of data from subgroups of people who are too rarely represented in a national general population survey to permit reliable conclusions.

It is clear from the foregoing that to maximize the importance of an international project's outcomes, collaboration should start as early as possible. This applies not only to methodological aspects but also to the identification of shared theoretical and practical interests and aims. Although setting up completely identical surveys may not always be possible, this should at least be aspired to, and optimal use of all the available possibilities has to be sought.

The survey data presented in this volume are based on what people reported about their behaviour, since direct observation in this area is not possible. The problem of the validity and reliability of the data collected in this type of survey has been examined many times (Catania *et al.*, 1990; Boulton, 1994). As in any survey on whatever subject, reporting is likely to be influenced by social norms. Given the different norms surrounding male and female sexual behaviour, a gender-related response bias can be expected. For instance, some men might consider it more in line with their social status to report varied sexual activity, while women might consider it more self-enhancing to report close relationships. Differential reporting might also be related to age and generation. It might be more important for young men than for older men to assert their masculinity by reporting more varied and intense sexual activity. People in younger age cohorts, who presumably began their sexual lives in a more open sexual climate, may find it easier to report certain practices than people from older generations. This might also apply to more highly educated people or urban populations. This response bias might correlate to the extent to which people subscribe to sex role stereotypes and in a more general way to the socio-cultural climate, although we have no information to assess this (except indirectly by looking at the 'no answer' rates to some questions, as has been done in a few chapters). Consequently, the impacts of these reporting biases will differ between countries. Interestingly, the impact of gender-related bias on reporting also seems to be related to the time period under examination: when this period is shorter, the gap in reporting between men and women narrows, suggesting that social norms have a stronger impact when people are asked to search in their memories.

Major Findings

In describing people's sexual behaviours we focused on four basic questions, that is, when do people start to have sex; whom do they have sex with; what do they do when they have sex; and how many sexual partners have they had? The answers to these questions depend on a variety of factors, some of which will be mentioned below, although most of them will be discussed more extensively in a later section. With regard to the specific issue of the sexual transmission of HIV, we shall focus on risky sexual behaviours, responses to risk and knowledge of HIV and AIDS.

It is clear that one cannot describe people's sexual behaviour as if it did not occur in a specific historical context. Some age-related differences between respondents can be understood only as a consequence of historical changes, rather than reflecting a developmental process. This is exemplified by some of the age-related differences in the data we described, which are explained by the fact that the sexual careers of today's younger people started and are unfolding in the context of AIDS.

In general, differences between countries were assessed by checking for overlapping confidence intervals. Based on these established differences, the particularities of the various countries emerge. The frequency with which a country could stand out depends, of course, on the number of comparisons the country was involved in. So the suggestion that a specific population does not seem to have many specific sexual characteristics can also be a consequence of a lack of comparison points. The reader should also keep in mind that it was not possible to mention each and every country when describing the comparisons' outcomes.

Sexual Initiation

A major finding regarding the start of people's sexual careers, that is, age at first intercourse, is that this is not stable over generations. The general trend all over Europe is a decrease in the age at first intercourse for younger samples, especially for women, although the rate of decrease tends to slow down in the younger generations. Of course, differences between countries still remain. Accordingly, we find that men in Athens[2] and Portugal in all age cohorts started their sexual careers fairly early (medians of 16 and 17 years, respectively), compared with other European countries, while women in Athens and Portugal were relatively late starters (22 and 23 years old, respectively). Finally, in Denmark, Iceland and Norway women in all age cohorts started their sexual careers relatively early, sometimes even earlier than men.

Despite the general decrease in age of sexual initiation seen in all countries, different patterns of change that are dependent on the points of departure in the various countries can be discerned. The drop in age is larger in countries where the older generations started at a relatively older age than in the other countries. This is the case for men in Belgium and the Netherlands, where the trend has swung from relatively late starts in the past to relatively early starts today. The data for former West Germany likewise reveal that sexual initiation occurred relatively late in older cohorts and relatively early in younger cohorts in comparison with other countries. French women in older age cohorts started their sexual careers at a relatively older age. While younger French women start earlier, from a European perspective they are still relatively late starters, as are the younger women in Athens, Belgium and Portugal. The difference between age cohorts is smaller in countries such as Denmark, Finland, Iceland and Norway, where people in older cohorts started their sex lives at a relatively early age.

A common thread running through the various patterns is that in countries in which there was a wide gap between the men and women in the older generations, the change over the course of successive generations has been more substantial for women than for men. As a result, men and women's ages at first intercourse now tend to converge in the younger generations, ranging from 16.3 to 19 (median age) for women and from 16.4 to 18.4 for men.

Finally, the relational context in which young people have their first sexual intercourse seems to have changed, likewise pointing to the way in which the genders relate socially is changing. Younger women seem to have had their first sexual experiences less often with a steady partner than older women did. Younger women are also less often in love with their first sexual partners and the initiative to engage in sexual activity is taken more equally by both men and women in younger cohorts rather than predominantly by men. Younger cohorts also report having used contraception the first time they had sex more often than people in older cohorts. Another generational difference is that younger people discuss sexuality more often with significant others than older people do.

Homosexual and Heterosexual Experiences

People's sexual partners are most often of the opposite sex. On the other hand, surveys revealed significant inter-country differences with regard to homosexual experiences. Relatively few men and women in Athens reported homosexual experiences over their lifetimes (respectively 1.7 per cent and 0.6 per cent of the sexually active people). Finnish women had a relatively high same-sex report rate (5.8 per cent on a lifetime basis). The highest rates of male homosexual experiences for both lifetime and the preceding year were reported by Dutch men (respectively 13.4 per cent and 6.3 per cent). The data also showed that people who had ever had sexual contact with someone of the same sex quite often also had had sex with someone of the opposite sex. Indeed, exclusively homosexual life histories were relatively rare and even less frequently observed than bisexual life histories, at least in general population surveys. *Exclusive* homosexuality, both lifetime and in the preceding year, was reported most often by Dutch men.

If people reported having had same-sex experiences, these experiences were quite often not recent: most homosexual experiences occurred before the age of 25. From the few surveys where sexual behaviour could be compared with people's stated sexual attraction towards men or women, it becomes clear that the two do not match completely, for a stated attraction did not exclude sexual contacts that were not in accordance with this attraction. Dutch men reported being sexually attracted to men more frequently than did French and Finnish men.

Aspects of Sexual Practices

The frequency with which people reported having sex in a steady relationship differs between the various countries, but is close to two times a week on average. Men and women in Athens, France, Portugal and Spain declared having sex more frequently than the average, and men and women in Belgium and the Netherlands least frequently. The percentage of men and women involved in a long-lasting relationship (at least one year) who had sex with one or more other persons in the preceding year ranged from 5.6 per cent (Great Britain) to 10.3 per cent (Norway) for men and from 2.3 per cent (Great Britain) to 5.6 per cent (Norway) for women.

There is a clear hierarchy of common and less common sexual practices across Europe, structured as follows: sexual techniques such as oral sex and especially anal sex and oral–anal contact are less common in all countries. In addition, people who have ever practised one of these less common sexual techniques are more likely to have practised other less common sexual techniques as well. Genital fondling and intercourse are practised by almost all people in each country at some time in their lives. If people reported having ever practised these latter two techniques, they often practised them recently, too. This is not true for the less common sexual practices, suggesting that at least for some people practising techniques such as oral sex is bound to specific phases in their sexual careers. On the other hand, the fact that younger people more often reported having performed oral sex suggests that what people do sexually is also dependent upon the time period in which they are sexually socialized.

Having had sex with more than one person on a lifetime basis, regardless of current relationship status, was reported by from 46.1 per cent (Norway) to 63.8 per cent (Spain) of the male respondents and from 36.2 per cent (Spain) to 53.9 per cent (Norway) of the female respondents. The frequency of having had only one sexual partner ranges from 12.4 per cent (Finland) to 20.2 per cent (Norway) for men and 20.8 per cent (Finland) and 44.4 per cent (Spain) for women. The finding that people with same-sex partners, on average, reported more lifetime sexual partners was remarkably consistent across Europe.

Risk-related Behavioural Aspects

To assess the occurrence of potential risk of HIV transmission, several aspects of sexual behaviour were examined. These included the number of partners, experiences of paid sex, condom use, and a history of STDs.

Multipartnership

From 2.0 per cent (France and West Germany) to 7.0 per cent (Finland) and from 0.2 per cent (West Germany) to 3.3 per cent (Finland) of the sexually active male and female respondents, respectively, reported having had more than five sexual partners in the preceding year.

Paid Sex

The number of men who reported having ever paid for sex ranges from 6.6 per cent in Great Britain to 38.6 per cent in Spain. The number of men who reported paying for sex in the preceding year ranges from 1.1 per cent in France to 11.0 per cent in Spain. Paying for sex was found to be more common among the men who had had sex with another man at least once than among men with exclusively heterosexual contacts. In the countries where these data were available, very few respondents reported knowingly having had sex with injecting drug users in the preceding year or in more recent intervals.

Condom Use

Lifetime experience of condoms either as a birth control method or to prevent HIV transmission is relatively high in Europe: between 51 per cent and 88 per cent of the various populations have used condoms at least once in their lives. Lifetime condom use is relatively low in Athens and Portugal and high in former West Germany, Netherlands and Switzerland. Respondents who reported more than five partners in the preceding year tended to report more frequent use of condoms, while the small number of men who reported having paid for sex in the preceding year quite frequently reported using condoms during these episodes.

History of STDs

Having had an STD is a good indicator of risky sexual behaviour. However, measuring STD prevalence in general population surveys is difficult because exposure to risk and access to testing, which are specific to each country, are almost always lumped together. A history of an STD was reported by around 20 per cent of the men and women in Norway and Finland. This is two to three times higher than the rates in East Germany, West Germany and the Netherlands. Older men and younger women reported the highest frequencies of diagnosed STDs in their respective gender categories. STDs were clearly more often reported by men who paid for sex at least once and by people who reported more sexual partners. Not only men but also women who reported same-sex partners were more likely to have had an STD at least once in their lives, although these women most probably contracted the STD through their male partners.

Behaviour Change and Testing

At least one-fifth of the population in the different European countries reported having changed their behaviour in response to the HIV epidemic, although these reports do not necessarily reflect actual behaviour and the stated behaviour changes may not necessarily have been sufficient to prevent HIV transmission. Behavioural adjustments in response to HIV risk were reported most frequently in the Netherlands and former West Germany; they were lowest in Portugal and Spain. These behaviour changes are not limited to the adoption of condom use. The various surveys show that individuals deal with the risk of sexual transmission of HIV in a variety of ways, such as the selection or reduction in the number of partners, discussing risks and past sexual life with their partners, and adopting safer sex practices. In most countries, preventive behaviour that relied on partner selection was mentioned as often as, sometimes even more often than, condom use. Abstinence and giving up specific risky sexual practices in response to HIV were rarely mentioned. In general, younger people stated having done something in the preceding year to prevent HIV transmission, in particular using condoms and being more selective in their choice of partners, more often than older people.

In absolute terms, testing for HIV, which can be undertaken for a variety of reasons, seems to be a widespread practice in Europe, although the promotion of HIV testing has so far been rather limited, and was even discouraged in some countries when the surveys were being conducted. The across-the-board testing rate was more than 10 per cent in all countries, with HIV-testing being reported more often by younger people than by older people. Testing for HIV was reported relatively frequently by people in Germany and relatively rarely in the Netherlands.

Knowledge about AIDS and Discriminatory Attitudes

Most respondents in the various countries were aware that HIV could be transmitted through sex and injecting drug use involving contaminated needles. More than 97 per cent of the respondents in eight out of the nine surveys recognized these two routes of viral transmission. Notwithstanding this high figure, relatively large numbers of respondents believed that transmission was also possible via routes that from a medical perspective do not seem to carry any risk, such as kissing someone with HIV/AIDS, using public toilets, and sharing glasses or plates. The potential for direct HIV infection, for example through the exchange of saliva and possible contact with blood during a kiss, seemed to trigger more fear or doubt than the potential for indirect transmission via a toilet seat or bowl in one case, or by a plate or cooking utensil in the other case. The numbers of people who did not reject out of hand such practices as coitus interruptus, washing after sexual intercourse, even taking the pill, as affording protection from HIV and those who believed that an AIDS vaccine existed are far from negligible.

In general, it seems that younger people are more knowledgeable about HIV transmission and prevention than older people. More young people know that condoms are an effective means to prevent HIV transmission and that HIV cannot be transmitted by kissing or using public toilets. On the other hand, more older people than younger people know that HIV cannot be transmitted by sharing a cup and that coitus interruptus and washing after intercourse are not effective preventive measures.

In the few countries where this could be assessed, it seems that segregationist attitudes towards people with HIV and AIDS are especially strong in persons who have more inaccurate knowledge about the virus's transmission routes and means of protection. This does not necessarily mean that the former is a direct consequence of the latter, however, for inaccurate knowledge and a desire for segregation may feed off each other and be part of a more general way of building identity through distancing oneself from other groups.

Differences between Countries

The various differences between the countries can be understood only if several kinds of factors, effective at a variety of levels, are taken into account concurrently. In this study, differences in data were interpreted predominantly after they had been established. In future cross-national comparisons of sexuality, attempts should be made to include possibly explanatory factors in the project's design.

Several between-country differences are quite likely reinforced by differences in male and female sex roles, which reflect the social positions of men and women in these societies. The sexual behaviour patterns of men and women diverged more in countries with relatively big male/female role differences, such as Portugal and Spain, than in countries where the roles are less far apart, such as in the northern European countries (Hofstede, 1991). It is quite likely that these differences are mediated by gender-related differences in sexual scripts (Gagnon and Simon, 1973). In some countries the sexual scripts of men and women diverge more than in others. While male/female equality might be something people aspire to in some countries, male/female differences might be valued more strongly in other countries. As a consequence, gender-related differences in age at first sexual intercourse may be stronger in countries with more traditional gender roles than in countries with more egalitarian systems. Country-to-country disparities in gender-related differences support the idea that at least some gender-related differences are due to gender-specific socialization patterns as well as biological differences.

Countries differ more with respect to their sexual climates, with some being more generally permissive than others. Sexual climate is also reflected in the country's legal situation. For instance, countries with more permissive climates may have legislation against discrimination based on sexual orientation. The relationship between the legal situation and social climate is, however, not simple. To understand fully how legal aspects are related to sexual climate, we need also to look at the ways in which various legal codes have come about.

That sexual climate affects sexuality is clear from the findings presented about homosexual behaviour. The Netherlands, which is generally seen as a sexually open society (Ester, Halman and De Moor, 1994), has the highest proportion of reported male homosexuality. How, and to what extent, a country's sexual climate affects its people's sexual behaviour is less clear. The Dutch and Belgians reported the lowest average frequency of sexual activity within a current steady relationship, suggesting that the effect of the sexual climate upon behaviour is at least differential. The data single out Finland as being sexually rather diverse. What is remarkable is that various findings apply not only to Finnish men, but to Finnish women as well. This is in sharp contrast to France, for instance, where we also find much sexual variety, but much more so for men than for women.

Part of a country's sexual climate is linked to the way contraception has been handled historically, and the extent to which young people are informed about and have access to birth control. This might explain the relatively low rates of condom use in Athens and Portugal and the high rates in former West Germany, the Netherlands and Switzerland. Countries also differ in terms of the health services available and systems of STD control. In this respect, the higher rates of STDs reported by people in the Nordic countries quite likely also reflect more broad-based screening programmes, which are particularly well developed in Scandinavia.

Several differences between the countries are quite likely AIDS-related, in the broadest sense of the term. Whilst in southern European countries more people have been infected via injecting drug use, in northern countries most people have been infected via homosexual transmission. These epidemiological differences have given rise to major differences in AIDS education (Moerkerk, 1990; Wellings and Field, 1996), ranging from its being relatively absent in most southern European countries to fairly intense education efforts in countries such as the Netherlands (Sandfort, 1998). This could explain why we found that behavioural adjustments in response to HIV risk were reported the least frequently in Portugal and Spain and much more frequently in the Netherlands and former West Germany.

Countries differ with respect to the priority given to HIV testing as a way to contain the epidemic, although the present data seem to suggest that national screening policies have not made much of a difference. The fact that the official policy in the Netherlands has until recently actively discouraged HIV testing does, however, help explain the rather low frequency of testing observed in this country. Another policy difference has to do with the emphasis given to using condoms as a means of protecting against HIV, which has probably been the strongest in Switzerland (Dubois-Arber *et al.*, 1997).

Historical Changes

A number of intergenerational differences can be observed across Europe. These differences may result partly from reporting bias, for it is possible that it is easier for the younger generations, who have been socialized in a more 'tolerant' sexual climate, to report their sexual behaviour and, more specifically, sexual behaviour not related to procreation. Still, it is unlikely that reporting bias can account for all the differences, since observed variations are too systematic for that.

A combination of factors can account for the intergenerational changes. Biological factors, such as the earlier onset of biological puberty – a development that has been going on for at least the last two centuries (Wysak and Frisch, 1982) – may play a role in lowering the age of sexual initiation. But social factors play an important role as well. One of these social factors is the narrowing of the gap between male and female roles that followed the spread of oral contraceptives, the enhanced educational opportunity for women, and the growing participation of women in the labour market. Economic development and growing prosperity have also created more space for leisure activities and individualism, while religion has become less important as a structuring factor. The changing normative context, as well as changing sexual behaviour itself, will in turn have affected each other in a gradual, long-term process rather than through sudden change such as that implied by the so-called 'sexual revolution'.

Although various AIDS-related aspects have been described, the impact of AIDS does not yet seem to have affected the main dimensions of sexual behaviour investigated in these surveys. AIDS does not seem to have reversed the decrease in age at first intercourse, or even stopped it, nor does the average number of partners appear to have fallen. It should, however, be realized that AIDS-related changes *per se* could not actually be measured in the surveys included here, since almost all were cross-sectional rather than longitudinal in design. We do know from other studies, such as those of Dubois-Arber *et al.* (1997), De Vroome *et al.* (1994) and Herlitz and Strandell (1997), that behavioural changes have occurred, especially in specific subgroups of the population such as young people and people with multiple partners. It is encouraging to see that, especially in these subpopulations, condom use is relatively high. If AIDS affects the sexual behaviour of the general population it might take more time to become visible. Recent figures from the US National Center for Health Statistics show that the mean age at first intercourse in the United States is rising. Although it is unclear to what extent this trend is caused by AIDS and related prevention activities, the finding at least suggests that the ongoing decrease in age at first intercourse (regardless of how it is evaluated) is not an irreversible process and similar changes might be observed in follow-up surveys in Europe as well.

Factors Structuring Sexual Behaviour

The authors of various chapters in this volume cross-tabulated reported sexual behaviours with several common variables. These cross-tabulations showed several differences between subcategories of people. As in other studies (Cleland and Ferry, 1995; Laumann *et al.*, 1994), differences in sexual behaviour were observed in relation to gender, age, level of education, place of residence, cohabitation status, and aspects of sexual career such as age at first intercourse and the number of sexual partners in various time periods. We shall now summarize and try to interpret the major differences, bearing in mind that the observed trends were statistically significant in most but not necessarily all countries. Furthermore, the trends described were not necessarily found in each country included in the overview, and on a few occasions they were based on observations in only the few countries in which the respective issue had been studied.

Gender

Men and women in all European countries differ systematically in their reports of several aspects of their sexual behaviour, with men generally reporting more varied sexual activity. More women than men never masturbate and those who do masturbate do so less frequently than men. Men generally report having had their first sexual intercourse at an earlier age than women, especially in southern European countries. Men also report more often that their first sex partner was younger and that they perceived this first relationship as less serious than later ones, whereas women more often report that their first intercourse occurred with a steady partner with whom they were in love. Men usually have had more sexual partners before they start a steady relationship.

Men report having had sexual experiences with someone of the same gender, having had more sexual partners in their lives, and having more frequent sex with their steady partners more often than women do. When they are involved in a steady relationship, they also report having had sex outside the relationship in the preceding year, and that significant others approve of this behaviour, and do so more strongly, more often than women do. Practising specific sexual techniques such as oral and anal sex is also more prevalent among men.

Men more often report having used a condom, regardless of the time frame. As mentioned above, older men and younger women reported the highest frequencies of diagnosed STDs over life in their respective gender categories. Looking at a more recent period, women more often than men report having had an STD, regardless of the number of partners they report. Women report more often than men talking about sexuality with significant others.

Gender-related differences can be explained in various ways aside from methodological bias. The differential reporting of STDs might reflect more active screening and testing in women induced by STDs' potential negative consequences on female fertility. These differences might also be caused by biomedical factors. Other gender differences might be a consequence of dominant social representations: it is possible that women may remain in part 'silent' about the extent of their condom use because of prevailing images of female sexuality, in which priority is given to stable relationships that are propitious to the development of emotional closeness, while condoms are associated more with frivolity (Bajos *et al.*, 1997). It is also possible that since men are the ones who wear condoms, women simply may not interpret using condoms as being *their* behaviour.

For other observed differences in sexual behaviour between men and women, two opposing perspectives are usually put forward (Baldwin and Baldwin, 1997): a psycho-evolutionary perspective suggesting that gender-related differences in sexual behaviour are based on men and women's different reproductive roles, and a sex role socialization perspective suggesting that men and women acquire different norms about sexual behaviour as part of the learning process. Both perspectives offer acceptable explanations for some of the differences observed here. That socialization effects play a role – although the precise processes involved still have to be explored – is suggested by some of the differences. The main reason is that gender trends are not fixed but change over time, and from one country to the next. Furthermore, women do not form a homogeneous group. The existence of intragroup differences must be explained by different learning experiences, which may in turn depend on variations in social autonomy.

Age

Most of the observed age differences should quite likely be interpreted as consequences of changes over time in the sexual climate, affecting younger and older age cohorts differently. However, a few age-related differences are quite likely consequences of individual maturation and aging. In general, younger people masturbate and have sex with their steady partners more often than older people do. They also report more sexual partners in the preceding year than older people do. Finally, younger people more often report having had an STD in a recent period, which is probably connected to their more active sex lives.

Level of Education

People's sexual behaviour is systematically related to their level of education. Although it could not be taken into account in analyzing the data, it is important to state that level of education is not constant across generations, and the general rise in average level of education in the younger generations will have affected sexual behaviour in society accordingly. Having said this, we see that people with a higher level of education have their first sexual intercourse at a later age and more often report having had same-sex experiences, masturbating and having practised the less common sexual techniques, such as oral sex. Anal sex, however, seems to be more common among people with lower levels of education. Men with lower levels of education also report having sex with their steady partners more frequently than men with higher levels of education do, whereas no such correlation appears for women. Having had sex with someone outside the steady relationship is reported more frequently by more educated than less educated women.

More highly educated people more often report a recent STD episode, but no general lifetime trends are observed. They are more knowledgeable about transmission of HIV and its prevention, and also more often report having done something to prevent HIV transmission. Finally, condom use and HIV testing are more widespread among people with higher levels of education.

The impact of people's level of education on various aspects of sexuality can be understood in various ways. Spending more years in school may delay the acquisition of independence and consequently sexual initiation. Extended education, on the other hand, implies better access to information and might also broaden people's normative horizons, making them more responsive to new sexual opportunities and more likely to engage in practices such as oral sex. In contrast, young people who leave school early will become independent more quickly and escape parental control and the restricting influence of the school or the university. They can thus be expected to operate autonomously.

Place of Residence

Sexual behaviour seems also to be related to the degree of urbanization of the place of residence. Men and women who live in urban areas report masturbating more frequently, having practised the less common sexual techniques, having had same-sex experiences, and having had more sexual partners more frequently than rural inhabitants. In line with these differences, city dwellers also report a higher incidence of STDs. On the other hand, the frequency with which people in steady relationships have sex is not related to their place of residence. People living in urban areas more often report having had sex outside their steady relationship. However, they do not expect significant others to be more positive about sexual contacts outside the steady relationship. City dwellers also report higher rates of HIV testing and knowing somebody who is HIV-infected or has AIDS than their rural counterparts.

Where people live might induce differences similar to these associated with level of education. Rural areas may be stricter about people's sexual behaviours, while urban centres not only give people more room to develop their own behavioural patterns, but also present them with the opportunity for greater sexual variety. It should also be realized that where people are currently living does not always reflect where they were born. It is, for instance, well-known that gay men tend to move from rural to urban areas, most probably in order to find an environment with more opportunities to develop their lifestyles. This might be the case for other people as well, implying that the connections between place of residence and sexual behaviour are at least bidirectional.

Cohabitation Status

There are several differences in the expression of sexuality between people who live with their steady partners and those who do not, although these differences will be confounded by age. People who do not live with their steady partner more often report masturbating and having ever practised the less common sexual techniques. There is no systematic difference in the frequency with which people have sex depending on whether they live together or separately. Finally, there is a general tendency for people who do not live with a steady partner to report having adjusted their sexual behaviour to the risk of AIDS by using condoms or by giving up penetrative sex more often than those who cohabit.

Level of Sexual Interest

It has already been shown that the younger age cohorts are characterized by the earlier onset of sexual careers. Regardless of these historical changes, people differ according to their age at sexual initiation. People who start their sexual career earlier than others more often report having had sexual contact with someone of the same sex, masturbating more often, having practised the less common sexual techniques, having had more sexual partners and, if they have one, more frequent sex with their steady partners. The age at which people first have sexual intercourse seems to be an important predictor of subsequent sexual activity.

The number of partners people reported having had is related to other aspects of people's sexual behaviour as well: same-sex experiences and STDs were more widespread among people who reported having had more sexual partners. This group adjusted their behaviour more frequently in response to HIV, especially by using condoms and choosing their partners more selectively. They were also more frequently tested for HIV and more often knew a person with HIV or AIDS.

The differences presented here may reflect both consequences of socialization resulting in higher levels of sexual interest and inherited differences in temperament, giving some people a stronger sexual interest than others.

Lessons for HIV Prevention

To some extent the data reported in this chapter can be interpreted as feedback on HIV prevention activities in the various countries. Although the cross-sectional design of the studies forces us to be cautious, AIDS does not seem to have affected the main parameters of sexual behaviour, at least not at the times these surveys were carried out. Given the fact that a behavioural response to the risk of HIV is not relevant for the total population, the number of people who reported changes in their sexual behaviour is high, while the prevalence of condom use by young people and people with multiple partners that was detected in most of the European countries investigated here is encouraging. Moreover, people have not responded to the risk of HIV only by using condoms; other, not necessarily always completely effective, responses have been reported as well. From an epidemiological perspective it is important to emphasize that a substantial proportion of survey respondents with multiple partners reported never having used condoms and never having been tested for HIV. These are the very people who may play an important role in the further development of the AIDS epidemic.

Knowledge about HIV transmission and prevention is relatively good. However, still not all the knowledge people have is in line with the available preventive information. What is more, what people know about HIV is not a purely cognitive phenomenon, but also a function of anxieties elicited by the disease and pre-existing representations about illnesses in general, which are partially dependent upon gender.

The data presented here prompt several suggestions for further policies as well. There is still a need for continued and more specific information about HIV. Several misunderstandings that might easily lead to discrimination against people with HIV/AIDS still seem to exist. Recent developments in AIDS treatment, the resulting changes in the character of the disease, and the changing relevance of knowing one's serostatus add to the importance of informing people. For the purposes of information campaigns, however, one must recognize that people are not clean slates. People already have ideas about what sickness is, may mistrust experts and sources of information and so on, and process all new information in this context. Thus, the point is probably not to reiterate the same messages but to refine message contents and work on the relations between their senders and receivers. Less educated people, who, as the surveys show, tend to be less well informed about HIV transmission and ways of prevention, might constitute a major challenge in this respect.

The fact that much homosexual behaviour is practised by people who do not identify themselves as 'gay' indicates that the prevention of HIV transmission in same-sex sexual encounters must be extended beyond the gay communities (although these communities' roles remain vital for the spread and maintenance of safer sexual practices) by addressing same-sex transmission in general prevention campaigns as well. Furthermore, the data presented underline the importance of integrating various kinds of information in the development of HIV prevention policies in order to be as effective as possible. First of all, it is important to acknowledge that sexuality is already structured by various social factors; the impact of AIDS and of AIDS prevention comes on top of these factors. As a consequence, HIV/AIDS prevention should be placed within the larger scheme of sex education. In order to reduce communication difficulties, sex education should also address mutual ignorance and differences in men's and women's expectations about sexual interactions. From a more general perspective, it is important to work on sexual norms as well so that it becomes socially acceptable for women to request the use of condoms for the purpose of prevention.

The data also support the notion that education has to start early, as has already been stressed for the prevention of unwanted pregnancies. Early sex education seems to be all the more important as age at first intercourse has proven to be a powerful predictor of various adult sex life characteristics. Programmes should, however, allow for normative and sexual diversity, for the range of sexual experiences at any given age is extremely hetereogeneous. The fear that early sex education would encourage young people to start exploring their sexuality even earlier appears to be unwarranted. On the contrary, studies have shown that sex education seems to have a slight delaying effect on age at first intercourse (Mellanby *et al.*, 1995; Wellings *et al.*, 1995) and to increase the rate of contraceptive use at first intercourse markedly (Aggleton, Baldo and Slurkin, 1993; Greydanus, Pratt and Dannison, 1995).

For the prevention of HIV transmission to be effective, it is also important to be in keeping with each nation's traditions in the area of contraception. Furthermore, it should be acknowledged that condom use is not the only way of adapting to HIV risk. People may adapt to AIDS differently according to their position in the life cycle and the types of relationship in which they are engaged. As long as these practices are effective enough to limit HIV transmission, they should be supported, either by general campaigns or in smaller scale actions, depending on what is most effective and produces the least counterproductive effects.

Less educated people might deserve specific attention, not only because of greater gaps in their knowledge of HIV/AIDS but because they also tend to embark on their sexual careers relatively early, which, as we have seen, is correlated with various indicators of sexual risk. They also use condoms less often, get tested for HIV less often, and are less likely to have changed their sexual behaviour in order to prevent HIV transmission. Reaching these people will be a major challenge for prevention throughout Europe.

Suggestions for Future Research

As has been shown, there is not a one-to-one relationship between reported and actual behaviour. People are not always able to present the information in the format researchers would like to have, due, for instance, to an inability to reconstruct the information or because the required information is too specific. People also do not always know the things researchers would like to know. For instance, since several STDs are asymptomatic, people do not necessarily always know whether they have had an STD. Furthermore, people have various conscious or unconscious motives to distort information, to play things down or to boast. Unfortunately it is seldom possible to disentangle the effects of reporting bias and of 'real' factors. In this respect, higher levels of reported condom use will be a reflection of actual use and a greater willingness to report about condom use, as well as a striving to meet socially desirable norms. This greater willingness will result from a more liberal climate towards condom use, which itself will be the result of more condom use as well as actually inducing more condom use.

It is important to acknowledge that the effects of social desirability stem not only from respondents themselves, but from an interaction between the respondent and the instrument used to collect data. For instance, questions might be asked in such a way that people interpret them as not applying to their situations; in this sense, same-sex sexual experiences might be 'forgotten' when they are referred to using the term 'homosexual', since these people did not categorize these experiences as such, or do not label themselves as homosexual. Likewise, if women are asked plainly about the use of condoms they may under-report actual use because they might not think of themselves as using condoms, since they do not actually wear them. Furthermore, answer formats may give people clues as to what is expected of them or in which normative range their answers should fall. These methodological influences upon the quality of the elicited data have been demonstrated several times in this book. To be able to improve the quality of surveys about sexual behaviour, more studies should be done about the impact of these methodological issues and the way they affect survey data quality.

The various chapters in this book contain a wealth of information on a variety of topics. The findings underline the importance of the social sciences' contributions to the theoretical and practical understanding of sexuality and preventive behaviours. Each chapter shows the importance of future social science research both nationally and internationally. Some of the issues included here should be explored in greater depth in the future. Other issues that were omitted from this overview should become part of such a project as well. Future cross-national comparisons should include information on attitudes and norms and values as they relate to sexuality. Given the rather diverse ways in which attitudes have been addressed in the various surveys examined here, it was practically impossible to include attitudinal data in this overview. A better understanding of differences between nations as well as other subcategories of people might, however, be gained by investigating how people think about sex in terms of intimacy, reproduction, or lust. These kinds of attitudinal data can be compared independently. Their meaning can also be explored in relation to various behavioural aspects. Understanding of the differences between countries can also be improved by conducting ethnographic studies to see how environmental and cultural factors affect sexuality in different countries.

The various changes in sexuality over the generations stress the need to follow up these developments. Since the effects of factors which structure sexual behaviour, such as gender, are not fixed, it is important to continue to monitor them, too. It would be interesting to see, in this respect, whether differences in sexuality between men and women continue to diminish or whether some characteristics persist. Further understanding of how sexual initiation patterns change over time can be obtained by looking at characteristics of people's first sexual partners. Furthermore, sexual initiation should be studied in relation to age at first marriage or cohabitation. A rise in mean age at first marriage with a continued decline in mean age at first intercourse would clearly indicate a relaxation in sexual mores.

It might be informative to look at other units of measurements than the individual. A relational perspective might help to understand how people adjust to the risk of HIV in relation to the different types of and moments in their relationships. This should also be done in relation to other aspects, such as STD prevention and birth control. By including normative orientations, such an approach could also generate a typology of intimate and sexual involvement.

The finding that sexuality is structured by various factors has elicited interest in the way in which these factors actually work. It might be revealing to study how population movements between urban and rural areas affect people's sexual values and behaviours. It would also be interesting to find out which factors mediate education's impact on sexual behaviour. Since the start of the sexual career seems to be a powerful predictor of various characteristics of adult sex life, it is important to explore which factors determine sexual initiation and how these experiences affect people's further sexual development.

It has been suggested that since many homosexual contacts seem to take place outside gay and lesbian lifestyles, there is need for a better understanding of the circumstances in which homosexual contacts occur. Furthermore, the finding that same-sex experiences (on a lifetime basis) is a risk indicator for STDs for women as well as men suggests the need to explore the sexual careers of women with same-sex experiences. A further, more representative exploration of how bisexuals, gay men and lesbians live their lives and how these circumstances influence their mental as well as physical well-being is relevant for the promotion of healthier lifestyles. This information might be helpful in designing specific prevention efforts to reach their targets more effectively.

Sexual interactions in which toys or accessories are used, or involving three or more people, could be studied as well. As suggested, it would be interesting to find out how the various sexual techniques relate to one another and to specific relational contexts with different levels of commitment. Are the less common techniques practised independently or are they practised as foreplay to vaginal intercourse? Furthermore, it would be interesting to adopt a developmental perspective and to understand what prompts people to engage in or stop practising specific sexual techniques.

The different rates of reported STDs should be studied in relation to available health services if they are to be interpreted more reliably. The data suggest that asymptomatic STDs are more widely diagnosed in countries that are known to have intensive screening programmes than in countries without such services.

More information is needed to understand the inter-country differences in condom use. Further comparative research should investigate in greater depth the different patterns of condom use by type and stage of relationship and the rationales for their use. The interrelations among the various motives for condom use should also be studied. The role of the condom as a contraceptive in the AIDS era is still unclear. While some believe that it is necessary to recommend taking the pill in addition to using condoms, others feel that this 'belt and braces' approach is not advisable. More research is needed in this area if policy is to be based on fact rather than opinion. Furthermore, the use of condoms should also be studied in relation to other ways of adapting to the risk of HIV and the policies in effect in the various countries.

People's sexuality and AIDS-related aspects have been studied here as individualized phenomena. We should like to stress, however, that sexual behaviour and risk behaviour are more complex phenomena. For a more complete understanding of these behaviours economic and political factors should be considered as well. As has been shown in many areas, these kinds of factors are important factors of people's health behaviours as well as their health (Evans, Barer and Marmor, 1994).

In this overview, AIDS-related aspects were studied less in depth and less systematically than various aspects of sexual behaviour. Further cross-national research should address more systematically how various subsamples of people perceive AIDS, what they know about AIDS (and the background of the misinformation that exists), and how people respond to AIDS, either with respect to their own potential risk or to people with HIV/AIDS. This should be studied against the background of differences in countries' respective epidemiological patterns, general AIDS policies, the changing nature of the illness, and the specific prevention campaigns that have been carried out. Have these national characteristics affected people's knowledge of AIDS and perceptions of the epidemic and risky sexual behaviour differently? Other factors, such as sex role stereotypes, sexual attitudes and legal regulations, should be included in these analyses as well. Such cross-national comparisons might improve our understanding of what goes on in each specific country. The outcomes of such comparisons, while interesting from an academic perspective, might also help policy makers to focus their national HIV prevention policies more effectively. Finally, developments in the treatment of AIDS and the consequently changing face of the disease underline the relevance of the constant monitoring of sexuality and its relationship with AIDS.

Notes

1 Designing and implementing such a common protocol is precisely the purpose of a new European Concerted Action, funded by the EU Europe Against AIDS programme, that continues this project and focuses on the study of new sexual encounters as well as on general indicators of sexual behaviour and prevention.

2 For Greece, data are available on Athens residents only. Given the differences in sexual behaviour related to urbanization, the findings for Athens cannot be generalized to the Greek population.

References

AGGLETON, P., BALDO, M. and SLUTKIN, G. (1993) 'Sex education leads to safer behavior', *Global AIDS News*, **4**, pp. 1–20.

BAJOS, N., DUCOT, B., SPENCER, B. and SPIRA, A. (1997) 'Sexual risk taking, socio-sexual biographies and sexual interaction: elements of the French national survey on sexual behaviour', *Social Science and Medicine*, **44**, 1, pp. 25–40.

BALDWIN, J.D. and BALDWIN, J. (1997) 'Gender differences in sexual interest', *Archives of Sexual Behavior*, **26**, 2, pp. 181–210.

BOULTON, M. (Ed.) (1994) *Challenge and Innovation. Methodological Advances in Social Research on HIV/AIDS*, London: Taylor & Francis.

CATANIA, J., GIBSON, D., CHITWOOD, D. and COATES, T. (1990) 'Methodological problems in AIDS behavioural research: influences on measurement error and participation bias in studies of sexual behaviour', *Psychological Bulletin*, **108**, pp. 339–62.

CLELAND, J. and FERRY, B. (Eds) (1995) *Sexual Behaviour and AIDS in the Developing World*, London: Taylor & Francis.

DUBOIS-ARBER, F., JEANNIN, A., KONINGS, E. and PACCAUD, F. (1997) 'Increased condom use without other major changes in sexual behavior among the general population in Switzerland', *American Journal of Public Health*, **87**, 4, pp. 558–66.

ESTER, P., HALMAN, L. and DE MOOR, R. (Eds) (1994) *The Individualizing Society. Value Change in Europe and North America*, Tilburg: Tilburg University Press.

EVANS, R.G., BARER, M.L. and MARMOR, T.R. (Eds) (1994) *Why Are Some People Healthy and Others Not? The Determinants of Health of Populations*, New York: Aldine de Gruyter.

GAGNON, J.H. and SIMON, W. (1973) *Sexual Conduct*, Chicago: Aldine Publishing Company.

GREYDANUS, D., PRATT, H. and DANNISON, L. (1995) 'Sexuality education programs for youth: current state of affairs and strategies for the future', *Journal of Sex Education and Therapy*, **4**, pp. 238–54.

HERLITZ, C. and STRANDELL, A. (1997) 'Public reactions to AIDS in Sweden', *European Journal of Public Health*, **7**, 2, pp. 193–8.

HOFSTEDE, G. (1991) *Cultures and Organizations. Software of the Mind*, London: HarperCollins.

LAUMANN, E.O., GAGNON, J.H., MICHAEL, R.T. and MICHAELS, S. (1994) *The Social Organization of Sexuality. Sexual Practices in the United States*, Chicago: Chicago University Press.

MELLANBY, A.R., PHELPS, F.A., CRICHTON, N.J. and TRIPP, J.H. (1995) 'School sex education: an experimental programme with educational and medical benefit', *British Medical Journal*, **311**, pp. 414–17.

MOERKERK, H. (1990) 'AIDS prevention strategies in European countries', in PAALMAN, M.E.M. (Ed.) *Promoting Safer Sex*, Amsterdam: Swets & Zeitlinger.

SANDFORT, T.G.M. (Ed.) (1998) *The Dutch Response to HIV: Pragmatism and Consensus*, London: UCL Press.

DE VROOME, E.M.M., PAALMAN, M.E.M., DINGELSTAD, A.A.M., KOLKER, L. and SANDFORT, T.G.M. (1994) 'Increase in safe sex among the young and nonmonogamous: knowledge, attitudes and behavior regarding safe sex and condom use in The Netherlands from 1987 to 1993', *Patient Education and Counseling*, **24**, pp. 279–88.

WELLINGS, K. and FIELD, B. (1996) *Stopping AIDS. AIDS/HIV Public Education and the Mass Media in Europe*, London and New York: Longman.

WELLINGS, K., WADSWORTH, J., JOHNSON, A., FIELD, J., WHITAKER, L. and FIELD, B. (1995) 'Provision of sex education and early sexual experience: the relation examined', *British Medical Journal*, **311**, pp. 417–20.

WYSHAK, G. and FRISCH, R.E. (1982) 'Evidence for a secular trend in age of menarche', *The New England Journal of Medicine*, **306**, pp. 1033–5.

Notes on Contributors

Nathalie Bajos is a social demographer with a PhD in public health. After having carried out several research projects on medical emergency services and occupational diseases, she is currently a researcher in public health at the National Institute of Health and Medical Research (Institut National de la Santé et de la Recherche Médicale – INSERM) in Paris, where she was one of the principal coordinators of the national survey on sexual behaviour in France (the ACSF-survey). She is the author or co-author of a lot of publications resulting from this survey, among which *Sexual Behaviour and AIDS* (edited with Alfred Spira and the ACSF Group, Aldershot, Avebury, 1994) and *La sexualité aux temps du sida* (edited with Michel Bozon, Alexis Ferrand, Alain Giami and Alfred Spira, Paris, Presses Universitaires de France, 1998). She is currently engaged in an evaluation of the enforcement of the abortion law in France.

Nathalie Beltzer, PhD in economics, is a researcher at the National Institute of Health and Medical Research (INSERM) in Paris. Her current work focuses on decision models such as the Production Function Model or the Expected Utility Theory applied to risk perception, individual management of the HIV risk, and the individual choice of preventive strategies. She has worked on the national survey on sexual behaviour in France (ACSF, 1992), and since 1990 belongs to the KABP team.

Henny Bos was until December 1997 a research assistant at the Department of Gay and Lesbian Studies at Utrecht University, predominantly focusing on gay and lesbian health issues. Nowadays she works at the Netherlands Institute of Social Sexual Research (NISSO), doing a study about homosexuality in the workplace.

Michel Bozon is a sociologist and Director of Research at the National Institute for Population Studies (Institut National d'Etudes Démographiques (INED), Paris, France). He has organized several quantitative surveys on mating, youth and the family. His current work focuses on the sociology of human sexuality, specifically in a cross-cultural perspective. He is one of the co-organizers of the French survey on sexual behaviour (ACSF). His recent publications include *Sexuality and the Social Sciences. A French Survey on Sexual Behaviour* (edited with Henri Leridon, Aldershot, Dartmouth, 1996) and *La sexualité aux temps du sida* (edited with Nathalie Bajos, Alexis Ferrand, Alain Giami and Alfred Spira, Paris, Presses Universitaires de France, 1988).

Mitchell Cohen is Executive Director of the Partnership for Community Health (New York), an associate at the HIV Center for Clinical and Behavioral Studies, Columbia University, and an associate consultant for the International HIV/AIDS Alliance located in London. He splits his time between developing models for HIV/AIDS prevention and care and providing technical assistance in establishing and evaluating HIV/AIDS prevention and care programmes.

Françoise Dubois-Arber, MD in internal medicine and MSc in public health, has done work on implementing primary health care programmes in South America (Peru and Nicaragua, 1983–86). Since 1987 she has been specializing in evaluation research. She is currently head of the Prevention Programmes Evaluation Unit at the University Institute for Social and Preventive Medicine in Lausanne, Switzerland, and is in charge of the evaluation of the national AIDS prevention strategy. In this context she has directed several trend surveys and qualitative research on sexual behaviour in the general population and various other groups.

Alexis Ferrand is a professor of sociology and head of the Institute of Sociology, at the Université des Sciences et Technologies in Lille, France. He is a member of the ACSF, the group that conducted the national survey on sexual behaviours in France (1992). After developing research on sociability and friendship he became interested in analyzing the dynamics of elective relationships and the structure of personal networks. In this area he has published several papers including 'Social networks and normative tensions' (with T.A.B. Snijders, in *Sexual interactions and HIV risk*, Luc Van Campenhoudt *et al.*, Eds, London, Taylor and Francis, 1997) and 'La structure des systèmes de relations' (*L'Année Sociologique*, 1, 1997).

Elina Haavio-Mannila is a professor of sociology and head of the department at the University of Helsinki, Finland. Her field of studies include the history of Finnish sociology, medical sociology and gender studies. She has compared women in politics, work and family in the Nordic and Eastern European countries. She is currently comparing sexual attitudes and behaviour on the basis of survey data and sexual autobiographies in Finland, St. Petersburg (Russia) and Estonia. She has published a large number of sociological books and articles including *Sexual Pleasures: Enhancement of Sex Life in Finland, 1971–1992* (with Osmo Kontula, Aldershot, Dartmouth, 1995).

Michael Haeder is a sociologist and project director at ZUMA (Center for Survey Research and Methodology) in Mannheim. He currently divides his research interests between methodological studies and a project to observe the transformation process in former East Germany. He was in charge in 1989–90 of the survey on sexual behaviour and AIDS in East Germany about which he published several reports and papers.

Michel Hubert, sociologist, is a professor at the Facultés universitaires Saint-Louis (FUSL) in Brussels where he teaches social sciences research methodology. After having worked in the field of urban sociology, he has been involved in several research projects, both qualitative and quantitative, on sexual behaviour and HIV risk at the Center for sociological studies (Centre d'études sociologiques – CES). With J. Marquet he coordinated the Belgian national survey on sexual behaviour and attitudes towards HIV/AIDS. He was also the project leader of the European Union Concerted Action on Sexual Behaviour and Risks of HIV Infection within the Biomedical and Health Research Programme (BIOMED), of which this book is one of the outcomes, and is now coordinating a European project on the study of HIV risk in new relationships.

Philippe Huynen is a sociologist and a specialist in data management and processing. He teaches Computer Sciences for the Social Sciences at FUSL in Brussels. As a member of the CES research team he is responsible for data collection and statistical analysis for the various projects in which he is involved.

Elizabeth Ioannidi is a sociologist-researcher at the Department of Sociology, National School of Public Health in Athens. She has been involved in AIDS research programmes since 1989 and her experience is mainly on sexual behaviour and AIDS. Her current work focuses on qualitative methods and more specifically the biographical – interpretive method. Additional fields of interest are inequalities in health in relation to the refugee problem in Europe.

André Jeannin is a sociologist and senior researcher at the Prevention Programmes Evaluation Unit of the University Institute of Social and Preventive Medicine in Lausanne, Switzerland, and has been a member of the team in charge of the evaluation of the Swiss AIDS prevention strategy since 1992. He specializes in general population surveys for the evaluation of AIDS prevention programmes.

Osmo Kontula PhD is Senior Lecturer in Sociology at the University of Helsinki and Senior Researcher at the Population Research Institute, The Family Federation of Finland. He has broad research experience on sexuality and has published many books on sexual issues and many papers in books and journals. The books include *Sexual Pleasures: Enhancement of Sex Life in Finland,*

1971–1992 (with Elina Haavio-Mannila, Aldershot, Dartmouth, 1995). He is also the chairman of the Finnish Association of Sexology.

Henri Leridon is Director of Research at INED and Editor-in-Chief of the journal 'Population'. He has worked on various aspects of fertility and on the transformations of the family, mainly in developed countries; he has also participated in the French national survey on sexual behaviour (ACSF). His publications include *Human Fertility. The Basic Components* (University of Chicago Press, 1977) and several books published in the INED series. He has also co-edited *Natural Fertility/Fécondité Naturelle* (with J. Menken, Ordina ED., 1979), *Biomedical and Demographic Determinants of Human Reproduction* (with R. Gray and A. Spira, Oxford University Press, 1993), *Sexuality and the Social Sciences* (with Michel Bozon, Aldershot, Dartmouth, 1996).

Per Magnus is head of the Section of Epidemiology at the National Institute of Public Health in Oslo, Norway, and is a professor in community medicine at the University of Oslo. He has published a series of academic papers in the fields of genetic, perinatal and infectious disease epidemiology. In addition to performing population based studies of sexual behaviour in Norway, he has worked with cohort studies of HIV-positive people with the aim of identifying factors that can postpone disease development, and with mathematical modelling to understand the potential for the spread of sexually transmitted diseases in different populations.

Jacques Marquet is a professor of sociology at the Catholic University of Louvain (UCL) in Louvain-la-Neuve and at FUSL in Brussels. With Michel Hubert, he coordinated the Belgian national survey on sexual behaviour and attitudes towards HIV/AIDS. Beside sexual behaviour and AIDS, his main research interests and publications are in the sociology of the family and social sciences methods.

Danièle Peto is a research assistant in sociology at FUSL. Her main research subjects are the sociological aspects of AIDS prevention and the sociology of intimacy and sexuality. Her publications include *Sida: l'amour face à la peur* (with Jean Remy, Luc Van Campenhoudt and Michel Hubert, Paris, L'Harmattan, 1992) and 'Relationships between Sexual Partners and Ways of Adapting to the risk of AIDS: Landmarks for a Relationship-Oriented Conceptual Framework' (with Benoît Bastard, Laura Cardia-Vonèche and Luc Van Campenhoudt in Luc Van Campenhoudt, *et al.* (Eds), *Sexual Interactions and HIV Risk*, London, Taylor & Francis, 1997).

Theo Sandfort, social psychologist, is an appointed researcher at the Faculty of the Social Sciences (Utrecht University) and directs research at the Netherlands Institute for Social Sexological Research (NISSO, Utrecht). The research he directs focuses on the determinants of HIV-preventive behaviour of gay men and the general population. He is also involved in studies monitoring behavioural changes and assessing the impact of small and large scale interventions aimed at promoting safer sex. Next to HIV/AIDS-related issues he studies aspects of gay and lesbian lives, including coming out processes, life styles, relationships and discrimination. He is the former Director of the Department of Gay and Lesbian Studies at Utrecht University and has been a member of the Prevention and Education Section of the Dutch National Committee on AIDS Control (NCAB). His most recent publication as an editor is *The Dutch response to HIV: Pragmatism and consensus* (London, UCL Press, 1998).

Brenda Spencer is a social scientist employed as research manager at the University Institute of Social and Preventive Medicine in Lausanne, Switzerland. Her research career began in the UK where she worked on a large range of subjects in the field of sexual and reproductive health. She obtained her doctorate in the Department of Community Medicine at the University of Manchester. In 1988 she moved to INSERM, in France, where she became involved in AIDS-related research, including the national survey on sexual behaviour (ACSF). She took up her current position in Lausanne in 1996 where she is engaged in research programmes designed to evaluate the Swiss AIDS prevention strategy and the federal measures taken to reduce the problems related to drug use. She has acted as international consultant on AIDS prevention programmes in a number of African countries and is author of *The Condom Effectiveness Matrix: An analytical tool for defining condom research priorities* (Paris, Les Editions INSERM, 1994).

Jon Martin Sundet is a psychologist, educated at the University of Oslo, Norway. At present, he is a professor at the Institute of Psychology at the University of Oslo. He was affiliated with the National institute of Public Health in Oslo from 1987 to 1989. His main research work is focused on two fields: 1) twin research, investigating the relative contributions of genes and environmental factors to intelligence and personality (currently his main research area) and 2) sexual behaviour (he was one of the principal investigators of the Norwegian survey on sexual behaviour in 1987). Earlier research interest was visual perception. He has published many papers, mainly in international journals.

Luc Van Campenhoudt is a professor in sociology at FUSL in Brussels, where he is the Director of CES. He is also professor at the Catholic University of Louvain (UCL), Belgium. His publications include *Manuel de recherche en sciences sociales* (with Raymond Quivy, Paris, Dunod, 1988 and 1995); *Sida: l'amour face à la peur* (with Danièle Peto, Jean Remy and Michel Hubert, L'Harmattan, 1992); and *Sexual Interaction and HIV-Risk. New Conceptual Perspectives in European Research* (edited with Mitchell Cohen, Gustavo Guizzardi and Dominique Hausser, Taylor & Francis, 1997).

Gertjan van Zessen PhD, is a clinical psychologist currently in a private sexology practice. He has been involved in sex research and HIV/AIDS since 1984. He was involved in the Netherlands general population studies among adults (1989) and young people (1990, 1995) and in a series of qualitative studies among prostitutes and their clients, expatriates, heterosexuals and bisexuals with multiple partners, and young people – the latter in the context of a European Communities Concerted Action (with Roger Ingham). Current work is focused on compulsive sexuality.

Josiane Warszawski is an epidemiologist in INSERM, Paris. She is involved in methodological research for improving screening programs and epidemiological surveillance of sexually transmitted diseases, and, more generally, the use of complex sampling surveys for public health objectives. She is the author of many papers in this field.

Ester Zantedeschi is a medical doctor and epidemiologist trained at La Sapienza University's School of Medicine, Rome. She has been a research fellow at the Italian Ministry of Health for epidemiological studies on HIV risk associated with sexual behaviour of young people. At present she teaches at the School of Hygiene and Preventive Medicine, La Sapienza University, Rome. She also worked at FUSL in 1994 in the Center for Sociological Studies. Dr Zantedeschi has published many papers on public health, knowledge of AIDS, sexual behaviour and HIV risk.

Index

Note: Page numbers followed by *t* or *f* refer to tables or figures